KETO CHAFFLES RECIPES

COOKBOOK

---

650 Quick, Easy, and Super-Tasty Waffles to Lose Weight and Boost Your Ketogenic Diet

Jessica Meal

Table of Contents

CHAPTER 8. WAFFLE MEAT RECIPES

CHAPTER 12. SIMPLE WAFFLE RECIPES 250

INTRODUCTION

The ketogenic diet, also known as "keto," has been many people's go-to way of eating for weight control. It can help people experience healthy and sustainable weight loss to promote optimal health. A relatively new addition to the wide variety of diets that are out there, keto became popular in recent years due to its emphasis on low-carbohydrate intake and high fat intake. This lifestyle approach forces the body to rely on breaking down fats instead of carbohydrates for energy, instead of its typical mode of using carbohydrates to make glucose. While a carbohydrate-rich diet is usually recommended for its ability to allow the body to power itself easily, without much effort, a keto diet calls for cutting back on carbs and turning instead to fat intake. A person becomes "keto-adapted" when their body makes ketones in sufficient amounts and they can fuel their brain with them. This phenomenon happens when the body starts releasing stored fat and uses it as the main source of fuel for energy rather than glucose from carbohydrates.

Although a keto diet is still not recommended for people with diabetes or those who are on low-carb diets, the keto diet is generally less restrictive than other popular diets such as Atkins and South Beach. It's important to do your research and consult a medical professional before deciding whether or not to give it a try.

The keto diet is a high-fat, moderate-protein, and low-carb eating plan. It's called "ketogenic" because the body starts releasing fatty acids from your fat tissue when metabolism is elevated. This state of "ketosis" causes the body to start making ketones that burn up stored fat in your liver to produce energy. The goal of a ketogenic diet is to force the body into ketosis so that you burn fat instead of carbohydrates.

The keto diet, or ketogenic diet, has been around for decades but was first used widely as a therapy for children with uncontrolled epilepsy. As science progressed, more research was done on the effects of this low-carb, high-fat eating plan. The benefits were proven effective for those who were looking to lose weight and also improve their health in doing so. It has also been shown to aid in insulin sensitivity and also help prevent metabolic syndrome and diabetes type 2 by reducing inflammation.

Another important thing to remember: You can end the day with a much higher amount of fat in your body than what you started it with! This is called net carbs. The total amount of carbs consumed in any given day doesn't matter much; the weight lost at the end of the day will be triggered by how many grams of fat are consumed. The general rule is to consume fewer carbs during the day and more fat at night. It's okay to have high-carb foods like fruit at night.

To sum it all up, the ketogenic diet is a weight loss plan that features high levels of fat, moderate amounts of protein, and very few carbohydrates. When compared with other popular diets such as Atkins or South Beach, keto has been found by many experts to be easier to follow and more sustainable in the long run. It is also thought to be more beneficial to long-term weight loss as it allows the body to become "keto-adapted" and use fat as its primary energy source.

It is important to note that the keto diet should only be followed under strict medical supervision. There have been many instances where people have followed this diet without any supervision and ended up in the hospital with pancreatitis or acidosis, both of which can be serious medical conditions. This diet should be neither used nor followed without a thorough understanding of its effects on the body.

CHAPTER 1. THE BENEFITS OF THE KETOGENIC DIET

While the ketogenic diet is widely recognized as a "rapid diet for fat loss," the crucial role that it plays in healthy living goes beyond weight loss. In reality, higher energy rates and weight loss are side attractions compared with other huge benefits that can be obtained from the diet. Scientific studies have proven these advantages.

First of all, it should be noted that carbohydrate diets with their high quantity of sugar and other processed components do not offer any health benefits. These are common calories, and the majority of processed foods deny the body the nutrients needed for a healthy life. Below are the benefits for energy conversion derived from low carbohydrates and higher fat intake.

CONTROL OF BLOOD SUGAR

Low body sugar levels are important to the treatment and prevention of diabetes. Keto diets have been known to be a very effective tool for diabetes prevention. Many patients with diabetes have enormous body weight, making weight loss a necessity. Meanwhile, in addition to what the keto diet does, carbohydrates are converted into sugar, which is very harmful to patients with diabetes because it causes an increase in sugar levels. Therefore, low-carbohydrate consumption virtually prevents such a spike in sugar and also regulates blood sugar levels.

MENTAL FOCUS

The keto diet is related to low-carbohydrate regulation and increased fat and protein. As discussed, the body is forced to depend on fats as its main source of fuel generation. It differs from the traditional Western diet that is less nutritional, especially in fatty acids that are much required for good brain function.

When people experience deficiencies and cognitive disorders such as Alzheimer's, this implies insufficient glucose for brain use. The loss of insulin allows the energy level to decline, thereby increasing the brain's performance. The keto diet, however, prevents this deficiency as it provides additional energy to the brain.

The study also revealed that the keto diet could improve the memory capacity of people with Alzheimer's disease. The memory capacity of people affected by Alzheimer's is also proportional to the number of ketones in the body.

An average individual's interpretation of this information is that the keto diet improves brain functionality, memory capacity, and overall brain health. This is due to the presence of fatty acids, namely fish omega 3 and omega 6. The brain tissue mainly consists of fatty acids (which is why fish are referred to as "Brainfood"), which means that the use of such fatty acids will improve the brain's health. Our body does not produce fatty acids alone; only through our diet can we obtain them. And the keto diet is full of fatty acids.

When on a diet with a higher quantity of carbohydrates, the result can be a muddled brain, where it becomes less possible to focus on thoughts. However, increased energy in comparison to keto diets makes it easier to focus. In reality, for better brain performance, people who do not want weight loss follow keto diets.

INCREASED ENERGY

Poor carbohydrate-filled diets often result in weakness and fatigue following daily activities. Meanwhile, fatty acids are a better efficient source of energy, constantly renewing the body system, making one feel more energized and strengthened in comparison with the feelings of a "sugar" rush.

ACNE

It appears surprising to many people when they get to know that the keto diet also helps with healthy skin and the elimination of skin acne. This is because it is not a pronounced benefit and not well-documented. While acne is a relatively common skin disease among adults, it is more prominent among teens as about ninety of them suffer from it. Acne, over time, has been perceived to be a result of poor diet; however, controlled research studies are ongoing to establish the authenticity of the claim. It has been proven that individuals on the keto diet have clearer skin, which is free from acne. The logical explanation for this is that a 1972 study proved that a large amount of insulin causes skin acne, which is being prevented by keto diets as it keeps insulin at a low and moderate level needed for healthy living, hence, improved skin health.

Also, inflammation causes acne. Meanwhile, keto diets reduce inflammation, which in turn helps the body in reducing the outbursts of acne. Fatty acids have been proven to be an effective anti-inflammatory, and they are abundant in fishes. Although research is ongoing on keto diets and their benefits, it has been established that the keto diet is essential for clearer, improved, and radiant skin.

KETO AND ANTI-AGING

Naturally, aging comes with many diseases. Although there is no study on the effect of a keto diet on human brain cells, studies on mice proved that brain cells improve when on a keto diet.

Many scientific studies have shown that the keto diet has positive effects on people suffering from Alzheimer's disease. It is recognized that diets with a good proportion of good nutrients, healthy fats, low-carbohydrate, high protein content, low sugar content, and also abundant in antioxidants help to improve our well-being while these diets also shield us from harmful substances from poor diets.

Research has also proven that an efficient way of slowing down the aging process is by consuming more fatty acids which the body converts to energy rather than heavy reliance on sugar as the primary energy source.

Also, the consumption of a moderate quantity of calories and eating less is one of the basic health principles which help to reduce our susceptibility to obesity and its consequences.

Although studies on keto diets are relatively small, however, the few but thrilling benefits derived from the ketogenic diet on our well-being emphasize the effectiveness of the diet in aiding natural growth while keeping the natural effects of aging in check. A regular Western diet with high sugar content and processed foods are not suitable for the easy aging process.

KETO AND HUNGER

1 of the reasons that many people avoid dieting is because many traditional diets make people feel hungry, allowing them to feel deprived, which makes them easily give up. However, due to its low-carbohydrate and low-calorie content, the keto diet plugs this gap, which makes people feel filled and happy.

KETO AND EYESIGHT

It is known that high blood sugar levels increase the likelihood of cataracts developing. Keto diets help keep good eyesight and also protect against cataracts due to their effective control of the body's sugar level.

KETO AND AUTISM

Although keto diets increase the brain's flexibility, a recent study of autistic patients has shown that the keto diet actually deals with autism. The study, which showed positive effects of keto diets on autism, revealed that students exhibited improved autistic behavior, especially those with lower autism.

MACRONUTRIENTS AND MICRONUTRIENTS

The benefits of a ketogenic diet, as mentioned earlier, are not limited to weight loss, but the diet comes with a range of health benefits. The positive reviews for the aforementioned diet have increased significantly, and this rise in popularity has prompted researchers and scientists to perform additional controlled trials to test its long-term effectiveness. The primary reason this diet helps in weight loss is the decreased appetite, which naturally makes keeping the low-calorie intake quite easy. If you over-consume calories, no matter the quality of your macronutrients, it will inhibit weight loss in your body.

A macronutrient's mass and ratio define how much one can consume of the macronutrient. Based on the diet regimen the amount of each macronutrient in low-carb diets will differ. The macronutrient composition is as follows when it comes to the ketogenic diet, macronutrient composition = 5 percent carbs + 15 percent protein + 80 percent fats.

A traditional ketogenic diet needs you to eat 20–30 g. of carbs in a day while fat intake depends on protein and carbs intake. A few examples of macronutrient-rich foods are:

Fats (coconut oil, olive oil, macadamia nuts, avocado, brazil nuts)

Protein (eggs, cheese, yogurt, milk, chicken, fish)

Carbohydrates (sweets, sugary snacks, bread, cereals, pasta, potatoes)

Carbohydrates

Dietary carbohydrates also called carbs are responsible for energy generation in your body. The human body uses carbohydrates to generate energy. Experts say however that carbs are not the main energy source. The body can make energy out of dietary fat and protein.

When you follow a ketogenic diet, the carb intake is extremely low, which is a complete contrast to the current Western diet. People who follow the modern Western diet today derive their dietary calories from the carbs they eat. Your body releases insulin when you consume carbohydrates and this, in turn, hinders the production of ketones in the liver making it impossible for the body to get into ketosis. Therefore, when you are on a keto diet, it's important to monitor and control your carb intake. A standard keto diet recommends reducing your carb intake to or below 5 percent.

A properly planned and well-designed ketogenic diet will have fiber intake along with fats as the crucial component. Fiber is important for keeping your gut healthy and keeping you satiated as it increases the bulk of the food. Including fiber-rich cruciferous vegetables and leafy greens is crucial for a proper ketogenic diet. The total carbohydrates minus the total fiber will be your net carb consumption, and it is this measure that will help you track your carb intake.

You need to understand that an increase in fiber intake does not affect blood ketone levels and blood glucose levels as well. Fibers are immune to digestion, which can provide you with a satiated sensation that reduces your appetite.

Proteins

Proteins are large molecular structures that consist of long and tiny amino acid chains. They are responsible for:

Glucose conversion through gluconeogenesis

Charging the intermediates in different metabolic pathways such as the Krebs Cycle

Building the functional and structural components of the cells

Although the body can use protein as a source of energy, that is not its primary function. Hence, it is important to have an adequate protein balance in your body to maintain muscle mass while following the keto diet. You must ensure that the calories from protein intake do not exceed 20–25 percent or else the protein gluconeogenesis process may hinder ketone production.

Let your protein intake be somewhere between 0.8–1.2 g. per kg. of your body weight when you begin with the ketogenic diet. This can help you balance your protein requirements against the potential for unnecessary gluconeogenesis.

Fats

Obesity has always been in the spotlight on the wrong side. Many people have confused this with being the reason for increased weight and heart problems. Fat is the only macronutrient possessing molecules of triglycerides. The main functionality of fat as nutrition in your food is to provide you with additional levels of energy and make up your system's key structural and functional parts.

Nutrient fat is often confused with fat. The fat in your cells and the different types of available fat molecules are not identical.

CHAPTER 2. WHAT IS A CHAFFLE

Waffles have gotten too well known in the keto network recently and in light of current circumstances. Waffles is a very adaptable bread swap that can be utilized for a vast assortment of things. They can be used as a pizza outside layer (clearly), as sandwich bread, or even as a sweet!

Chaff is genuinely anything you need it to be, with a couple of adjustments. We have utilized chaffs in various manners, as to make a Keto Peanut Butter Cup Waffle, Best Oreo Keto Waffles, or even a Keto Pumpkin Cheesecake Waffle. What's more, obviously, we have idealized the first waffle with our Easy Traditional Keto Waffle Recipe.

EXQUISITE WAFFLES VS. SWEET WAFFLES

There are fundamentally two sorts of waffles: delicate and cute. It's difficult to state on the off chance that one kind is superior to the next since they are both so delicious, so we will simply discuss the incredible things that every sort of waffle brings to the table.

As we previously referenced, flavorful waffles are utilized in (you got it) exquisite desserts. There are now and then uses as bread when making a sandwich, they are being used as a pizza covering, or they are utilized in some other delicious dish you like.

Perhaps the best thing about appetizing waffles is that they will, in general, be somewhat more straightforward and faster to make. The most fundamental waffle is simply cheddar and eggs, which means making it is as simple as splitting an egg and blending it in with some cheddar. We're talking about 30 sec. worth of work to make dinner. It doesn't beat that!

Sweet waffles are undoubtedly simple to make as well. However, once in a while, require a couple of extra fixings. In any case, however, making a sweet waffle is as simple as combining a few fixings and tossing it on a waffle iron.

Sweet waffles can be utilized to make a wide range of things. 1 of our most loved waffle desserts is a strawberry shortcake waffle, and it is so delicious! It sincerely tastes precisely like the strawberry shortcake you get at a celebration!

WOULD YOU BE ABLE TO MAKE WAFFLES AHEAD AND FREEZE?

While we don't generally suggest freezing a previously made pizza waffle, you can surely freeze the waffles themselves and defrost them to make a waffle pizza. Waffles freeze very well and make for a great dinner prep nourishment.

There are two essential manners by which you can freeze waffles. The primary method to freeze your waffles is to wrap them separately in aluminum foil and freeze them that way. This requires the least number of steps; however, it can take more time. The second, and presumably the least demanding all-around approach to freeze waffles is to streak freeze them in the cooler on a heating sheet and, afterward, include them all into a plastic ziplock cooler bag.

However, if the waffles are still warm, the steam will eventually turn to water and cause all of your chaffles to freeze together. This will make it difficult to defrost one by one.

CHAPTER 3. TIPS ON HOW TO MAKE PERFECT WAFFLES

Making the perfect keto waffles is quite easy if you follow a few simple steps.

1. BLEND THE BATTER

My number one tip for the perfect waffles is to blend the batter. It's a game-changer. Ever since I shared some of these tips, they went viral on social media, and many people have been using them to make the fluffiest, most tasty waffles!

I discovered the blending trick when I was working on my Keto Waffles Book. I tested with several different versions of the waffle dough, which I then used in over seventy-five waffle recipes.

For best results, I make use of a small Bamix blender which is perfect for blending a small quantity of the batter, although you could double the batch and use the usual food processor, or even a stick blender will do just fine.

Blending the batter will really do the magic for you—I don't make waffles any other way. Here are some of the reasons:

When you blend the batter before pouring it into the waffle maker, it makes the batter thicker and less likely to leak out.

The flavor is much better when the batter is blended.

Also, blending makes the perfect fluffy texture with no cheese bits and no eggy taste after.

2. USE A KITCHEN SCALE

To get perfect results every time, it's better if you make use of a kitchen scale for most of your ingredients. Ideally, when it comes to keto baking, cup measurements are not a hundred percent reliable as product density may vary.

3. AVOID USING BAKING POWDER IN WAFFLES

Using baking powder will give the waffles volume and make them fluffier and less dense.

If you can't find gluten-free baking powder, you can make use of a mixture of baking soda and cream of tartar. You will only need an equivalent of 1/8 tsp. baking powder, so it may be difficult to measure out if you only make one batch. To get 1 tsp. gluten-free baking powder, simply use 1/2 tsp. cream of tartar and 1/4 tsp. baking soda. If you don't have a cream of tartar, then you can use the same amount of lemon juice or apple cider vinegar.

Endeavor to stick with the recommended amounts of baking powder. You will need less baking powder when making sweet waffles than you will in savory waffles because most sweeteners also act as a raising agent. If you make use of excess baking powder, the batter will likely overflow, and your waffle maker will get messed up.

4. DO NOT OVERFILL YOUR WAFFLE MAKER

Endeavor not to overfill your waffle maker and follow the recommended quantity per waffle. What may appear like a small quantity will expand several times once you begin to heat it.

5. THE SIZE OF THE EGG MATTERS

A big egg should weigh about 50 g. (1.8 oz.). A large egg white will weigh approximately 33 g./1.2 oz., but you may get 10–20% more or less, even if it's a big egg.

The recipe will still come out good with a slightly larger egg, but the batter might likely leak out of your waffle maker, so always monitor it and gently lift it up if, eventually, the batter starts to overflow. This will minimize the pressure on the batter, and it will be less likely to spill.

6. ALWAYS KEEP MONITORING YOUR WAFFLE MAKER

You will be working with a small quantity of the batter when using a mini waffle maker, so there will always be the tendency of overflowing. For that reason, always watch the batter and if it's about to overflow, gently lift the lid to minimize the pressure on the batter. This should make the leak stop. You can also use a plastic or wooden spatula to gently push back any batter that is about to leak out.

Another way to avoid leaking is to add the batter in 2 parts per waffle. To do this, spoon part of the batter into the waffle maker. Then close the lid and cook for about a minute. Open the lid and add more batter in. Gently close the lid and cook for another 2–4 min.

7. WHAT YOU NEED TO DO IF THE BATTER IS TOO RUNNY

The batter will be too runny when you blend the cheese, eggs, and sweetener. To prevent that from happening, pour in the sweetener after you might have blended the cheese with the egg by simply using a spoon to mix it.

Finally, if you're working on your own recipe and the batter seems too runny, you can add 1–2 tsp. coconut flour or up to 1 tsp. psyllium husk powder. This will make the batter thicken, and the tendency of overflowing will be less likely.

8. ALLOW THE WAFFLES TO COOL DOWN BEFORE SERVING

Hot waffles fresh from the waffle maker will be soft, and there are some types of sweet waffles that may be fragile. That's why it's wise to first open the cover of your waffle maker and let the waffle cool slightly (approximately 15–30 sec.) before using a wooden or plastic spatula to gently scoop them to a cooling rack.

As the waffles cool down, they will become harden and crisp up. Base on the batter and the cheese you used, you will get slightly different textures. The cooking time for waffles varies between 2–5 min. or might take a long time if you prefer your waffles crispier.

Note that some types of cheese like shredded mozzarella and some other ingredients like cacao powder or chocolate chips might get burnt, so make sure to check the waffles after 2 min. and every other minute.

CHAPTER 4. BREAKFAST AND BRUNCH WAFFLE RECIPES

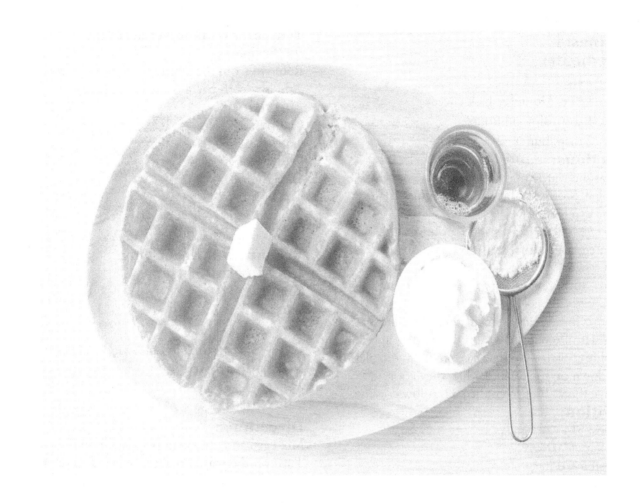

1. BREAKFAST WAFFLE SANDWICH

Preparation time: 5 min.
Cooking time: 15 min.
Servings: 1
Ingredients:

- 1 egg
- 1/2 c. Monterey Jack cheese
- 1 tbsp. almond flour
- 2 tbsp. butter

Directions:

Preheat the waffle maker for 5 min.

Combine Monterey Jack cheese, almond flour, and the egg in a bowl.

Take 1/2 of the batter and pour it into the preheated waffle maker. Allow cooking for 3–4 min.

Repeat the previous step for the remaining batter.

Melt the butter on a small pan. Just like you would with French toast, add the waffles and let each side cook for 2 min. To make them crispier, press down on the waffles while they cook.

Remove the waffles from the pan. Allow cooling.

Nutrition:

Calories: 514
Total Fat: 47 g.
Cholesterol: 0 mg.
Sodium: 0 mg.
Total Carbs: 0 g.
Sugar: 0 g.
Protein: 21 g.

2. HALLOUMI CHEESE WAFFLES

Preparation time: 5 min.
Cooking time: 10 min.
Servings: 1
Ingredients:

- 3 oz. halloumi cheese
- 2 tbsp. pasta sauce

Directions:

Make 1/2-in. thick slices of halloumi cheese.

With the waffle maker still turned off, place the cheese slices on it.

Turn on the waffle maker and let the cheese cook for 3–6 min.

Remove from the waffle maker and let it cool.

Add low-carb pasta or marinara sauce.

Nutrition:

Calories: 333
Total Fat: 26 g.
Saturated Fat: 0 g.
Cholesterol: 0 mg.
Total Carbs: 2 g.
Protein: 22 g.

3. BREAKFAST WAFFLE

Preparation time: 5 min.
Cooking time: 5 min.
Servings: 2
Ingredients:

- 2 eggs
- 1/2 c. shredded mozzarella cheese

For the toppings:

- 2 ham slices
- 1 fried egg

Directions:

Mix eggs and cheese into a small bowl.

Turn on the waffle maker to heat and oil it with cooking spray. Onto the waffle maker, add half of the batter.

Cook for 2–4 min., remove, and repeat with the remaining batter. Place egg and ham between two waffles to make a sandwich.

Nutrition:

Carbs: 1 g.
Fat: 8 g.
Protein: 9 g.
Calories: 115

4. HOT DOG WAFFLES

Preparation time: 15 min.
Cooking time: 14 min.
Servings: 2
Ingredients:

- 1 egg, beaten
- 1 c. finely grated cheddar cheese
- 2 hot dog sausages, cooked
- Mustard dressing for topping
- 8 pickle slices

Directions:

Preheat the waffle iron.

In a medium bowl, mix the egg and cheddar cheese.

Open the iron and add half of the mixture. Close and cook until crispy, 7 min.

Transfer the waffle to a plate and make a second waffle in the same manner.

To serve, top each waffle with a sausage, swirl the mustard dressing on top, and then divide the pickle slices on top.

Nutrition:

Calories: 231
Total Fat: 18.29 g.
Saturated Fat: 0 g.
Cholesterol: 0 mg.
Total Carbs: 2.8 g.
Protein: 13.39 g.

5. OMELETE

Preparation time: 8 min.
Cooking time: 17 min.
Servings: 2
Ingredients:

- 7 oz. spinach (frozen)
- 6 large eggs
- 2 tbsp. milk
- 2 tsp. oil
- 1 tbsp. herbs
- 1/4 c. grated sharp cheddar
- 1/4 c. grated parmesan cheese
- 1/4 c. crumbled, mild feta cheese
- 1 handful of kale, chopped
- 1/2 c. ricotta cheese
- Pepper for taste

Directions:

Ensure there is no liquid in your spinach.

Chop the spinach finely then do the same with the kale.

Add the parmesan cheese along with cheddar, eggs, and milk and mix well.

Mix the herbs, feta, and ricotta in a separate bowl, and then season with pepper.

Place the bowl to the side.

Heat a single teaspoon of olive oil in a non-stick pan

Pour in half of the egg mix you made.

On medium-high heat fry until just set.

Add half of the ricotta mix on top before folding the omelet over.

Place a lid over the pan and then cook for another minute so that your filling is warmed.

Repeat for the second omelet.

Nutrition:

Calories: 522
Total Fat: 34.7 g.
Saturated Fat: 0 g.
Cholesterol: 0 mg.
Total Carbs: 10.3 g.
Fiber: 2.4 g.
Protein: 44 g.

6. PANDAN ASIAN WAFFLES

Preparation time: 3 min.
Cooking time: 8 min.
Servings: 2
Ingredients:

- 1/2 c. cheddar cheese, finely shredded
- 1 egg
- 3 drops of pandan extract
- 1 tbsp. almond flour
- 1/3 tsp. garlic powder

Directions:

Warm up your mini waffle maker.

Mix the egg, almond flour, garlic powder with cheese into a small bowl.

Add pandan extract to the cheese mixture and mix well.

For a crispy crust, add 1 tsp of shredded cheese to the waffle maker and cook for 30 sec.

Pour and cook the mixture in the waffle maker for 5 min.

Repeat with the remaining batter.

Serve with fried chicken wings with BBQ sauce.

Nutrition:

Calories: 170

Total Fat: 13 g.

Saturated Fat: 0 g.

Cholesterol: 0 mg.

Total Carbs: 2 g.

Protein: 11 g.

7. HAM AND JALAPENOS WAFFLE

Preparation time: 5 min.

Cooking time: 9 min.

Servings: 3

Ingredients:

- 2 lb. cheddar cheese, finely grated
- 2 large eggs
- 1/2 jalapeno pepper, finely grated
- 2 oz. ham steak
- 1 medium scallion
- 2 tsp. coconut flour

Directions:

Shred the cheddar cheese using a fine grater.

Deseed the jalapeno and grate using the same grater.

Finely chop the scallion and ham.

Pour all the ingredients into a medium bowl and mix well.

Spray your waffle iron with cooking spray and heat for 3 min.

Pour 1/4 of the batter mixture into the waffle iron.

Cook for 3 min., until crispy around the edges.

Remove the waffles from the heat and repeat until all the batter is finished.

Once done, allow them to cool and enjoy.

Nutrition:

Calories: 120

Total Fat: 10 g.

Saturated Fat: 0 g.

Cholesterol: 0 mg.

Total Carbs: 2 g.

Protein: 12 g.

8. HOT HAM WAFFLES

Preparation time: 5 min.

Cooking time: 4 min.

Servings: 4

Ingredients:

- 1/2 c. mozzarella cheese, shredded
- 1 egg
- 1/4 c. ham, chopped
- 1/4 tsp. salt
- 2 tbsp. mayonnaise
- 1 tsp. Dijon mustard

Directions:

Preheat your waffle iron.

In the meantime, add the egg into a small mixing bowl and whisk.

Mix in the ham, cheese, and salt.

Scoop half the mixture using a spoon and pour into the hot waffle iron.

Close and cook for 4 min.

Remove the waffle and place it on a large plate.

Repeat the process with the remaining batter.

In another bowl, add the mustard and mayo. Mix together until smooth.

Slice the waffles in quarters and use the mayo mixture as the dip.

Nutrition:

Calories: 110

Total Fat: 12 g.

Saturated Fat: 0 g.
Cholesterol: 0 mg.
Total Carbs: 6 g.
Protein: 12 g.

9. BACON AND EGG WAFFLES

Preparation time: 5 min.
Cooking time: 10 min.
Servings: 2
Ingredients:

- 2 eggs
- 4 tsp. collagen peptides, grass-fed
- 2 tbsp. pork panko
- 3 slices crispy bacon

Directions:

Warm-up your mini waffle maker.
Combine the eggs, pork panko, and collagen peptides. Mix well. Divide the batter into two small bowls.
Once done, evenly distribute 1/2 of the crispy chopped bacon on the waffle maker.
Pour one bowl of the batter over the bacon. Cook for 5 min. and immediately repeat this step for the second waffle.
Plate your cooked waffles and sprinkle with extra panko for an added crunch.

Nutrition:

Calories: 266
Total Fat: 17 g.
Saturated Fat: 0 g.
Cholesterol: 0 mg.
Total Carbs: 11.2 g.
Protein: 27 g.

10. CHEESE-FREE BREAKFAST WAFFLE

Preparation time: 4 min.
Cooking time: 12 min.
Servings: 1
Ingredients:

- 1 egg
- 1/2 c. almond milk ricotta, finely shredded.
- 1 tbsp. almond flour
- 2 tbsp. butter

Directions:

Mix the egg, almond flour, and ricotta into a small bowl.
Separate the waffle batter into two and cook each for 4 min.
Pour the melted butter on top of the waffles.
Put them back in the pan and cook on each side for 2 min.
Remove from the pan and allow them to set for 2 min.
Enjoy while still crispy.

Nutrition:

Calories: 530
Total Fat: 50 g.
Saturated Fat: 0 g.
Cholesterol: 0 mg.
Total Carbs: 3 g.
Protein: 23 g.

11. BACON WAFFLE OMELETTES

Preparation time: 5 min.
Cooking time: 10 min.
Servings: 2
Ingredients:

- 2 slices bacon, raw
- 1 egg
- 1 tsp. maple extract, optional
- 1 tsp. all spices

Directions:

Put the bacon slices in a blender and turn it on.
Once ground up, add in the egg and all spices.
Go on blending until liquefied.
Heat your waffle maker on the highest setting and spray with non-stick cooking spray.
Introduce half the omelet into the waffle maker and cook for 5 min. max.
Remove the crispy omelet and repeat the same steps with the rest of the batter.
Enjoy warm.

Nutrition:
Calories: 59
Total Fat: 4.4 g.
Saturated Fat: 0 g.
Total Carbs: 1 g.
Protein: 5 g.

12. KETO WAFFLE TOPPED WITH SALTED CARAMEL SYRUP

Preparation time: 15 min.
Cooking time: 10 min.
Servings: 2
Ingredients:

- 1 egg
- 1/2 c. mozzarella cheese
- 1/4 c. cream
- 2 tbsp. collagen powder
- 1 1/2 tbsp. almond flour
- 1 1/2 tbsp. unsalted butter
- Pinch of salt
- 3/4 tbsp. powdered erythritol
- Pinch of baking powder

Directions:
Preheat your waffle machine
Whisk together the waffle ingredients that include the egg, mozzarella cheese, almond flour, and baking powder.
Pour the mixture on the waffle machine. Let it cook until golden brown.
To make the caramel syrup, turn on the flame under a pan to medium heat. Melt the unsalted butter on the pan.
Then turn the heat low and add collagen powder and erythritol to the pan and whisk them. Gradually add the cream and remove it from the heat. Then add the salt and continue to whisk.
Pour syrup onto the waffle and enjoy.

Nutrition:
Calories: 605

Fat: 45 g.
Protein: 48 g.
Carbohydrates: 5.1 g.

13. KETO WAFFLE BACON SANDWICH

Preparation time: 15 min.
Cooking time: 10 min.
Servings: 2
Ingredients:

- 1 egg
- 1/2 c. shredded mozzarella cheese
- 2 tbsp. almond flour
- 2 strips of pork or beef bacon
- 1 slice of any type of the cheese
- 2 tbsp. coconut oil

Directions:
Preheat your waffle machine.
In a bowl, beat 1 egg, 1/2 c. mozzarella cheese, and almond flour. Pour the mixture on the waffle machine. Let it cook until it is golden brown. Then remove in a plate.
Warm coconut oil in a pan over medium heat. Then place the bacon strips in the pan. Cook until crispy over medium heat. Assemble the bacon and cheese on the waffle.

Nutrition:
Calories: 580
Fat: 52 g.
Carbohydrates: 3 g.

14. CRISPY ZUCCHINI WAFFLE

Preparation time: 15 min.
Cooking time: 5 min.
Servings: 3
Ingredients:

- 2 eggs
- 1 fresh zucchini
- 1 c. shredded or grated cheddar cheese
- 2 pinches of salt

- 1 tbsp. onion (chopped)
- 1 clove of garlic

Directions:
Preheat the waffle maker.
Start by dicing onions and mashing the garlic. Then grate the zucchini.
Add 2 eggs and the grated zucchini into a bowl.
Also, add the onions, salt, and garlic for extra flavor. You can also add other herbs to give your waffle more flavor. Then sprinkle 1/2 c. cheese on top of the waffle machine.
Add the mixture from the bowl to the waffle machine. Add the remaining cheese on top of the waffle machine and close the waffle machine. Make sure the waffle cooks for about 3–5 min. until it turns golden brown.
By the layering method, you will achieve the perfect crisp. Take out your zucchini waffles and serve them hot and fresh.

Nutrition:
Calories: 170
Fat: 12 g.
Carbohydrates: 4 g.
Protein: 11 g.

15.PEANUT BUTTER WAFFLE

Preparation time: 15 min.
Cooking time: 10 min.
Servings: 3
Ingredients:
- 1 egg
- 1/2 c. cheddar cheese
- 2 tbsp. peanut butter
- Few drops of vanilla extract

Directions:
Grate some cheddar cheese.
Add one egg, cheddar cheese, 2 tbsp. peanut butter, and a few drops of vanilla extract and mix thoroughly.

Then sprinkle some shredded cheese as a base on the waffle maker. Pour the mixture on top of the waffle machine.
Sprinkle more cheese on top of the mixture and close the waffle machine. Ensure that the waffle is cooked thoroughly for about a few minutes until they are golden brown. Then remove it and enjoy your deliciously cooked waffles.

Nutrition:
Calories: 363
Fat: 29 g.
Protein: 22 g.
Carbohydrates: 4 g.

16.BEST KETO WAFFLE

Preparation time: 10 min.
Cooking time: 5 min.
Servings: 4
Ingredients:
- 2 eggs
- 1 c. shredded cheddar cheese
- 1 scoop of Perfect Keto Flavored Collagen

Directions:
Heat the mini waffle iron.
While the waffle iron is heating, mix all the ingredients in a medium-sized bowl.
Spoon 1/4 c. mix into the waffle maker and cook for 3–4 min. or until waffles are crisp.
Serve and enjoy!

Nutrition:
Calories: 326
Fat: 24.75 g.
Carbohydrates: 2 g. (net: 1 g.)
Fiber: 1 g.
Protein: 25 g.

17. HAM CHEDDAR WAFFLES

Preparation time: 15 min.
Cooking time: 14 min.
Servings: 2
Ingredients:

- 1 c. finely shredded parsnips, steamed
- 2 eggs, beaten
- 8 oz. ham, diced
- 1 1/2 c. grated cheddar cheese
- 1/2 tsp. garlic powder
- 2 tbsp. chopped fresh parsley leaves
- 1/2 tsp. dried thyme
- 1/4 tsp. smoked paprika
- Salt and black pepper to taste

Directions:

Preheat the waffle iron.

Mix all the ingredients into a bowl. Then, add half of the batter to the waffle iron. Close and cook for 6–7 min. or until crispy.

Put the waffle on a plate and make a second one. Serve warm!

Nutrition:

Calories: 373
Fat: 15.68 g.
Carbohydrates: 24.38 g. (net: 1 g.)
Fiber: 3.9 g.
Protein: 34.05 g.

18. BACON ZUCCHINI WAFFLE

Preparation time: 10 min.
Cooking time: 8 min.
Servings: 4
Ingredients:

- 4 eggs
- 1 1/4 c. mozzarella cheese, shredded
- 1/2 c. almond flour
- 1/4 tsp. baking powder
- 1/4 tsp. garlic powder
- 1 tsp. onion powder
- 2 tbsp. spring onion, sliced
- 3 bacon slices, cooked and diced
- 1 medium zucchini, grated
- Pepper
- Salt

Directions:

In a medium bowl, whisk the eggs.

Add spring onion, baking powder, garlic powder, onion powder, bacon, zucchini, pepper, and salt and stir until well combined.

Add the shredded cheese and almond flour and stir to combine.

Heat the waffle iron. Pour 1/4 of the egg mixture in a hot waffle iron and cook until golden brown.

Serve and enjoy.

Nutrition:

Net Carbs: 4.2 g.
Calories: 191
Total Fat: 14.2 g.
Saturated Fat: 3 g.
Protein: 12.2 g.
Carbs: 6.5 g.
Fiber: 2.3 g.
Sugar: 2 g.
Fat: 67%
Protein: 25%
Carbs: 8%

19. CINNAMON BLUEBERRY WAFFLE

Preparation time: 10 min.
Cooking time: 16 min.
Servings: 4
Ingredients:

- 2 eggs
- 1/2 tsp. baking powder
- 1/2 c. blueberries
- 1 tsp. cinnamon
- 2 tsp. Swerve
- 3 tbsp. almond flour
- 1 c. mozzarella cheese, shredded

Directions:

Heat the waffle maker.

In a mixing bowl, mix together eggs, cheese, almond flour, Swerve, cinnamon, and baking powder until well combined.

Add blueberries and stir well.

Pour 1/4 of the batter into the hot waffle maker and cook for about 4–5 min. or until cooked.

Make the remaining batter waffles using the same process.

Serve and enjoy.

Nutrition:

Net Carbs: 4.7 g.

Calories: 96

Total Fat: 6.1 g.

Saturated Fat: 1.6 g.

Protein: 6.1 g.

Carbs: 6 g.

Fiber: 1.3 g.

Sugar: 2.2 g.

Fat: 56%

Protein: 25%

Carbs: 19%

20. VANILLA PROTEIN WAFFLE

Preparation time: 10 min.
Cooking time: 12 min.
Servings: 3
Ingredients:

- 2 eggs
- 1/8 tsp. vanilla
- 1 tbsp. Swerve
- 1/2 c. mozzarella cheese, shredded
- 1/2 scoop vanilla protein powder

Directions:

Heat the waffle maker.

In a mixing bowl, mix together eggs, vanilla, Swerve, cheese, and protein powder.

Pour 1/3 of the batter into the hot waffle maker and cook for 4 min. or until cooked.

Serve and enjoy.

Nutrition:

Net Carbs: 2.4 g.

Calories: 92

Total Fat: 4.6 g.

Saturated Fat: 1.7 g.

Protein: 10 g.

Carbs: 2.4 g.

Fiber: 0 g.

Sugar: 0.8 g.

Fat: 46%

Protein: 43%

Carbs: 11%

21. PERFECT PROTEIN WAFFLE

Preparation time: 10 min.
Cooking time: 8 min.
Servings: 2
Ingredients:

- 1 egg
- 1/4 tsp. baking powder
- 1 scoop whey protein powder
- 1/2 c. mozzarella cheese, shredded

Directions:

Mix all the ingredients.

Heat the waffle maker and lightly grease.

Pour 1/2 of the batter into the hot waffle maker and cook for 3–4 min.

Make the remaining batter waffle.

Serve and enjoy.

Nutrition:

Net Carbs: 2.6 g.

Calories: 112

Total Fat: 4.4 g.

Saturated Fat: 1.9 g.

Protein: 15.8 g.

Carbs: 2.6 g.

Fiber: 0 g.

Sugar: 0.6 g.

Fat: 35%

Protein: 56%

Carbs: 9%

22. ZUCCHINI COCONUT WAFFLE

Preparation time: 10 min.
Cooking time: 10 min.
Servings: 2
Ingredients:

- 2 eggs
- 1/4 c. coconut flour
- 1/4 tsp. garlic powder
- 3 tbsp. parmesan cheese, grated
- 1/2 c. cheddar cheese, shredded
- 1 medium zucchini, shredded
- 1/4 tsp. salt

Directions:
Add all the ingredients into the mixing bowl and mix until well combined.
Spray the waffle iron using the cooking spray.
Heat the waffle iron. Pour 1/4 of the mixture in a hot waffle iron and cook until golden brown.
Serve and enjoy.

Nutrition:
Net Carbs: 3.5 g.
Calories: 220
Total Fat: 15.3 g.
Saturated Fat: 8.4 g.
Protein: 15.6 g.
Carbs: 5.2 g.
Fiber: 1.7 g.
Sugar: 2.4 g.
Fat: 64%
Protein: 29%
Carbs: 7%

23. HEALTHY BREAKFAST WAFFLE

Preparation time: 10 min.
Cooking time: 8 min.
Servings: 2
Ingredients:

- 1 tbsp. cream cheese
- 2 tbsp. coconut flour
- 1/4 c. mozzarella cheese, shredded
- 2 1/2 tbsp. water
- 1 tbsp. flaxseed meal
- Pinch of salt

Directions:
Heat the waffle maker and lightly grease.
In a bowl, mix together all the ingredients.
Pour half of the batter into the hot waffle maker and cook for 4 min.
Serve and enjoy.

Nutrition:
Net Carbs: 2.3 g.
Calories: 76
Total Fat: 4.2 g.
Saturated Fat: 2.1 g.
Protein: 3 g.
Carbs: 6.3 g.
Fiber: 4 g.
Sugar: 0.1 g.
Fat: 64%
Protein: 20%
Carbs: 16%

24. JALAPENO CHEDDAR WAFFLE

Preparation time: 10 min.
Cooking time: 8 min.
Servings: 2
Ingredients:

- 1 egg
- 8 slices deli jalapeno
- 1/2 c. cheddar cheese, shredded

Directions:
Heat the waffle maker and lightly grease.
In a small bowl, mix together egg, cheese, and jalapeno slices.
Pour 1/2 of the egg mixture into the waffle maker and cook for 3–4 min.
Serve and enjoy.

Nutrition:
Net Carbs: 0.6 g.
Calories: 146
Total Fat: 11.6 g.
Saturated Fat: 6.6 g.
Protein: 9.8 g.
Carbs: 0.8 g.
Fiber: 0.2 g.
Sugar: 0.3 g.
Fat: 72%
Protein: 26%
Carbs: 2%

25. CRISPY ZUCCHINI BREAKFAST WAFFLE

Preparation time: 10 min.
Cooking time: 20 min.
Servings: 4
Ingredients:

- 2 eggs, lightly beaten
- 1 c. cheddar cheese, grated
- 1 small zucchini, grated and squeeze out excess liquid
- 1 garlic clove, minced
- 1 1/2 tbsp. onion, minced

Directions:
Heat the waffle maker and lightly grease.
In a bowl, mix eggs, garlic, onion, zucchini, and cheese until well combined.
Pour 1/4 c. batter into the hot waffle maker and cook for 5 min. or until golden brown.
Make the remaining batter waffles.
Serve and enjoy.

Nutrition:
Net Carbs: 1.7 g.

Calories: 153
Total Fat: 11.6 g.
Saturated Fat: 6.7 g.
Protein: 10.3 g.
Carbs: 2.1 g.
Fiber: 0.4 g.
Sugar: 1 g.
Fat: 69%
Protein: 26%
Carbs: 5%

26. SIMPLE AND PERFECT BREAKFAST WAFFLE

Preparation time: 10 min.
Cooking time: 6 min.
Servings: 2
Ingredients:

- 1 egg, lightly beaten
- 1/2 c. mozzarella cheese, shredded

Directions:
Add the egg into a small bowl and whisk with a fork. Add the shredded cheese and stir to combine.
Spray the waffle iron with cooking spray.
Pour half egg mixture into the hot waffle iron and cook for 2–3 min. Remove the waffle and cook the remaining batter.
Serve and enjoy.

Nutrition:
Net Carbs: 0.4 g.
Calories: 51
Total Fat: 3.4 g.
Saturated Fat: 1.4 g.
Protein: 4.8 g.
Carbs: 0.4 g.
Fiber: 0 g.
Sugar: 0.2 g.
Fat: 60%
Protein: 37%
Carbs: 3%

27. BACON CHEESE WAFFLE

Preparation time: 10 min.
Cooking time: 12 min.
Servings: 4
Ingredients:

- 2 eggs, lightly beaten
- 1/4 tsp. garlic powder
- 1/4 tsp. onion powder
- 3/4 c. cheddar cheese, shredded
- 2 bacon slices, cooked and chopped

Directions:
Heat the waffle maker and lightly grease.
In a bowl, mix eggs, garlic powder, onion powder, bacon, and cheese.
Pour 1/4 of the batter into the hot waffle maker and cook for 3 min. or until cooked.
Serve and enjoy.
Nutrition:
Net Carbs: 0.8 g.
Calories: 126
Total Fat: 10 g.
Saturated Fat: 5.3 g.
Protein: 8.4 g.
Carbs: 0.9 g.
Fiber: 0.1 g.
Sugar: 0.4 g.
Fat: 72%
Protein: 25%
Carbs: 3%

28. ASIAN BREAKFAST WAFFLE

Preparation time: 10 min.
Cooking time: 8 min.
Servings: 2
Ingredients:

- 1 egg
- 1 bacon slice, cooked and chopped
- 2 tbsp. green onion, sliced
- 1 tbsp. mayonnaise
- 1/2 c. mozzarella cheese, shredded

Directions:
Heat the waffle maker and lightly grease.
In a bowl, whisk together egg, cheese, mayonnaise, green onion, and bacon.
Pour half of the egg mixture into the hot waffle maker and cook for 4 min.
Serve and enjoy.
Nutrition:
Net Carbs: 2.6 g.
Calories: 90
Total Fat: 6.6 g.
Saturated Fat: 1.9 g.
Protein: 5.2 g.
Carbs: 2.8 g.
Fiber: 0.2 g.
Sugar: 0.8 g.
Fat: 66%
Protein: 23%
Carbs: 11%

29. BREAKFAST CAULIFLOWER WAFFLE

Preparation time: 10 min.
Cooking time: 10 min.
Servings: 2
Ingredients:

- 1 egg, lightly beaten
- 1/2 c. cauliflower rice
- 1 tbsp. almond flour
- 1/4 c. Mexican cheese, shredded
- Pepper
- Salt

Directions:
Heat the waffle maker and lightly grease.
Add all the ingredients into the bowl and mix until well combined.
Pour 1/2 of the batter into the hot waffle maker and cook for 5 min. or until golden brown.
Serve and enjoy.
Nutrition:
Net Carbs: 1.3 g.

Calories: 258
Total Fat: 22 g.
Saturated Fat: 12.8 g.
Protein: 18 g.
Carbs: 2.3 g.
Fiber: 1 g.
Sugar: 0.9 g.
Fat: 74%
Protein: 24%
Carbs: 2%

30.PERFECT BREAKFAST WAFFLE

Preparation time: 10 min.
Cooking time: 8 min.
Servings: 2
Ingredients:

- 1 egg
- 1/8 tsp. baking powder
- 1 tbsp. mayonnaise
- 1 tsp. water
- 1 tbsp. almond flour
- Pinch of salt

Directions:
Heat the waffle maker.
Add all the ingredients into the small bowl and mix until well combined.
Pour half of the batter into the hot waffle maker and cook for 3–4 min. or until golden brown.
Serve and enjoy.
Nutrition:
Net Carbs: 2.4 g.
Calories: 80
Total Fat: 6.4 g.
Saturated Fat: 1.2 g.
Protein: 3.6 g.
Carbs: 2.8 g.
Fiber: 0.4 g.
Sugar: 0.8 g.
Fat: 71%
Protein: 17%

Carbs: 12%

31.EASY BREAKFAST WAFFLE

Preparation time: 10 min.
Cooking time: 8 min.
Servings: 2
Ingredients:

- 1 egg, lightly beaten
- 1/4 tsp. garlic powder
- 1/2 c. mozzarella cheese, shredded
- 1/2 tsp. psyllium husk powder

Directions:
Heat the waffle maker and lightly grease.
Whisk the egg in a bowl with the remaining ingredients until well combined.
Pour 1/2 of the batter into the hot waffle maker and cook until golden brown.
Serve and enjoy.
Nutrition:
Net Carbs: 0.7 g.
Calories: 55
Total Fat: 3.4 g.
Saturated Fat: 1.4 g.
Protein: 4.8 g.
Carbs: 1.3 g.
Fiber: 0.6 g.
Sugar: 0.3 g. Fat: 57%
Protein: 36%
Carbs: 7%

32.CHEESE CABBAGE WAFFLE

Preparation time: 10 min.
Cooking time: 8 min.
Servings: 2
Ingredients:

- 1 egg, lightly beaten
- 2 tbsp. cabbage, chopped
- 2 tbsp. almond flour
- 1/3 c. mozzarella cheese, grated
- 1/2 bacon slice, chopped

- 1 1/2 tbsp. green onion, sliced
- Pepper
- Salt

Directions:
Heat the waffle maker and lightly grease.
Add all the ingredients into a bowl and stir to combine.
Pour half of the batter into the hot waffle maker and cook until golden brown.
Serve and enjoy.

Nutrition:
Net Carbs: 1.5 g.
Calories: 91
Total Fat: 6.9 g.
Saturated Fat: 1.5 g.
Protein: 5.9 g.
Carbs: 2.5 g.
Fiber: 1 g.
Sugar: 0.7 g.
Fat: 68%
Protein: 25%
Carbs: 7%

33.CHEESE HAM WAFFLE

Preparation time: 10 min.
Cooking time: 8 min.
Servings: 2
Ingredients:
- 1 egg, lightly beaten
- 1/2 c. cheddar cheese, shredded
- 1/4 c. ham, chopped

1/4 tsp. garlic salt
For dip:
- 1 tbsp. mayonnaise
- 1 1/2 tsp. Dijon mustard

Directions:
Heat the waffle maker and lightly grease.
Whisk the eggs in a bowl.
Stir in ham, cheese, and garlic salt until combine.
Pour half of the batter into the hot waffle maker and cook for 3–4 min.

For dip:
In a small bowl, mix mustard and mayonnaise.
Serve waffle with dip.

Nutrition:
Net Carbs: 3 g.
Calories: 205
Total Fat: 15.6 g.
Saturated Fat: 7.5 g.
Protein: 12.9 g.
Carbs: 3.4 g.
Fiber: 0.4 g.
Sugar: 0.9 g.
Fat: 69%
Protein: 26%
Carbs: 5%

34.FLAVORFUL BAGEL WAFFLE

Preparation time: 10 min.
Cooking time: 10 min.
Servings: 2
Ingredients:
- 1 egg, lightly beaten
- 3/4 c. mozzarella cheese, shredded
- 1/2 tsp. baking powder, gluten-free
- 1 tbsp. almond flour
- 1/4 tsp. garlic powder
- 1/4 tsp. onion powder
- 1 1/2 tsp. bagel seasoning

Directions:
Heat the waffle maker and lightly grease.
In a bowl, mix egg, bagel seasoning, baking powder, onion powder, garlic powder, and almond flour until well combined.
Add the cheese and stir well.
Pour 1/2 of the batter into the hot waffle maker and cook for 5 min.
Serve and enjoy.

Nutrition:
Net Carbs: 1.9 g.
Calories: 85
Total Fat: 5.8 g.

Saturated Fat: 1.9 g.
Protein: 6.6 g.
Carbs: 2.4 g.
Fiber: 0.5 g.
Sugar: 0.5 g.
Fat: 61%
Protein: 31%
Carbs: 8%

35. CRISPY WAFFLE
Preparation time: 10 min.
Cooking time: 10 min.
Servings: 2
Ingredients:

- 1 egg
- 2 tbsp. butter, melted
- 1/8 tsp. baking powder
- 1 tsp. coconut flour
- 1/4 c. almond flour
- Pinch of salt

Directions:
Preheat the waffle maker and lightly grease. Add all the ingredients into the mixing bowl and mix until well combined.
Pour 1/2 of the batter into the hot waffle maker and cook for 4–5 min.
Serve and enjoy.

Nutrition:
Net Carbs: 1 g.
Calories: 159
Total Fat: 15.6 g.
Saturated Fat: 8.2 g.
Protein: 3.8 g.
Carbs: 1.9 g.
Fiber: 0.9 g.
Sugar: 0.3 g.
Fat: 88%
Protein: 9%
Carbs: 2%

36. EVERYTHING WAFFLE
Preparation time: 8 min.
Cooking time: 10 min.
Servings: 2
Ingredients:

- 1 large egg
- 1 oz. 6 cheese Italian blend cheese, finely shredded
- 3 tbsp. almond flour
- 1 pinch salt
- Butter flavored non-stick cooking spray

For the topping:

- 2 oz. Cream Cheese
- 2 tsp. Everything Bagel Seasoning

Directions:
Plugin the mini waffle maker and preheat it. There is a light for many waffle makers to indicate when it is preheated. Be sure that it is completely heated before continuing for the best results.
Crack the large egg into a small bowl and beat vigorously with a fork until well-mixed yolk and white.
Chop the shredded Italian cheese into smaller pieces using a small chopping board and medium-sized knife. It ensures that the cheese can be distributed more evenly throughout the egg mixture.
Add the egg mixture with the butter, almond flour, and salt and whisk with a fork until all is well mixed.
Sprinkle the waffle maker with non-stick cooking spray flavored with butter.
Put 1/2 of the mixture in a miniature waffle maker's grill center. Stretch the mixture to the grill edges and close the waffle maker.
Cook the waffle for 5 min. or till brown and cook through until toasty.
Gently remove the waffle using a small fork and place it to cool on a sheet of paper towels.

Spray the waffle maker with non-stick cooking spray flavored with butter and cook the remaining mixture of the waffle the same as the first.

When they cool down, the waffles will become crisper.

Layer cream cheese and waffles and sprinkle with bagel seasoning.

Nutrition:
Calories: 249
Carbohydrates: 5 g.
Protein: 11 g.
Fat: 22 g.
Saturated Fat: 7 g.
Cholesterol: 116 mg.
Sodium: 169 mg.
Potassium: 91 mg.
Fiber: 2 g.
Sugar: 1 g.
Iron: 1 mg.

37.ALMOND MAYO WAFFLES
Preparation time: 10 min.
Cooking time: 14 min.
Servings: 2
Ingredients:
- 1 egg, beaten
- 2 tsp. water
- 4 tbsp. mayonnaise
- 2 tsp. sugar-free maple syrup
- 1/2 c. grated Swiss cheese
- 3 tbsp. almond flour
- 1/4 tsp. baking powder

Directions:
Preheat the waffle iron.

Meanwhile, in a medium bowl, combine all the ingredients.

Then, open the iron, add half of the batter, close the iron, and cook for 6–7 min. or until crispy.

Transfer the waffle onto a plate and make another waffle with the remaining ingredients. Enjoy!

Nutrition:
Calories: 300
Carbohydrates: 4.72 g.
Protein: 15.7 g.
Fat: 24.55 g.
Cholesterol: 116 mg.
Sodium: 327 mg.
Potassium: 227 mg.

38.CAJUN SHRIMP AND AVOCADO WAFFLE
Preparation time: 10 min.
Cooking time: 15 min.
Servings: 2
Ingredients:
- 2 slices of bacon
- 1/2 c. cheddar cheese (shredded)
- 1 tbsp. avocado oil
- 1 egg
- 1/2 c. onions (sliced)
- 2 tsp. Cajun seasoning
- 1 tbsp. almond flour
- 1 lb. shrimps
- Salt and pepper to taste

Directions:
Heat the avocado oil in a pan placed over low-medium heat. Add the bacon and cook for 3 min. per side or until crispy brown. Remove the pieces from the oil and pat dry with a paper towel. Set aside the oil used.

Put the shrimp in a bowl, add Cajun seasoning, avocado oil, salt, and pepper. Allow it to marinate for 15 min.

Place the used oil on medium heat and fry the shrimp for 2 min. per side. Remove and dry with a paper towel.

To make the waffle bread, preheat the waffle machine. In a bowl, combine egg, cheddar cheese, almond flour, and Cajun seasoning. Cook in your waffle machine.

Assemble your sandwich and serve.

Nutrition:
Calorie: 390
Carbs: 2.5 g.,
Fats: 16 g.,
Protein: 19 g.

39. BEACON AND CHEESE WAFFLE SANDWICH

Preparation time: 5 min.
Cooking time: 10 min.
Servings: 1
Ingredients:

- 2 beacon strip
- 1 egg
- 1 slice of cheddar cheese
- 1/2 c. mozzarella cheese (shredded)
- 1/2 tsp. baking powder
- 2 tbsp. almond oil
- 2 tbsp. almond flour
- 1 tsp. Italian herbs

Directions:

In a bowl, add almond flour, egg, mozzarella cheese, Italian herbs, and baking powder. Mix thoroughly.

Preheat the waffle machine, sprinkle some cheese, and leave for a few seconds. Pour the mixture and sprinkle more cheese.

Cook for 3–4 min. or until it turns golden brown. Place a pan over low-medium heat, add almond oil, then add your bacon and cook for 2 min. per side or until it turns golden brown.

Assemble the sandwich with bacon and cheese.

Nutrition:
Calorie: 929
Carbs: 2.2 g.
Fats: 30 g.
Protein: 24 g.

40. CORN BREAD WITH HOT DOG WAFFLE

Preparation time: 10 min.
Cooking time: 10 min.
Servings: 1
Ingredients:

- 2 tsp. almond flour
- 1/2 c. cheddar cheese (shredded)
- 1 sausage
- 2 tbsp. unsalted butter
- 1 tbsp. diced jalapeno
- 1 egg

Cornbread flavoring:
1 small onion (diced)
1/4 tsp. baking powder
1/4 tsp. salt
Tomato Ketchup (unsweetened)
Mustard sauce

Directions:

To prepare the cornbread, preheat the waffle-maker. In a bowl, add egg, 1/2 tbsp. jalapenos, almond flour, baking powder, and cheddar cheese. Mix.

Pour the mixture into the machine and cook for 3–4 min. or until it turns golden brown. Set aside.

Fill a pot with water, place over high-medium heat, and allow to boil. Add the sausage and boil for 3–5 min., remove and set aside.

Place a pan over medium heat, add unsalted butter and fry your sausage. Place the fried sausage inside the cornbread, add onions, cheddar cheese, jalapeno, ketchup, and mustard sauce. Serve.

Nutrition:
Calorie: 243
Carbs: 2.9 g.
Fats: 14 g.
Protein: 13.7 g.

41. WAFFLE BACON SANDWICH

Preparation time: 15 min.
Cooking time: 10 min.
Servings: 2
Ingredients:

- 1/2 c. mozzarella cheese
- 2 strips of bacon (either pork or beef)
- 2 tbsp. coconut flour
- 2 tbsp. coconut oil
- 2 slice of cheddar cheese
- 1 egg

Directions:

In a bowl, add egg, mozzarella, and flour. Mix the ingredients.

Preheat the waffle machine, sprinkle cheese, and allow it to melt. Pour the mixture and cook for 3–4 min.

In a pan, heat coconut oil, add your bacon, and fry for 2–3 min. per side, or until it is crispy.

Arrange the bacon and cheese on your waffle, enjoy.

Nutrition:
Calorie: 295
Carbs: 2.6 g.
Fats: 24.2 g.
Protein: 30

42. SAUSAGE BALL WAFFLE

Preparation time: 10 min.
Cooking time: 10 min.
Servings: 1
Ingredients:

- 1 egg
- 1/2 lb of Italian sausage
- 1/4 c. parmesan cheese
- 2 tbsp. flour
- 1 c. cheddar cheese (grated)
- 1 tsp. baking powder

Directions:

In a bowl, combine the egg, flour, cheddar, baking powder, and Italian sausage. Mix well.

Preheat the waffle-maker, sprinkle parmesan cheese, and allow cooking for about 30 sec.

Pour in the sausage mixture, close, and allow cooking for 3–4 min. or until it turns golden brown.

Serve hot.

Nutrition:
Calorie: 245
Carbs: 1.1 g.
Fats: 13.4 g.
Protein: 19.1 g.

43. PARMESAN CHICKEN FILLED WAFFLE

Preparation time: 10 min.
Cooking time: 5 min.
Servings: 2
Ingredients:

- 2 slices of parmesan cheese
- 1/2 c. chicken breast (shredded)
- 1/4 c. parmesan cheese
- 1 tbsp. pizza sauce
- 1 egg
- 1/4 c. mozzarella cheese
- 1 tsp. thick cream cheese
- 1/4 tsp. garlic powder
- 1/4 tsp. Italian seasoning

Directions:

In a bowl, combine the shredded chicken, garlic powder, Italian seasoning, mozzarella, parmesan, cream cheese, egg, and mix until smooth.

Preheat your waffle-maker, sprinkle some cheese on top. Leave for seconds, pour the chicken mixture, and sprinkle some cheese. Close the waffle-maker.

Cook the waffle for 3–5 min. or until it turns golden brown. Remove and spread pizza sauce on top, add the parmesan cheese slice (make sure the waffle is hot when adding the cheese to allow it to melt).

Serve hot.

Nutrition:

Calorie: 225

Carbs: 2.1 g.

Fats: 8.3 g.

Protein: 9.3 g.

44.KETO CHOCOLATE WAFFLE RECIPE

Preparation time: 10 min.

Cooking time: 5 min.

Servings: 2

Ingredients:

- 1 tsp. vanilla extract
- 1 egg
- 1 tsp. cocoa powder
- 3/4 oz. cream cheese
- 1–1/2 tbsp.coconut flour

Directions:

In a bowl, add all the ingredients and mix thoroughly.

Preheat the waffle-maker, pour the mixture and allow cooking for 3–4 min. or until it turns golden brown.

Serve hot.

Nutrition:

Calorie: 230

Carbs: 4 g.

Fats: 10 g.

Protein: 13 g.

45.SALAMI SANDWICH

Preparation time: 30 min.

Cooking time: 15 min.

Servings: 2

Ingredients:

1 egg

2 salami patties

1/2 c. mozzarella cheese (shredded)

1 slice of cheddar cheese

1/2 tsp. salt

2 slices of tomatoes

2 tbsp. coconut oil

2 slices of lettuce

1 tsp. Italian seasoning

Directions:

Heat coconut oil in a pan, add the salami patties and allow them to fry for 2 min. per side. Remove and pat dry with a paper towel, set aside.

In a bowl, add egg, mozzarella cheese, and Italian seasoning. Mix well.

Preheat the waffle-maker, sprinkle cheese, and allow it to melt. Pour the mixture into the waffle-maker and allow it to cook for 3–4 min. This is the sandwich base.

Assemble the sandwich with tomatoes, lettuce, and cheddar. Enjoy.

Nutrition:

Calorie: 270

Carbs: 3.1 g.

Fats: 15 g.

Protein: 11.9 g.

46.JALAPENO CHICKEN POPPER WAFFLES

Preparation time: 10 min.

Cooking time: 5 min.

Servings: 2

Ingredients:

- 1/2 c. chicken (shredded)
- 1/4 c. mozzarella cheese
- 1/4 tsp. garlic powder
- 1/4 c. parmesan cheese
- 1/4 tsp. onion powder
- 1 fresh jalapeno (diced)
- 1 egg
- 1 tsp. cream cheese

Directions:

Preheat the waffle-maker.

In a bowl, add all the ingredients and mix thoroughly.

Sprinkle cheese on the waffle-maker and heat for 20 sec. Pour the mixture on top and allow it to cook for 3–4 min.

Serve with any sauce or toppings of choice

Nutrition:

Calorie: 231.4

Carbs: 4.5 g.

Fats: 10.6 g.

Protein: 19.2 g.

47.JICAMA HASH BROWN WAFFLE

Preparation time: 5 min.

Cooking time: 10 min.

Servings: 2

Ingredients:

- 1 jicama root (peeled and shredded)
- 2 eggs
- 1 c. shredded cheddar cheese
- 1 tbsp. onions (minced)
- 1 clove garlic (pressed)
- Salt and pepper to taste

Directions:

Place the shredded jicama in a bowl, sprinkle with salt, and mix. Squeeze out excess water. Place in the microwave for 4–6 min.

Add all the ingredients to a bowl, including the jicama root. Mix thoroughly.

Preheat the waffle-maker, sprinkle with cheese and allow to melt. Pour the batter over the cheese and sprinkle more cheese.

Allow the batter to cook for about 3–4 min.

Serve fresh and hot.

Nutrition:

Calorie: 164

Carbs: 5 g.

Fats: 10.4 g.

Protein: 11.4 g.

48.CARNIVORE WAFFLES

Preparation time: 3 min.

Cooking time: 5 min.

Servings: 2

Ingredients:

- 1/2 c. pork rind (crushed)
- 1/2 c. cheddar cheese (shredded)
- 1 egg
- 1/4 tsp. salt.
- 1/4 tsp. onion powder
- 1/4 tsp. garlic powder

Directions:

Preheat the waffle-maker.

Add all the ingredients together in a bowl and whisk thoroughly.

Pour the waffle batter on the waffle-maker and top with some cheese.

Cook for 4–5 min. or until it turns golden brown.

Serve hot

Nutrition:

Calorie: 192

Carbs: 1 g.

Fats: 18 g.

Protein: 21.6 g.

49.BLT WAFFLE SANDWICH

Preparation time: 3 min.

Cooking time: 7 min.

Servings: 2

Ingredients:

- 2 slice bacon strips
- 1/2 c. cheddar cheese
- 1 slice of tomatoes
- 1 egg
- 1/2 tsp. Italian seasoning
- Slices of lettuce
- 1 tbsp.diced onions
- 2 tbsp. coconut oil

Directions:

Preheat the waffle-maker.

In a bowl, mix the egg, cheese, and Italian seasoning. Sprinkle some cheese on the waffle maker and allow it to melt. Pour the mixture and top with more cheese. Cook for 3–4 min.

Place a pan over medium heat, add coconut oil and fry your beacon for 2–3 min. per side, or until it turns golden brown and crispy.

Arrange your sandwich with tomatoes, onions, and lettuce.

Nutrition:
Calorie: 287
Carbs: 4 g.
Fats: 28 g.
Protein: 32 g.

50. FRIED PICKLE WAFFLE STICK

Preparation time: 6 min.
Cooking time: 4 min.
Servings: 2
Ingredients:
- 6 sliced pickles
- 1/2 c. mozzarella cheese
- 1 egg
- 1 tbsp. pickle juice
- 1/4 c. pork panko

Directions:
Drain excess juice from the pickle. Mix all the other ingredients.

Preheat the waffle-maker, sprinkle some cheese, and allow it to melt. Pour the mix on the cheese, add the sliced pickle, and another layer of the mix.

Cook for 3–4 min.

Serve with any sauce of choice.

Nutrition:
Calorie: 265
Carbs: 3.4 g.
Fats: 22.7 g.
Protein: 16.6 g.

51. BEACON-CHEESE-BISCUIT WAFFLE

Preparation time: 5 min.
Cooking time: 10 min.
Servings: 2
Ingredients:
- 2 beacon strips
- 1 tbsp. diced onions
- 2 tbsp. unsalted butter
- 1/2 c. cheddar cheese (shredded)
- 1/2 c. almond flour
- 2 tbsp. parmesan cheese
- 1 tbsp. fresh parsley (chopped)
- 1 tsp. baking powder
- 2 tbsp. sour cream
- Salt and pepper to taste
- 1 egg

Directions:
Preheat the waffle-maker.

Place a pan over medium heat and add the butter. Add the bacon strip and cook for 2–3 min. per side or until crispy. Blot dry with a paper towel and chop onto smaller pieces.

In a bowl, add cream, parmesan cheese, cheddar cheese, bacon, and egg. Whisk thoroughly, set aside. In another bowl, combine almond flour, onions, baking powder, parsley, salt, and pepper. Mix.

Add the egg mixture to the flour mixture and mix.

Sprinkle cheese on the waffle-maker and allow to melt, pour the mixture and cook for 3–4 min., repeat for the remaining batter.

Serve hot.

Nutrition:
Calorie: 172.6
Carbs: 3.3 g.
Fats: 12.7 g.
Protein: 10.8 g.

52.MUSHROOM STUFFED WAFFLES

Preparation time: 15 min.
Cooking time: 25 min.
Servings: 2
Ingredients:
For the waffle:

- 2 egg
- 1/2 c. mozzarella cheese (shredded)
- 1/2 tsp. onion powder
- 1/4 tsp. garlic powder
- 1/4 tsp. salt or as per your taste
- 1/4 tsp. black pepper or as per your taste
- 1/2 tsp. dried poultry seasoning

For stuffing:

- 1 small onion, diced
- 4 oz. mushrooms
- 3celery stalks
- 4 tbsp. butter
- 3 eggs

Directions:
Preheat a mini waffle maker if needed and grease it
In a mixing bowl, add all the waffle ingredients and mix them well
Pour the mixture to the lower plate of the waffle maker and spread it evenly to cover the plate properly; close the lid
Cook for at least 4 min. to get the desired crunch
Remove the waffle from the heat and keep it aside
Make as many waffles as your mixture and waffle maker allow
Take a small frying pan and melt the butter in it on medium-low heat
Sauté celery, onion, and mushrooms to make them soft
Take another bowl and tear waffles down into small pieces

Add the eggs and the veggies to it
Take a casserole dish, and add this new stuffing mixture to it
Bake it at 350 °F for around 30 min. and serve hot

Nutrition:
Calorie: 544
Carbs: 10.96 g.
Fats: 39.85 g.
Protein: 34.89 g.

53.JAPANESE STYLED BREAKFAST WAFFLE

Preparation time: 5 min.
Cooking time: 5 min.
Servings: 2
Ingredients:

- 1 egg
- 1/2 c. mozzarella cheese (shredded)
- 1 slice of bacon
- 2 tbsp. Kewpie mayo
- 1 green onion stalk

Directions:
Preheat a mini waffle maker if needed and grease it
In a mixing bowl, beat an egg and put 1 tbsp. Kewpie Mayo
Chop green onion and put half of it in the mixing bowl and half aside
Cut the bacon into pieces of 1/4 in. and add in the mixing bowl and mix well
Sprinkle around 1/8 c. shredded mozzarella cheese to the lower plate of the waffle maker and pour the mixture over it
Again sprinkle 1/8 c. shredded mozzarella cheese to the top of the mixture
Cook for at least 4 min. to get the desired crunch
Remove the waffle from the heat and drizzle Kewpie mayo

Serve by sprinkling the remaining green onions

Make as many waffles as your mixture and waffle maker allow

Nutrition:
Calorie: 209
Carbs: 3.22 g.
Fats: 14.89 g.
Protein: 15.22 g.

54. TURKEY WAFFLE

Preparation time: 5 min.
Cooking time: 5 min.
Servings: 2
Ingredients:
For the waffle:
- 2 egg
- 2 tbsp. cream cheese
- 1 tbsp. vanilla extract
- 2 tbsp. almond flour
- 1 tsp. heavy cream
- 1 tsp. cinnamon powder
- 1 tbsp. swerve sweetener

For For the assembling:
- 2 slices of the cheese
- 2 slices of ham
- 2 slices of turkey

Directions:
Preheat a mini waffle maker if needed and grease it

In a mixing bowl, add all the waffle ingredients and mix them well

Pour the mixture into the lower plate of the waffle maker and spread it evenly to cover the plate properly

Cook for at least 4 min. to get the desired crunch

Remove the waffle from the heat and keep it aside for around 1 min.

Make as many waffles as your mixture and waffle maker allow

Serve with a cheese slice, a turkey, and a ham

You can also serve with any of your favorite low-carb raspberry jam on top

Nutrition:
Calorie: 355
Carbs: 12.2 g.
Fats: 23.5 g.
Protein: 19.87 g.

55. ZUCCHINI NUT BREAD WAFFLE

Preparation time: 5 min.
Cooking time: 5 min.
Servings: 2
Ingredients:
For the waffle:
- 1 egg:
- 1 c. zucchini (shredded)
- 2 tbsp. cream cheese, softened
- 1/2 tsp. cinnamon
- 1 tsp. erythritol blend
- 1 tbsp. nutmeg, (grounded)
- 2 tsp. butter
- 1/2 tsp. baking powder
- 3 tbsp. walnuts
- 2 tsp. coconut flour

For the frosting:
- 4 tbsp. cream cheese
- 1/4 tsp. cinnamon
- 2 tbsp. butter
- 2 tbsp. caramel (sugar-free)
- 1 tbsp. walnuts (chopped)

Directions:
Grate zucchini and leave it in a colander for 10 min.

Squeeze with your hands to drain the water

Preheat a mini waffle maker and grease it

In a mixing bowl, beat an egg, zucchini, and the other waffle ingredients

Pour the mixture to the lower plate of the waffle maker and spread it evenly to cover the plate properly and close the lid

Cook for at least 4 min. to get the desired crunch

Remove the waffle from the heat

Make as many waffles as your mixture and waffle maker allow

Whisk all the frosting ingredients together except for the walnuts and give a uniform consistency

Serve the waffles with frosting on top and chopped nuts

Nutrition:
Calorie: 562
Carbs: 29.4 g.
Fats: 43.3 g.
Protein: 17.07 g.

56. KETO "APPLE" FRITTER WAFFLES

Preparation time: 30 min.
Cooking time: 30 min.
Servings: 5
Ingredients:
For the filling:
- 2 c. diced jicama
- 1/4 c. + 1 tbsp. Swerve sweetener blend
- Butter
- 1 tsp. cinnamon
- 1/8 tsp. nutmeg
- Dash clove
- 1/2 tsp. vanilla
- 20 drops of Apple Flavor LorAnn Oils®

For the waffle:
- 2 eggs
- 1/2 c. grated mozzarella cheese
- 1 tbsp. almond flour
- 1 tsp. coconut flour
- 1/2 tsp. baking powder

For the glaze:
- 1 tbsp. butter
- 2 tsp. heavy cream
- 3 c. powdered sweetener such as swerve confectioners
- 1/4 tsp. vanilla essence

Directions:
For the filling:
Cut the jicama and cut into small dices.

In a medium-low heat pan, melt the butter and add the diced jicama and the sweetener.

Leave it to slowly simmer for 10–20 min., looking at it till the jicama is tender, stirring frequently. Avoid using high heat, or the sweetener will easily caramelize and burn. A light amber color should grow and thicken.

When the jicama is tender, remove from the heat and stir in the spices and flavorings.

For the waffle:
Preheat up to hot waffle iron.

Beat all the ingredients, except the milk, in a medium bowl. Stir the mixture of jicama into the eggs.

Put 1 tbsp. grated cheese on that waffle iron.

Spoon 2 tbsp. egg/jicama mixture into the waffle iron and finish with another tablespoon of the milk.

Open the waffle and cook for 5–7 min. until well browned and crispy.

Remove from the wire rack.

Repeat it 3–4 times.

For the filling:
Melt the butter in a small saucepan and add Swerve and heavy cream.

Simmer over medium heat for a few minutes or until lightly thickened.

Stir the vanilla.

Drizzle the hot frost over the cuffs. It's going to harden as it cools.

Nutrition:
Calories 186
Total Fat: 14.3 g.

Cholesterol 108.1 mg.
Sodium 117.7 mg.
Total Carbohydrate 8.5 g.
Dietary Fiber 3.4 g.
Sugars 1.5 g.
Protein: 7 g.
Vitamin A 148.2µg

57. WAFFLE GLAZED WITH RASPBERRY

Preparation time: 7 min.
Cooking time: 5 min.
Servings: 1
Ingredients:
For the waffle:

- 1 egg
- 1/4 c. mozzarella cheese, shredded
- 2 tsp. cream cheese, softened
- 1 tsp. sweetener
- 1tsp almond flour
- 1/2 tsp. baking powder
- Drops of glazed donut flavoring

For the filling:

- 1/4 c. raspberries
- 1 tsp. chia seeds
- 1 tsp. confectioners sweetener

For the glaze:

- 1 tsp. powdered sweetener
- Heavy whipping cream

Directions:
For the waffle:
Preheat your waffle maker.
Mix all the waffle ingredients.
Spray your waffle maker with cooking oil and add the batter mixture into the waffle maker.
Cook for 3 min. and set aside.
For the filling:
Mix all the ingredients under the filling section.
Place in a pot and heat on medium.

Gently mash the raspberries and set them aside to cool.
For the glaze:
Stir together the ingredients in a small dish.
For the assembling:
Lay your waffles on a plate and add the fillings mixture between the layers.
Drizzle the glaze on top and enjoy.
Nutrition:
Calories: 188
Fats: 23 g.
Carbs: 12 g.
Protein: 17 g.

58. LIGHT PARMESAN WAFFLES

Preparation time: 10 min.
Cooking time: 7 min.
Servings: 4
Ingredients:

- 1 egg, beaten
- 1/2 tsp. ground flaxseed
- 1/4 tsp. baking powder
- 1/3 c. finely grated cheddar cheese
- 1/4 c. finely grated Parmesan cheese

Directions:
Preheat the waffle iron.
Meanwhile, in a medium bowl, mix all the ingredients except the Parmesan cheese.
Open the iron and sprinkle a little of the Parmesan cheese in the bottom. Pour on 1/4 c. of the mixed ingredients and top with a little more of the Parmesan cheese.
Close the iron and cook until crispy, 6–7 min.
Remove the waffle onto a plate and set it aside.
Make three more waffles using the remaining ingredients in the same manner.
Allow cooling and serve.
Nutrition:
Calories 119
Fats 5.62 g.
Carbs: 7.36 g.

Protein: 9.72 g.

59. MINT CHOCOLATE WAFFLE

Preparation time: 5 min.
Cooking time: 4 min.
Servings: 2
Ingredients:

- 1 large egg
- 1 oz. cream cheese, softened
- 1 tbsp. chocolate chips
- 1 tbsp. Stevia sweetener
- 1 tbsp. low-carb mint extract
- 1/2 tbsp. cacao powder
- 1/4 tsp. baking powder

Directions:
Reheat the mini waffle maker until hot
Whisk the egg in a bowl, add the cheese, then mix well
Stir in the remaining ingredients (except toppings, if any).
Scoop 1/2 of the batter onto the waffle maker, spread across evenly
Cook until a bit browned and crispy, about 4 min.
Gently remove from the waffle maker and let it cool
Repeat with the remaining batter.
Serve and enjoy!

Nutrition:
Calories 241
Net carbs 2 g.
Fat 19 g.
Protein 13 g.

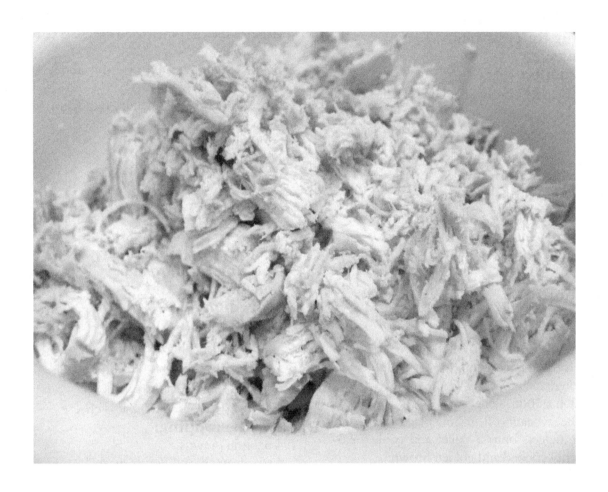

60. CHICKEN BITES WITH WAFFLES

Preparation time: 10 min.
Cooking time: 10 min.
Servings: 2
Ingredients:

- 1 chicken breasts cut into 2x 2 in. chunks
- 1 egg, whisked
- 1/4 c. almond flour
- 2 tbsps. onion powder
- 2 tbsps. garlic powder
- 1 tsp. dried oregano
- 1 tsp. paprika powder
- 1 tsp. salt
- 1/2 tsp. black pepper
- 2 tbsps. avocado oil

Directions:

Add all the dry ingredients together into a large bowl. Mix well.

Place the eggs into a separate bowl.

Dip each chicken piece into the egg and then into the dry ingredients.

Heat oil in a 10-in. skillet.

Once the avocado oil is hot, place the coated chicken nuggets onto a skillet and cook for 6–8 min. until cooked and golden brown.

Serve with waffles and raspberries.

Enjoy!

Nutrition:

Calories 401
Fats 219 g.
Protein: 32.35 g.
Net Carbs: 1.46 g.
Fiber 3 g.

61. WAFFLE EGG SANDWICH

Preparation time: 15 min.
Cooking time: 10 min.
Servings: 2
Ingredients:

- 2 slice cheddar cheese
- 1 egg omelet

Directions:

Prepare your oven to 400 °F.

Arrange the egg omelet and cheese slice between the waffles.

Bake in the preheated oven for about 4–5 min. until cheese is melted.

Once the cheese is melted, remove it from the oven.

Serve and enjoy!

Nutrition:

Protein: 144
Fat: 37
Carbohydrates: 14

62. WAFFLES WITH PRAWNS

Preparation time: 15 min.
Cooking time: 10 min.
Servings: 3
Ingredients:

- 1 large egg
- 1 tbsp. almond flour
- 1 tbsp. full-fat Greek yogurt
- 1/8 tsp. baking powder
- 1/4 c. shredded Swiss cheese

For the topping:

4 oz. grill prawns
4 oz. steamed cauliflower mash
1/2 zucchini sliced
3 lettuce leaves
1 tomato, sliced
1 tbsp. flax seeds

Directions:

Make 3 waffles with the given waffles ingredients.

For serving, arrange lettuce leaves on each waffle.

Top with zucchini slice, grill prawns, cauliflower mash, and a tomato slice.

Drizzle the flax seeds on top.

Serve and enjoy!

Nutrition:
Protein: 71
Fat: 75
Carbohydrates: 12

63.WAFFLE WITH CHEESE AND BACON

Preparation time: 15 min.
Cooking time: 15 min.
Servings: 2
Ingredients:

- 1 egg
- 1/2 c. cheddar cheese, shredded
- 1 tbsp. parmesan cheese
- 3/4 tsp. coconut flour
- 1/4 tsp. baking powder
- 1/8 tsp. Italian Seasoning
- Pinch of salt
- 1/4 tsp. garlic powder

For the topping:

- 1 bacon sliced, cooked, and chopped
- 1/2 c. mozzarella cheese, shredded
- 1/4 tsp. parsley, chopped

Directions: q
Preheat the oven to 400 °F.
Switch on your mini waffle maker and grease it with cooking spray.
Mix together the waffle ingredients in a mixing bowl until combined.
Spoon half of the batter in the center of the waffle maker and close the lid. Cook the waffles for about 3 min. until cooked.
Carefully remove the waffle from the maker.
Arrange the waffles in a greased baking tray.
Top with mozzarella cheese, chopped bacon, and parsley.
Bake in the oven for 4–5 min.
Once the cheese is melted, remove it from the oven.
Serve and enjoy!
Nutrition:
Protein: 90

Fat: 222
Carbohydrates: 3%

64.GRILL BEEFSTEAK AND WAFFLE

Preparation time: 15 min.
Cooking time: 10 min.
Servings: 1
Ingredients:

- 1 beefsteak rib eye
- 1 tsp. salt
- 1 tsp. pepper
- 1 tbsp. lime juice
- 1 tsp. garlic

Directions:
Prepare your grill for direct heat.
Mix together all spices and rub over beefsteak evenly.
Place the beef on the grill rack over medium heat. Cover and cook the steak for about 6–8 min. Flip and cook for another 5 min. until cooked through.
Serve with keto simple waffle and enjoy!
Nutrition:
Protein: 274
Fat: 243
Carbohydrates: 22

65.CAULIFLOWER WAFFLES AND TOMATOES

Preparation time: 15 min.
Cooking time: 15 min.
Servings: 2
Ingredients:

- 1/2 c. cauliflower
- 1/4 tsp. garlic powder
- 1/4 tsp. black pepper
- 1/4 tsp. salt
- 1/2 c. shredded cheddar cheese
- 1 egg

For the topping:

- 1 lettuce leave

- 1 tomato sliced
- 4 oz. cauliflower steamed, mashed
- 1 tsp. sesame seeds

Directions:

Add all the waffle ingredients into a blender and mix well.

Sprinkle 1/8 shredded cheese on the waffle maker and pour the cauliflower mixture in a preheated waffle maker and sprinkle the rest of the cheese over it.

Cook the waffles for about 4–5 min. until cooked For serving, lay lettuce leaves over the waffle top with steamed cauliflower and tomato.

Drizzle sesame seeds on top.

Enjoy!

Nutrition:

Protein: 49

Fat: 128

Carbohydrates: 21

66.CHICKEN CAULI WAFFLE

Preparation time: 27 min.

Cooking time: 12 min.

Servings: 2

Ingredients:

- 3–4 pieces of Chicken or 1/2 c. when done
- 2 garlic cloves (finely grated)
- 2 egg
- Salt, as per your taste
- 1 green onion stalk
- 1 tbsp. soy sauce
- 1 c. cauliflower rice
- 1 c. mozzarella cheese
- 1/4 tsp. black pepper or as per your taste
- 1/4 tsp. white pepper or as per your taste

Directions:

Melt the butter in an oven and set aside, then cook the chicken in a skillet using salt and a cup of water to boil. With the lid closed, cook for

18 min. Once done, put off the heat and shred the chicken into pieces, then discard all bones.

Using another mixing bowl prepare a mix containing peppers (white and black), soy sauce, cauliflower rice, grated garlic, beaten egg with the shredded chicken pieces. Mix evenly. Preheat and grease the waffle maker. Pour 1/8 c. mozzarella into the waffle maker with the mixture on the cheese, add another cup (1/8) of mozzarella on the waffle. With a closed lid, heat the waffle for 5 min. to a crunch, and then remove the waffle. Repeat for the remaining waffles mixture to make more batter. Serve by garnishing the waffle with chopped green onions and enjoy.

Nutrition:

Calories: 2109

Total Fat: 56.37 g.

Saturated Fat: 14.104 g.

Cholesterol: 1714 mg.

Total Carbs: 10.04 g.

Protein: 368.36 g.

67.CHICKEN WAFFLE

Preparation time: 12 min.

Cooking time: 6 min.

Servings: 2

Ingredients:

- 2 egg
- 4 tbsp. buffalo sauce (can be as desired)
- 1 c. chicken
- 1 c. cheddar cheese
- 1/4 c. whipped cream cheese
- 1 tsp. butter

Directions:

Melt some butter in a pan with the shredded chicken added to it.

Add 2 tbsp. buffalo sauce into the heated mix.

Using a mixing bowl, prepare a mixture containing eggs with whipped cream cheese, cheddar cheese, and the cooked chicken, then mix evenly.

Preheat and grease a waffle maker.

Sprinkle some cheddar cheese at the base of the waffle maker, then spread the mixture evenly on the waffle maker with a bit of the cheese.

Heat to a crispy form for 5 min. and repeat the process for the remaining batter.

Serve the dish with some buffalo sauce to enjoy.

Nutrition:

Calories: 770

Total Fat: 32.45 g.

Saturated Fat: 12 g.

Cholesterol: 958 mg.

Total Carbs: 4.48 g.

Protein: 108.7 g.

68.CHICKEN MOZZARELLA WAFFLE

Preparation time: 12 min.

Cooking time: 6 min.

Servings: 2

Ingredients:

- 1 c. chicken
- 1 c. + 4 tbsp. mozzarella cheese
- 1/2 tsp. basil
- 1 tsp. butter
- 2 egg
- 6 tbsp. tomato sauce
- 1/2 tbsp. garlic

Directions:

Melt some butter in a pan with the shredded chicken added into it and stir for few minutes. Add basil with garlic and set aside.

Using a mixing bowl, prepare a mixture containing eggs with cooked chicken and mozzarella cheese, then mix evenly.

Preheat and grease a waffle maker. Spread the mixture on the base of the mini-waffle maker evenly, then heat for 5 min. to a crispy form.

Repeat the process for the remaining batter.

On a baking tray, arrange the waffles with tomato sauce and grated cheese to garnish the top.

Heat the oven at 399 °F to melt the cheese then serve hot.

Nutrition:

Calories: 931

Total Fat: 32.45 g.

Saturated Fat: 8.71 g.

Cholesterol: 958 mg.

Total Carbs: 25.33 g.

Protein: 113.96 g.

69.CHICKEN BBQ WAFFLE

Preparation time: 32 min.

Cooking time: 11 min.

Servings: 2

Ingredients:

- 1/2 c. chicken
- 1 tbsp. bbq sauce (sugar-free)
- 1 egg
- 2 tbsp. almond flour
- 1/2 c. cheddar cheese
- 1 tbsp. butter

Directions:

Melt some butter in a pan with the shredded chicken added into it and stir for 11 min.

Using a mixing bowl, prepare a mixture containing all the ingredients with the cooked chicken, then mix evenly.

Preheat and grease a waffle maker.

Spread the mixture on the base of the waffle maker evenly, and then heat for 7 min. to a crispy form.

Repeat the process for the remaining batter.

Serve hot.

Nutrition:

Calories: 375

Total Fat: 15.73 g.

Saturated Fat: 5.34 g.

Cholesterol: 472 mg.

Total Carbs: 1.37 g.

Protein: 53.59 g.

70.CHICKEN SPINACH WAFFLE

Preparation time: 41 min.
Cooking time: 11 min.
Servings: 2
Ingredients:

- 1/2 c. spinach
- Pepper, as per your taste
- 1 tsp. basil
- 1/2 c. chicken, boneless
- 1/2 c. shredded mozzarella
- 1 tbsp. garlic powder
- Salt, as per your taste
- 1 egg
- 1 tbsp. onion powder

Directions:

Heat the chicken in water to boil, then shred it into pieces and keep aside.

Heat the spinach for 9 min. to strain.

Using a mixing bowl, prepare a mixture containing all the ingredients with the cooked chicken, then mix evenly.

Preheat and grease a waffle maker.

Spread the mixture on the base of the waffle maker evenly, and then heat for 7 min. to a crispy form.

Repeat the process for the remaining batter.

Serve crispy with your desired keto sauce.

Nutrition:

Calories: 138
Total Fat: 5.78 g.
Saturated Fat: 1.81 g.
Cholesterol: 312 mg.
Total Carbs: 14.39 g.
Protein: 7 .82 g.

71.CHICKEN PARMESAN WAFFLE

Preparation time: 30 min.
Cooking time: 5 min.
Servings: 2
Ingredients:

- 1/2 cup canned chicken breast or leftover shredded chicken
- 1/4 cup cheddar cheese
- 1/8 cup parmesan cheese
- 1 egg
- 1 teaspoon Italian seasoning
- 1/8 teaspoon garlic powder
- 1 teaspoon cream cheese, room temperature

For the topping:

- 2 slices of provolone cheese
- 1 tbsp. sugar-free pizza sauce (I like using Rao's sauces!)

Directions:

Preheat the mini waffle maker.

In a medium-size bowl, add all the ingredients and mix until they are fully incorporated.

Add 1 tsp. shredded cheese to the waffle iron for 30 sec. before adding the mixture.

This will create the best crust and make it easier to take this heavy waffle out of the waffle maker when it's done.

Pour half of the mixture into the mini waffle maker and cook it for a minimum of 4–5 min.

Repeat the above steps to cook the second Chicken Parmesan Waffle.

Top with a sugar-free pizza sauce and one slice of provolone cheese. I like to sprinkle the top with even more Italian Seasoning too!

Nutrition:

Calories: 213
Total Fat: 15.35 g.
Saturated Fat: 7.56 g.
Cholesterol: 339 mg.
Total Carbs: 5.59 g.
Protein: 12.64 g.

72.KETO CHICKEN WAFFLE

Preparation time: 15 min.
Cooking time: 10 min.
Servings: 2
Ingredients:

- 1 c. mozzarella cheese
- 2 eggs
- 1 c. cheddar cheese
- Salt to taste
- Black pepper to taste
- 17 g. almond flour
- 1 c. shredded chicken
- 1/2 c. frank's red-hot sauce
- 1/4 c. chopped celery

Directions:

Heat your waffle maker.

Always remember you heat your waffle maker till the point that it starts producing steam.

Remove the egg whites in a bowl and beat them to the point that they become fluffy.

Beat the egg yolks in a separate bowl.

Add in the egg yolks in the egg whites and delicately mix them with a spatula.

Combine the eggs, cheese, hot sauce, cheddar cheese, almond flour, and spices.

Add in the shredded chicken once the rest of the ingredients are well mixed.

When your waffle maker is heated adequately, pour in the mixture.

Close your waffle maker.

Let your waffle cook for 5-6 min. approximately.

When your waffles are done, dish them out.

Add the chopped celery on top of the waffles.

You can also serve some additional hot sauce alongside your waffles.

Your dish is ready to be served.

Nutrition:

Calories: 707
Total Fat: 18.5 g.
Saturated Fat: 4.58 g.
Cholesterol: 630 mg.
Total Carbs: 8.63 g.
Protein: 120.84 g

73.KETO CHICKEN PARMESAN WAFFLE

Preparation time: 15 min.
Cooking time: 10 min.
Servings: 2
Ingredients:

- 1 c. mozzarella cheese
- 2 eggs
- 1 c. parmesan cheese
- Salt to taste
- Black pepper to taste
- 17 g. almond flour
- 1 c. shredded chicken
- 17 g. garlic powder
- 34 g. Italian seasoning
- 2 slices of provolone cheese,
- 2 tbsp. sugar-free pizza sauce
- 1/4 c. chopped celery

Directions:

Heat your waffle maker.

Always remember you heat your waffle maker till the point that it starts producing steam.

Add the egg whites to a bowl and beat them to the point that they become fluffy.

Beat the egg yolks in a separate bowl.

Add in the egg yolks in the egg whites and delicately mix them with a spatula.

Combine the eggs and the rest of the ingredients except the pizza sauce, provolone cheese, and the chicken.

Add in the shredded chicken once the rest of the ingredients are well mixed.

When your waffle maker is heated adequately, pour in the mixture.

Close your waffle maker.

Let your waffle cook for 5–6 min. approximately.

When your waffles are done, dish them out.

Add the provolone cheese and the sugar-free pizza sauce on top of the waffles.

Your dish is ready to be served.

Nutrition:
Calories: 954
Total Fat: 35.78 g.
Saturated Fat: 14.61 g.
Cholesterol: 682 mg.
Total Carbs: 13.53 g.
Protein: 138.12 g.

74.KETO YOGURT WAFFLE

Preparation time: 15 min.
Cooking time: 10 min.
Servings: 2
Ingredients:

- 1 c. mozzarella cheese,
- 2 eggs
- 17 g. psyllium husk
- 34 g. yogurt
- 17 g. baking powder

Directions:

Heat your waffle maker.

Always remember you heat your waffle maker till the point that it starts producing steam.

Remove the egg whites in a bowl and beat them to the point that they become fluffy.

Beat the egg yolks in a separate bowl.

Add in the egg yolks in the egg whites and delicately mix them with a spatula.

Combine the eggs, mozzarella cheese, psyllium husk, yogurt, and baking powder.

When your waffle maker is heated adequately, pour in the mixture.

Close your waffle maker.

Let your waffle cook for 5–6 min. approximately.

When your waffles are done, dish them out.

Your dish is ready to be served.

Nutrition:
Calories: 144
Total Fat: 4.82 g.
Saturated Fat: 1.29 g.

Cholesterol: 320 mg.
Total Carbs: 2.49 g.
Protein: 22.39 g.

75.KETO CHEESY GARLIC BREAD WAFFLE

Preparation time: 25 min.
Cooking time: 15 min.
Servings: 2
Ingredients:

- 1 c. mozzarella cheese
- 2 eggs
- 20 g. chopped fresh cilantro
- 34 g. butter
- 17 g. chopped garlic
- Salt to taste
- 17 g. Italian seasoning
- 1/2 c. parmesan cheese

Directions:

Heat your waffle maker.

Always remember you heat your waffle maker till the point that it starts producing steam.

Remove the egg whites in a bowl and beat them to the point that they become fluffy.

Beat the egg yolks in a separate bowl.

Add in the egg yolks in the egg whites and delicately mix them with a spatula.

Combine the eggs and the rest of the ingredients except the chopped garlic, Italian seasoning, parmesan cheese, and butter.

Add in the shredded chicken once the rest of the ingredients are well mixed.

When your waffle maker is heated adequately, pour in the mixture.

Close your waffle maker.

Let your waffle cook for 5–6 min. approximately.

When your waffles are done, dish them out.

Mix the butter, chopped garlic, and Italian seasoning in a bowl.

Spread the butter mixture on the waffles with the help of a brush.

Add the shredded parmesan cheese on top.

Your dish is ready to be served.

Nutrition:
Calories: 290
Total Fat: 14.81 g.
Saturated Fat: 6.35 g.
Cholesterol: 353 mg.
Total Carbs: 5.96 g.
Protein: 32.7 g.

76.KETO JALAPENO POPPER WAFFLE

Preparation time: 15 min.
Cooking time: 10 min.
Servings: 2
Ingredients:

- 1 c. mozzarella cheese
- 2 eggs
- 20 g. chopped fresh cilantro
- 34 g. cream cheese
- Salt to taste
- 1 c. shredded chicken
- 17 g. Italian seasoning
- 1/2 c. jalapeno poppers

Directions:

Heat your waffle maker.

Always remember you heat your waffle maker till the point that it starts producing steam.

Remove the egg whites in a bowl and beat them to the point that they become fluffy.

Beat the egg yolks in a separate bowl.

Add in the egg yolks in the egg whites and delicately mix them with a spatula.

Combine the eggs and the rest of the ingredients except the cream cheese and cilantro.

Add in the shredded chicken once the rest of the ingredients are well mixed.

When your waffle maker is heated adequately, pour in the mixture.

Close your waffle maker.

Let your waffle cook for 5–6 min. approximately.

When your waffles are done, dish them out.

Add the cream cheese and cilantro on top.

Your dish is ready to be served.

Nutrition:
Calories: 220
Total Fat: 8.66 g.
Saturated Fat: 3.0 g.
Cholesterol: 334 mg.
Total Carbs: 7.71 g.
Protein: 27.1 g.

77.KETO PUMPKIN WAFFLE

Preparation time: 15 min.
Cooking time: 10 min.
Servings: 2
Ingredients:

- 1 c. mozzarella cheese
- 2 eggs
- 17 g. pumpkin spice
- 34 g. vanilla essence
- 17 g. baking powder
- 34 g. coconut flour
- 1/2 c. pumpkin puree
- Sugar-free syrup, as required

Directions:

Heat your waffle maker.

Always remember you heat your waffle maker till the point that it starts producing steam.

Remove the egg whites in a bowl and beat them to the point that they become fluffy.

Beat the egg yolks in a separate bowl.

Add in the egg yolks in the egg whites and delicately mix them with a spatula.

Combine the eggs, cheese, spices, puree, coconut flour, vanilla essence, baking powder, and coconut flour.

When your waffle maker is heated adequately, pour in the mixture.

Close your waffle maker.

Let your waffle cook for 5–6 min. approximately.

When your waffles are done, dish them out.

Add sugar-free syrup on top of the waffles.

Your dish is ready to be served.

Nutrition:
Calories: 333
Total Fat: 19.5 g.
Saturated Fat: 3.99 g.
Cholesterol: 320 mg.
Total Carbs: 10.65 g.
Protein: 31.94 g

78. KETO BUTTER CHICKEN WAFFLE WITH TZATZIKI SAUCE

Preparation time: 15 min.
Cooking time: 10 min.
Servings: 2
Ingredients:

- 1 c. mozzarella cheese
- 2 2 eggs
- 1 c. cheddar cheese
- Salt to taste
- Black pepper to taste
- 17 g. almond flour
- 1 c. shredded butter chicken
- 1/2 c. butter chicken sauce
- 1/4 c. tzatziki sauce
- 17 g. chopped cilantro

Directions:
Heat your waffle maker.
Always remember you heat your waffle maker till the point that it starts producing steam.
Remove the egg whites in a bowl and beat them to the point that they become fluffy.
Beat the egg yolks in a separate bowl.
Add in the egg yolks in the egg whites and delicately mix them with a spatula.
Combine the eggs and the rest of the ingredients except the chicken, cilantro, and tzatziki sauce.
Add in the shredded chicken once the rest of the ingredients are well mixed.
When your waffle maker is heated adequately, pour in the mixture.
Close your waffle maker.

Let your waffle cook for 5–6 min. approximately.
When your waffles are done, dish them out.
Add the chopped cilantro on top of the waffles.
You can also serve tzatziki sauce alongside your waffles.
Your dish is ready to be served.

Nutrition:
Calories: 195
Total Fat: 5.39 g.
Saturated Fat: 1.36 g.
Cholesterol: 320 mg.
Total Carbs: 13.48 g.
Protein: 24.97 g.

79. KETO PARMESAN GARLIC WAFFLE

Preparation time: 15 min.
Cooking time: 10 min.
Servings: 2
Ingredients:

- 1 c. mozzarella cheese,
- 2 eggs
- 20 g. chopped fresh cilantro
- 17 g. garlic powder
- Salt to taste
- 1 c. shredded chicken
- 17 g. Italian seasoning
- 1/2 c. parmesan cheese

Directions:
Heat your waffle maker.
Always remember you heat your waffle maker till the point that it starts producing steam.
Remove the egg whites in a bowl and beat them to the point that they become fluffy.
Beat the egg yolks in a separate bowl.
Add in the egg yolks in the egg whites and delicately mix them with a spatula.
Combine the eggs, cheese, garlic powder, and salt.
Add in the shredded chicken once the rest of the ingredients are well mixed.

When your waffle maker is heated adequately, pour in the mixture.

Close your waffle maker.

Let your waffle cook for 5–6 min. approximately.

When your waffles are done, dish them out.

Garnish it with a little parmesan and cilantro on top.

Your dish is ready to be served.

Nutrition:

Calories: 249

Total Fat: 11.78 g.

Saturated Fat: 5.1 g.

Cholesterol: 341 mg.

Total Carbs: 5.96 g.

Protein: 29.5 g.

80. KETO ROASTED BEEF WAFFLE SANDWICH

Preparation time: 20 min.

Cooking time: 15 min.

Servings: 2

Ingredients:

- 1 c. mozzarella cheese
- 2 eggs
- 34 g. mayonnaise
- 17 g. dijon mustard
- Salt to taste
- Black pepper to taste
- 50 g. beef
- 17 g. olive oil

Directions:

Heat your waffle maker.

Always remember you heat your waffle maker till the point that it starts producing steam.

Remove the egg whites in a bowl and beat them to the point that they become fluffy.

Beat the egg yolks in a separate bowl.

Add in the egg yolks in the egg whites and delicately mix them with a spatula.

Combine the eggs and the cheese as one.

When your waffle maker is heated adequately, pour in the mixture.

Close your waffle maker.

Let your waffle cook for 5–6 min. approximately.

In the meanwhile, cook your roast beef in a pan with olive oil.

Add in the salt and pepper on top of the eggs.

When done, dish them out on a plate.

Cut thin slices of roasted beef on top of your waffle.

When your waffles are done, dish them out.

Add on top of the waffles a little mayonnaise, the Dijon mustard sauce, and the roasted beef slice.

Make it a sandwich by placing another waffle piece.

Your dish is ready to be served.

Nutrition:

Calories: 153

Total Fat: 4.86 g.

Saturated Fat: 1.3 g.

Cholesterol: 320 mg.

Total Carbs: 4.61 g.

Protein: 22.84 g.

81. KETO REUBEN WAFFLE SANDWICH

Preparation time: 15 min.

Cooking time: 10 min.

Servings: 2

Ingredients:

- 1 c. mozzarella cheese
- 2 eggs
- 2 slices swiss cheese
- Salt to taste
- Black pepper to taste
- 50 g. corned beef
- 50 g. sauerkraut
- 17 g. butter

Directions:

Heat your waffle maker.

Always remember you heat your waffle maker till the point that it starts producing steam.

Remove the egg whites in a bowl and beat them to the point that they become fluffy.

Beat the egg yolks in a separate bowl.

Add in the egg yolks in the egg whites and delicately mix them with a spatula.

Combine the eggs and the rest of the ingredients except the cheese slices, sauerkraut, and corned beef slices.

When your waffle maker is heated adequately, pour in the mixture.

Close your waffle maker.

Let your waffle cook for 5–6 min. approximately. When your waffles are done, dish them out.

Add a little butter to a pan and then add a piece of the waffle on top of the butter.

Lay a slice of corned beef, Swiss cheese, and sauerkraut and place another waffle piece on top.

Cook your sandwich until the cheese melts by flipping it on both sides.

Your dish is ready to be served.

Nutrition:
Calories: 207
Total Fat: 8.76 g.
Saturated Fat: 3.8 g.
Cholesterol: 332 mg.
Total Carbs: 5.37 g.
Protein: 26.61 g.

82. KETO TERI AVOCADO WAFFLE SANDWICH

Preparation time: 25 min.
Cooking time: 20 min.
Servings: 2
Ingredients:

- 1 c. mozzarella cheese
- 2 eggs

For the patties:

- 20 g. chopped fresh cilantro
- 1 egg, one
- Salt to taste
- Black pepper to taste
- 1/2 lb. ground beef
- 17 g. pork rinds

For the garnish:

- 1/2 c. avocado slices
- Lettuce leaf

For the teriyaki sauce:

- 17 g. soy sauce
- 34 g. Japanese sake
- 17 g. swerve
- 5 g. xanthan gum

Directions:
Heat your waffle maker.

Always remember you heat your waffle maker till the point that it starts producing steam.

Remove the egg whites in a bowl and beat them to the point that they become fluffy.

Beat the egg yolks in a separate bowl.

Add in the egg yolks in the egg whites and delicately mix them with a spatula.

Combine the eggs and cheese for the waffle.

When your waffle maker is heated adequately, pour in the mixture.

Close your waffle maker.

Let your waffle cook for 5–6 min. approximately. When your waffles are done, dish them out.

In the meanwhile, mix all the ingredients for the Teriyaki sauce in a bowl.

Mix the ingredients for the patties.

Make 2 small patties and fry them in olive oil until they are done.

Lay a lettuce leaf on the waffle, add the patty and place the avocado slices on top.

Pour the teriyaki sauce on top and close your sandwich.

Your dish is ready to be served.

Nutrition:
Calories: 278
Total Fat: 15.18 g.
Saturated Fat: 3.4 g.
Cholesterol: 629 mg.
Total Carbs: 8.35 g.
Protein: 28.09 g.

83. KETO WESTERN BACON CHEESEBURGER WAFFLE

Preparation time: 25 min.
Cooking time: 20 min.
Servings: 2
Ingredients:

- 1 c. mozzarella cheese,
- 2 + 1 eggs
- 20 g. chopped fresh cilantro,
- Salt to taste
- Black pepper to taste
- 2 ground beef burger patty
- 4 pork strips

For the garnish:

- 4 onion rings
- 2 cheddar cheese slices
- 34 g. sugar-free barbeque sauce
- 17 g. olive oil

Directions:

Heat your waffle maker.

Always remember you heat your waffle maker till the point that it starts producing steam.

Remove the egg whites in a bowl and beat them to the point that they become fluffy.

Beat the egg yolks in a separate bowl.

Add in the egg yolks in the egg whites and delicately mix them with a spatula.

Combine the eggs and the rest of the ingredients for the waffle.

When your waffle maker is heated adequately, pour in the mixture.

Close your waffle maker.

Let your waffle cook for 5–6 min. approximately.

When your waffles are done, dish them out.

Fry the burger patty in olive oil until they are done.

Lay the burger patty on the waffle.

Pour the sugar-free barbeque sauce, and place the onion rings on top.

Close your sandwich.

Your dish is ready to be served.

Nutrition:
Calories: 382
Total Fat: 20.86 g.
Saturated Fat: 7.6 g.
Cholesterol: 677 mg.
Total Carbs: 6.62 g.
Protein: 40.85 g.

84. KETO WAFFLE CRAB ROLL

Preparation time: 25 min.
Cooking time: 15 min.
Servings: 2
Ingredients:

- 1 c. mozzarella cheese
- 2 eggs
- 50 g. shredded crab meat
- 17 g. garlic powder
- 17 g. bay seasoning

For the garnish:

- 20 g. chopped fresh cilantro
- 34 g. keto garlic mayonnaise
- 17 g. olive oil

Directions:

Heat your waffle maker.

Always remember you heat your waffle maker till the point that it starts producing steam.

Remove the egg whites in a bowl and beat them to the point that they become fluffy.

Beat the egg yolks in a separate bowl.

Add in the egg yolks in the egg whites and delicately mix them with a spatula.

Combine the eggs and cheese for the waffle.

When your waffle maker is heated adequately, pour in the mixture.

Close your waffle maker.

Let your waffle cook for 5–6 min. approximately.

When your waffles are done, dish them out.

Fry the shredded crab in olive oil until they are done.

Add the garlic powder and bay seasoning into the shredded crab.

Mix the garlic mayo and shredded crab together in a bowl.

Lay the crab mixture on the waffle.

Roll your waffle in the form of a taco.

Garnish the crab roll with the chopped cilantro.

Your dish is ready to be served.

Nutrition:

Calories: 144

Total Fat: 4.82 g.

Saturated Fat: 1.29 g.

Cholesterol: 320 mg.

Total Carbs: 2.49 g.

Protein: 22.39 g.

85. KETO FRIED FISH WAFFLE

Preparation time: 25 min.

Cooking time: 20 min.

Servings: 2

Ingredients:

- 1 c. mozzarella cheese
- 2 eggs

For the patties:

- 20 g. chopped fresh cilantro
- 1 egg
- Salt to taste
- Black pepper to taste
- 50 g. fish filet
- 17 g. all-purpose flour
- 17 g. bread crumbs

For the garnish:

- 1/2 c. avocado slices
- 2 lettuce leaf

For the mayo sauce:

- 17 g. soy sauce
- 34 g. cilantro
- 17 g. swerve
- 5 g. mayonnaise

Directions:

Heat your waffle maker.

Always remember you heat your waffle maker till the point that it starts producing steam.

Remove the egg whites in a bowl and beat them to the point that they become fluffy.

Beat the egg yolks in a separate bowl.

Add in the egg yolks in the egg whites and delicately mix them with a spatula.

Combine the eggs and cheese for the waffle.

When your waffle maker is heated adequately, pour in the mixture.

Close your waffle maker.

Let your waffle cook for 5–6 min. approximately.

When your waffles are done, dish them out.

In the meanwhile, mix all the ingredients for the mayo sauce in a bowl.

Mix the ingredients for the fried fish.

Fry the fish in olive oil until they are done.

Lay a lettuce leaf on the waffle, add the fried fish and place the avocado slices on top.

Pour the mayo sauce on top and close your sandwich.

Your dish is ready to be served.

Nutrition:

Calories: 338

Total Fat: 15.93 g.

Saturated Fat: 3.5 g.

Cholesterol: 629 mg.

Total Carbs: 19.47 g.

Protein: 30.09 g.

86. KETO LOBSTER ROLL WAFFLE

Preparation time: 25 min.

Cooking time: 15 min.

Servings: 2

Ingredients:

- 1 c. mozzarella cheese
- 2 eggs
- 50 g. shredded lobster meat
- 17 g. garlic powder
- 17 g. bay seasoning

For the garnish:

- 20 g. chopped fresh cilantro
- 34 g. keto garlic mayonnaise

- 17 g. olive oil

Directions:

Heat your waffle maker.

Remove the egg whites in a bowl and beat them to the point that they become fluffy.

Beat the egg yolks in a separate bowl.

Add in the egg yolks in the egg whites and delicately mix them with a spatula.

Combine the eggs and cheese for the waffle.

When your waffle maker is heated adequately, pour in the mixture.

Close your waffle maker.

Let your waffle cook for 5–6 min. approximately.

When your waffles are done, dish them out.

Fry the shredded lobster in olive oil until they are done.

Add the garlic powder and bay seasoning into the shredded salmon.

Mix the garlic mayo and shredded lobster together in a bowl.

Lay the lobster mixture on the waffle.

Roll your waffle in the form of a taco.

Garnish the lobster roll with the chopped cilantro.

Your dish is ready to be served.

Nutrition:

Calories: 144

Total Fat: 4.82 g.

Saturated Fat: 1.29 g.

Cholesterol: 320 mg.

Total Carbs: 2.49 g.

Protein: 22.39 g.

87.KETO SALMON WAFFLE TACOS

Preparation time: 25 min.

Cooking time: 15 min.

Servings: 2

Ingredients:

- 1 c. mozzarella cheese
- 2 eggs
- 50 g. shredded salmon meat

- 17 g. garlic powder
- 17 g. bay seasoning

For the garnish:

- 20 g. chopped fresh cilantro
- 34 g. keto garlic mayonnaise
- 17 g. olive oil

Directions:

Heat your waffle maker.

Always remember you heat your waffle maker till the point that it starts producing steam.

Remove the egg whites in a bowl and beat them to the point that they become fluffy.

Beat the egg yolks in a separate bowl.

Add in the egg yolks in the egg whites and delicately mix them with a spatula.

Combine the eggs and cheese for the waffle.

When your waffle maker is heated adequately, pour in the mixture.

Close your waffle maker.

Let your waffle cook for 5–6 min. approximately.

When your waffles are done, dish them out.

Fry the shredded salmon in olive oil until they are done.

Add the garlic powder and bay seasoning into the shredded salmon.

Mix the garlic mayo and shredded salmon together in a bowl.

Lay the salmon mixture on the waffle.

Roll your waffle in the form of a taco.

Garnish the salmon taco with the chopped cilantro.

Your dish is ready to be served.

Nutrition:

Calories: 144

Total Fat: 4.82 g.

Saturated Fat: 1.29 g.

Cholesterol: 320 mg.

Total Carbs: 2.49 g.

Protein: 22.39 g.

88. KETO TUNA MELT WAFFLE

Preparation time: 15 min.
Cooking time: 10 min.
Servings: 2
Ingredients:

- 1 c. mozzarella cheese
- 2 eggs
- 1 c. cheddar cheese
- Salt to taste
- Black pepper to taste
- 17 g. almond flour
- 1 c. shredded tuna
- 17 g. garlic powder
- 17 g. chopped cilantro
- Tzatziki sauce

Directions:

Heat your waffle maker.

Always remember you heat your waffle maker till the point that it starts producing steam.

Remove the egg whites in a bowl and beat them to the point that they become fluffy.

Beat the egg yolks in a separate bowl.

Add in the egg yolks in the egg whites and delicately mix them with a spatula.

Combine the eggs and the rest of the ingredients except the tuna, cilantro, and tzatziki sauce.

Add in the shredded tuna once the rest of the ingredients are well mixed.

When your waffle maker is heated adequately, pour in the mixture.

Close your waffle maker.

Let your waffle cook for 5–6 min. approximately.

When your waffles are done, dish them out.

Add the chopped cilantro on top of the waffles.

Your dish is ready to be served.

Nutrition:

Calories: 223
Total Fat: 5.9 g.
Saturated Fat: 1.48 g.
Cholesterol: 347 mg.
Total Carbs: 4.74 g.
Protein: 37.94 g.

89. EASY KETO FRIED CHICKEN WAFFLE

Preparation time: 25 min.
Cooking time: 20 min.
Servings: 2
Ingredients:

- 1 c. mozzarella cheese
- 2 eggs

For the fried chicken:

- 20 g. chopped fresh cilantro,
- 1 egg
- Salt to taste
- Black pepper to taste
- 50 g. chicken filet
- 17 g. all-purpose flour
- 17 g. bread crumbs

For the garnish:

- 1/2 c. avocado slices
- 2 lettuce leaf

For the mayo sauce:

- 17 g. soy sauce
- 34 g. cilantro
- 17 g. swerve
- 5 g. mayonnaise

Directions:

Heat your waffle maker.

Always remember you heat your waffle maker till the point that it starts producing steam.

Remove the egg whites in a bowl and beat them to the point that they become fluffy.

Beat the egg yolks in a separate bowl.

Add in the egg yolks in the egg whites and delicately mix them with a spatula.

Combine the eggs and cheese for the waffle.

When your waffle maker is heated adequately, pour in the mixture.

Close your waffle maker.

Let your waffle cook for 5–6 min. approximately.

When your waffles are done, dish them out.
In the meanwhile, mix all the ingredients for the mayo sauce in a bowl.
Mix the ingredients for the fried chicken.
Fry the chicken in olive oil until they are done.
Lay a lettuce leaf on the waffle, add the fried chicken and place the avocado slices on top.
Pour the mayo sauce on top and close your sandwich.
Your dish is ready to be served.

Nutrition:
Calories: 1122
Total Fat: 51.59 g.
Saturated Fat: 13.13 g.
Cholesterol: 986 mg.
Total Carbs: 19.47 g.
Protein: 138.46 g.

90.GARLIC AIOLI CHICKEN WAFFLE

Preparation time: 25 min.
Cooking time: 20 min.
Servings: 2
Ingredients:
- 1 c. mozzarella cheese
- 2 eggs

For the chicken:
- Salt to taste
- Black pepper to taste
- 50 g. rotisserie chicken

For the garnish:
- 1/2 c. avocado slices
- Lettuce leaf

For the sauce:
- 17 g. chopped garlic
- 34 g. cilantro
- 17 g. lemon juice
- 5 g. mayonnaise

Directions:
Heat your waffle maker.
Always remember you heat your waffle maker till the point that it starts producing steam.

Remove the egg whites in a bowl and beat them to the point that they become fluffy.
Beat the egg yolks in a separate bowl.
Add in the egg yolks in the egg whites and delicately mix them with a spatula.
When your waffle maker is heated adequately, pour in the mixture.
Close your waffle maker.
Let your waffle cook for 5–6 min. approximately.
When your waffles are done, dish them out.
Fry the chicken in olive oil until they are done.
In the meanwhile, mix all the ingredients for the garlic aioli sauce in a bowl.
Lay a lettuce leaf on the waffle, add the chicken and place the avocado slices on top.
Pour the garlic aioli sauce on top and close your sandwich.
Your dish is ready to be served.

Nutrition:
Calories: 748
Total Fat: 23.3 g.
Saturated Fat: 5.3 g.
Cholesterol: 630 mg.
Total Carbs: 9.5 g.
Protein: 120.67 g.

91.BARBECUE WAFFLE

Preparation time: 5 min.
Cooking time: 8 min.
Servings: 2
Ingredients:
- 1 egg, beaten
- 1/2 c. cheddar cheese, shredded
- 1/2 tsp. barbecue sauce
- 1/4 tsp. baking powder

Directions:
Plug in your waffle maker to preheat
Mix all the ingredients in a bowl
Pour half of the mixture into your waffle maker.
Cover and cook for 5–6 min.
Repeat the same steps for the remaining mixture.

Nutrition:
Calories 295

Total Fat: 23 g.
Saturated Fat: 13 g.
Cholesterol 223 mg.
Sodium 414 mg.
Potassium 179 mg.
Total Carbohydrate 2 g.
Dietary Fiber 1 g.
Protein: 20 g.
Total Sugars 1 g.

92.SIMPLE PIZZA WAFFLE

Preparation time: 15 min.
Cooking time: 7–9 min.
Servings: 4
Ingredients:
For the batter:

- 4 eggs
- 1 1/2 c. grated mozzarella cheese
- 1/2 c. grated parmesan cheese
- 2 tbsp. tomato sauce
- 1/4 c. almond flour
- 1 1/2 tsp.s baking powder
- Salt and pepper to taste
- 1 tsp. dried oregano
- 1/4 c. sliced salami

Other:

- 2 tbsp. olive oil for brushing the waffle maker
- 1/4 c. tomato sauce for serving

Directions:
Preheat the waffle maker.
Add the grated mozzarella and grated parmesan to a bowl and mix.
Add the almond flour and baking powder and season with salt and pepper and dried oregano.
Mix with a wooden spoon or wire whisk and crack in the eggs.
Stir everything together until the batter forms.
Stir in the chopped salami.
Brush the heated waffle maker with olive oil and add a few tablespoons of the batter. Close the lid and cook for about 7 minutes depending on your waffle maker.
Serve with extra tomato sauce on top and enjoy.

Nutrition:
Calories 319
Fat 25.2 g.
Carbs 5.9 g.
Sugar 1.7 g.
Protein: 19.3 g.
Sodium 596 mg.

93.CHICKEN BITES LUNCH WAFFLE

Preparation time: 15 min.
Cooking time: 10 min.
Servings: 2
Ingredients:

- 1 chicken breast cut into 2x 2 in. chunks
- 1 egg, whisked
- 1/4 c. almond flour
- 2 tbsps. onion powder
- 2 tbsps. garlic powder
- 1 tsp. dried oregano
- 1 tsp. paprika powder
- 1 tsp. salt
- 1/2 tsp. black pepper
- 2 tbsps. avocado oil

Directions:
Add all the dry ingredients together into a large bowl.
Mix well. Place the eggs into a separate bowl.
Dip each chicken piece into the egg and then into the dry ingredients.
Heat oil in a 10-in. skillet.
Once avocado oil is hot, place the coated chicken nuggets onto a skillet and cook for 6–8 min. until golden brown.
Serve with waffles and raspberries.

Nutrition:
Calories 401
Fats 219 g.
Protein: 32.35 g.

Net Carbs: 1.46 g.
Fiber 3 g.

94.BROCCOLI CHAME WAFFLE

Preparation time: 10 min.
Cooking time: 8 min.
Servings: 2
Ingredients:

- 1/3 c. raw broccoli, chopped finely
- 1/4 c. cheddar cheese, shredded
- 1 organic egg
- 1/2 tsp. garlic powder
- 1/2 tsp. dried onion, minced
- Salt and freshly ground black pepper, to taste

Directions:
Preheat a mini waffle iron and then grease it.
In a medium bowl, place all ingredients and, mix until well combined.
Place 1/4 of the mixture into the preheated waffle iron and cook for about 4 min. or until golden brown.
Repeat with the remaining mixture.
Serve warm.

Nutrition:
Calories: 9et
Carb: 1.5 g.
Fat: 6.9 g.
Saturated Fat: .7 g.
Carbohydrates: 2 g.
Fiber: 0.5 g.
Sugar: 0.7 g.
Protein: 6.8 g.

95.SALMON WAFFLES

Preparation time: 10 min.
Cooking time: 10 min.
Servings: 2
Ingredients:

- 1 large egg
- 1/2 c. shredded mozzarella
- 1 tbsp.cream cheese
- 2 slices salmon
- 1 tbsp.everything bagel seasoning

Directions:
Turn on the waffle maker to heat and oil it with cooking spray.
Beat the egg in a bowl, then add 1/2 c. mozzarella.
Pour half of the mixture into the maker and cook for 4 min.
Remove and repeat with the remaining mixture.
Let waffles cool, then spread cream cheese, sprinkle with seasoning, and top with salmon.

Nutrition:
Carbs: 3 g.
Fat: 10 g.
Protein: 5 g.
Calories: 201

96.WAFFLE KATSU SANDWICH

Preparation time: 15 min.
Cooking time: 20 min.
Servings: 4
Ingredients:
For the chicken:

- 1/4 lb. boneless and skinless thigh
- 1/8 tsp. salt
- 1/8 tsp. black pepper
- 1/2 c. almond flour
- 1 egg
- 3 oz. unflavored pork rinds
- 2 c. vegetable oil for deep frying

For the brine:

- 2 c. water
- 1 tbsp.salt

For the sauce:

- 2 tbsp.sugar-free ketchup
- 1 1/2 tbsp.Worcestershire Sauce
- 1 tbsp.oyster sauce
- 1 tsp. swerve/monk fruit

For the waffle:

- 2 egg
- 1 c. shredded mozzarella cheese

Directions:

Add the brine ingredients to a large mixing bowl. Add the chicken and brine for 1 hour.

Pat chicken dry with a paper towel. Sprinkle with salt and pepper. Set aside.

Mix Ketchup, oyster sauce, Worcestershire sauce, and swerve in a small mixing bowl.

Add the pork rinds into a food processor, making fine crumbs.

Fill one bowl with flour, a second bowl with beaten eggs, and a third with crushed pork rinds.

Dip and coat each thigh in flour, eggs, crushed pork rinds.

Add oil to cover 1/2 in. a frying pan, Heat to 375 °F.

Once the oil is hot, reduce heat to medium and add the chicken. The cooking time depends on the chicken's thickness.

Transfer to a drying rack.

Turn on the waffle maker to heat and oil it with cooking spray.

Beat the egg into a small bowl.

Place 1/8 c. the cheese on the waffle maker, then add 1/4 of the egg mixture and top with 1/8 c. cheese.

cook for 3–4 min.

Repeat tor remaining batter.

Top waffles with chicken katsu, 1 tbsp. sauce, and another piece of the waffle

Nutrition:

Carbs: 12 g.

Fat: 1 g.

Protein: 2 g.

Calories: 57

97. EASY CHICKEN PARMESAN WAFFLE

Preparation time: 15 min.
Cooking time: 5 min.
Servings: 2
Ingredients:
For the waffle:

- 1/2 c. canned chicken breast
- 1/4 c. cheddar cheese
- 1/8 c. parmesan cheese
- 1 egg
- 1 tsp. Italian seasoning
- 1/8 tsp. garlic powder
- 1 tsp. cream cheese, at room temperature

For the topping:

- 2 slices of provolone cheese
- 1 tbsp. sugar-free pizza sauce

Directions:

Preheat the mini waffle maker.

In a medium-size bowl, add all the ingredients and mix until it's fully incorporated.

Add 1 tsp. shredded cheese to the waffle iron for 30 sec. before adding the mixture. This will create the best crust and make it easier to take this heavy waffle out of the waffle maker when it's done.

Pour half of the mixture into the mini waffle maker and cook it for a minimum of 4–5 min.

Repeat the above steps to cook the second Chicken Parmesan Waffle.

Nutrition:

Total Fat: 21.8 g.

Cholesterol 134.6 mg.

Sodium 871 mg.

Total Carbohydrate 9.2 g.

Dietary Fiber 2.3 g.

Sugars 4.7 g.

Protein: 18.5 g.

98. PORK RIND WAFFLES

Preparation time: 20 min.
Cooking time: 10 min.
Servings: 2
Ingredients:

- 1 organic egg, beaten
- 1/2 c. ground pork rinds
- 1/3 c. mozzarella cheese, shredded
- Pinch of salt

Directions:

Preheat a mini waffle iron and then grease it.

In a bowl, place all the ingredients and beat until well combined.

Place half of the mixture into the preheated waffle iron and cook for about 5 min. or until golden brown.

Repeat with the remaining mixture.

Serve warm.

Nutrition:

Calories: 91
Carb: 0. 3 g.
Fat: 5.9 g.
Saturated Fat: 2.3 g.
Carbohydrates, 0.3 g.
Dietary Fat: 0 g.
Sugar: 0.2 g.
Protein: 9.2 g.

99. CHEDDAR PROTEIN WAFFLES

Preparation time: 25 min.
Cooking time: 40 min.
Servings: 8
Ingredients:

- 1/2 c. golden flax seeds meal
- 1/2 c. almond flour
- 2 tbsp. unsweetened whey protein powder
- 1 tsp. organic baking powder
- Salt and freshly ground black pepper, taste

- 1/4 c. cheddar cheese, shredded
- 1/3 c. unsweetened almond milk
- 2 tbsp. unsalted butter, melted
- 2 large organic eggs, beaten

Directions:

Preheat a mini waffle iron and then grease It.

In a large bowl, place flax seeds meal, flour, protein powder, and baking powder and mix well.

Stir in the cheddar cheese.

In another bowl, place the remaining ingredients and beat until well combined.

Add the egg mixture into the bowl with flax seeds meal mixture and mix until well combined.

Place the desired amount of the mixture into the preheated waffle iron and cook for about 4–5 min. or until golden brown.

Repeat with the remaining mixture.

Serve warm.

Nutrition:

Calories: 187
Net Carb: 1.8 g.
Fat: 1 4. 5 g.
Saturated Fat: 5 g.
Carbohydrates: 4.
Dietary Fiber: 3.1 g.

100. CHICKEN AND HAM WAFFLES

Preparation time: 10 min.
Cooking time: 16 min.
Servings: 4
Ingredients:

- 1/4 c. grass-fed cooked chicken, chopped
- 1-oz. sugar-free ham, chopped
- 1 organic egg, beaten
- 1/4 c. Swiss cheese, shredded
- 1/4 c. mozzarella cheese, shredded

Directions:

Pre-heat a mini waffle iron and then grease it.

In a medium bowl, place all ingredients and mix until well combined.

Place 1/4 of the mixture into the preheated waffle iron and cook for about 4 min. or until golden brown.

Repeat with the remaining mixture.

Serve warm.

Nutrition:

Calories: 71

Net Carb: 0.7 g.

Fat: 4.2 g.

Saturated Fat: 2 g.

Carbohydrates: 0.8 g.

Dietary Fiber: 0.1 g.

Sugar: 0.2 g.

Protein: 7.4 g.

101. CRUNCHY FISH AND WAFFLE BITES

Preparation time: 10 min.

Cooking time: 15 min.

Servings: 4

Ingredients:

For the cod:

- 1 lb. cod fillets, sliced into 4 slices
- 1 tsp. sea salt
- 1 tsp. pepper
- 1 tsp. garlic powder
- 1 egg, whisked
- 1 c. almond flour
- 2 tbsp. avocado oil

For the chaffle:

- 2 eggs
- 1/2 c. cheddar cheese
- 2 tbsps. almond flour
- 1/2 tsp. Italian seasoning

Directions:

Mix together the waffle ingredients in a bowl and make 4 squares.

Put the waffles in a preheated waffle maker.

Mix together the salt, pepper, and garlic powder in a mixing bowl.

Toss the cod cubes in this mixture and let sit for 10 min.

Then dip each cod slice into the egg mixture and then into the almond flour.

Heat oil in a skillet and cook the fish cubes for about 2–3 min., until browned.

Serve on the waffles and enjoy!

Nutrition:

Protein: 38% 121 g.

Fat: 59% 189 g.

Carbohydrates: 3% 11 g.

102. GRILL PORK WAFFLE SANDWICH

Preparation time: 10 min.

Cooking time: 15 min.

Servings: 2

Ingredients:

- 1/2 c. mozzarella, shredded
- 1 egg
- 1 pinch garlic powder

For the pork patty:

- 1/2 c. pork
- 1 tbsp. green onion, diced
- 1/2 tsp. Italian seasoning
- Lettuce leaves

Directions:

Preheat the square waffle maker and grease.

Mix together egg, cheese, and garlic powder in a small mixing bowl.

Pour the batter into a preheated waffle maker and close the lid. Make 2 waffles from this batter. Cook the waffles for about 2–3 min. until cooked through.

Meanwhile, mix together the pork patty ingredients in a bowl and make 1 large patty.

Grill the pork patty in a preheated grill for about 3–4 min. per side until cooked through.

Arrange the pork patty between two waffles with lettuce leaves. Cut the sandwich to make a triangular sandwich.

Enjoy!

Nutrition:
Protein: 48% 85
Fat: 48% 86
Carbohydrates: 4% 7

103. WAFFLE AND CHICKEN LUNCH PLATE

Preparation time: 10 min.
Cooking time: 15 min.
Servings: 1
Ingredients:

- 1 large egg
- 1/2 c. jack cheese, shredded
- 1 pinch salt

For serving:

- 1 chicken thigh
- Salt and pepper
- 1 tsp. garlic, minced
- 1 egg
- 1 tsp. avocado oil

Directions:
Heat your square waffle maker and grease it with cooking spray.
Pour the batter into the skillet and cook for about 3 min.
Meanwhile, heat oil in a pan, over medium heat. Once the oil is hot, add the chicken thigh and garlic; cook for about 5 min.
Flip and cook for another 3–4 min.
Season with salt and pepper and give them a good mix.
Transfer the cooked thigh to a plate.
Fry the egg in the same pan for about 1–2 min. according to your choice.
Once the waffles are cooked, serve with the fried egg and chicken thigh.
Enjoy!

Nutrition:
Protein: 31% 138
Fat: 66% 292
Carbohydrates: 2% kcal

104. WAFFLE DELI HAM SANDWICH

Preparation time: 15 min.
Cooking time: 10 min.
Servings: 2
Ingredients:

- 1 large egg
- 1/8 c. almond flour
- 1/2 tsp. garlic powder
- 3/4 tsp. baking powder
- 1/2 c. shredded cheese

For the filling:

- 2 slices deli ham
- 2 slices tomatoes
- 1 slice cheddar cheese

Directions:
Grease your square waffle maker and preheat it on medium heat.
Mix together the waffle ingredients in a mixing bowl until well combined.
Pour the batter into a square waffle and make two waffles.
Once the waffle is cooked, remove them from the maker.
For a sandwich, arrange deli ham, tomato slice, and cheddar cheese between two waffles.
Cut the sandwich from the center.
Serve and enjoy!

Nutrition:
Protein: 29% 70
Fat: 66% 159
Carbohydrates: 4% 10

105. WAFFLE CHEESE SANDWICH

Preparation time: 15 min.
Cooking time: 10 min.
Servings: 1
Ingredients:

- 2 square keto the waffle
- 2 slice cheddar cheese

- 2 lettuce leaves

Directions:

Prepare your oven at 400 °F.

Arrange lettuce leave and cheese slice between the waffles.

Bake in the preheated oven for about 4–5 min. until the cheese is melted.

Once the cheese is melted, remove it from the oven.

Serve and enjoy!

Nutrition:

Protein: 28% kcal

Fat: 69% 149

Carbohydrates: 3% 6

106. CHICKEN ZINGER WAFFLE

Preparation time: 20 min.

Cooking time: 15 min.

Servings: 2

Ingredients:

- 1 chicken breast, cut into 2 pieces
- 1/2 c. coconut flour
- 1/4 c. finely grated Parmesan
- 1 tsp. paprika
- 1/2 tsp. garlic powder
- 1/2 tsp. onion powder
- 1 tsp. salt and pepper
- 1 egg beaten
- Avocado oil for frying
- Lettuce leaves
- BBQ sauce

For the chaffle:

- 4 oz. cheese
- 2 whole eggs
- 2 oz. almond flour
- 1/4 c. almond flour
- 1 tsp. baking powder

Directions:

Mix together the waffle ingredients in a bowl.

Pour the waffle batter into the preheated and greased square waffle maker.

Cook the waffles for about 2 minutes until cooked through.

Make square waffles from this batter.

Meanwhile mix together coconut flour, parmesan, paprika, garlic powder, onion powder, salt, and pepper in a bowl.

Dip the chicken first in the coconut flour mixture then in the beaten egg.

Heat the avocado oil in a skillet and cook chicken from both sides, until lightly brown and cooked

Set the chicken zinger between two waffles with lettuce and BBQ sauce.

Enjoy!

Nutrition:

Protein: 30% 219

Fat: 60% 435

Carbohydrates: 9% 66

107. DOUBLE CHICKEN WAFFLES

Preparation time: 10 min.

Cooking time: 5 min.

Servings: 2

Ingredients:

- 1/2 c. boil shredded chicken
- 1/4 c. cheddar cheese
- 1/8 c. parmesan cheese
- 1 egg
- 1 tsp. Italian seasoning
- 1/8 tsp. garlic powder
- 1 tsp. cream cheese

Directions:

Preheat the Belgian waffle maker.

Mix together the waffle ingredients in a bowl and mix together.

Sprinkle 1 tbsp. cheese in a waffle maker and pour in the batter.

Pour 1 tbsp. cheese over the batter and close the lid.

Cook the waffles for about 4–5 min.

Serve with a chicken zinger and enjoy the double chicken flavor

Nutrition:
Protein: 30% 60
Fat: 65% 129
Carbohydrates: 5% 9

108. SALMON PIZZA WAFFLE

Preparation time: 5 min.
Cooking time: 6 min.
Servings: 4
Ingredients:
- 3 eggs, whisked
- 1/2 c. mozzarella, shredded
- 3 tbsp. heavy cream
- 1/2 c. smoked salmon, skinless, boneless, and flaked
- 1/2 c. baby spinach, torn
- 1/2 c. cherry tomatoes, cubed
- 2 tbsp. cream cheese, soft
- 3 tbsp. tomato passata

Directions:
In a bowl, mix the eggs with the cheese, cream, and cream cheese and stir well.

Preheat the waffle iron over medium-high heat, pour 1/4 of the waffle mix, cook for 6 min., and transfer to a plate.

Repeat with the rest of the batter, spread the passata over the waffles, divide the salmon and the other ingredients and serve.

Nutrition:
Calories 272
Fat 5.3 g.
Fiber 2.2 g.
Carbs 3 g.
Protein 7 g.

109. KALE AND MUSHROOM WAFFLE

Preparation time: 5 min.
Cooking time: 6 min.
Servings: 2
Ingredients:
- 2 eggs, whisked
- 2 tbsp. cream cheese, soft
- 2 tbsp. heavy cream
- 1/2 c. baby kale, torn
- 1/4 c. mushrooms, sliced
- 1 tbsp. cheddar, shredded
- 2 tbsp. tomato passata

Directions:
In a bowl, mix the eggs with the cream cheese and cream and stir.

Preheat the waffle iron over medium-high heat, pour half of the waffle mix, cook for 6 min. and transfer to a plate.

Repeat with the rest of the batter, sprinkle the passata, kale, mushrooms, and cheddar over the waffles, and serve.

Nutrition:
Calories 302
Fat 9.3 g.
Fiber 4.2 g.
Carbs 5 g.
Protein 11 g.

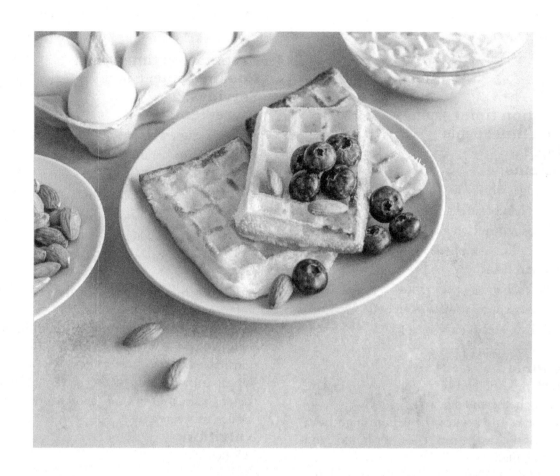

110. BUTTER AND CREAM CHEESE WAFFLES

Preparation time: 10 min.
Cooking time: 16 min.
Servings: 4
Ingredients:

- 2 tbsp. butter, melted and cooled
- 2 large organic eggs
- 2 oz. cream cheese, softened
- 1/4 c. powdered erythritol
- 1 1/2 tsp.s organic vanilla extract
- Pinch of salt
- 1/4 c. almond flour
- 2 tbsp. coconut flour
- 1 tsp. organic baking powder

Directions:
Preheat a mini waffle iron and then grease it.
In a bowl, add the butter and eggs and beat until creamy.
Add the cream cheese, erythritol, vanilla extract, and salt, and beat until well combined.
Add the flour and baking powder and beat until well combined.
Place 1/4 of the mixture into the preheated waffle iron and cook for about 4 min.
Repeat with the remaining mixture.
Serve warm.

Nutrition:
Calories 217
Total Fat: 18 g.
Cholesterol 124 mg.
Sodium 173 mg.
Total Carbs: 6.6 g.
Fiber 3.3 g.
Sugar 1.2 g.
Protein: 5.3 g.

111. PEANUT BUTTER WAFFLES

Preparation time: 5 min.
Cooking time: 8 min.
Servings: 2
Ingredients:

- 1 organic egg, beaten
- 1/2 c. mozzarella cheese, shredded
- 3 tbsp. granulated erythritol
- 2 tbsp. peanut butter

Directions:
Preheat a mini waffle iron and then grease it.
In a medium bowl, put all the ingredients and, with a fork, mix until well combined.
Place half of the mixture into the preheated waffle iron and cook for about 4 min.
Repeat with the remaining mixture.
Serve warm.

Nutrition:
Calories 145
Total Fat: 11.5 g.
Cholesterol 86 mg.
Sodium 147 mg.
Total Carbs: 3.6 g.
Fiber 1 g.
Sugar 1.7 g.
Protein: 8.8 g.

112. ALMOND BUTTER WAFFLES

Preparation time: 5 min.
Cooking time: 10 min.
Servings: 2
Ingredients:

- 1 large organic egg, beaten
- 1/3 c. mozzarella cheese, shredded
- 1 tbsp. erythritol
- 2 tbsp. almond butter
- 1 tsp. organic vanilla extract

Directions:
Preheat a mini waffle iron and then grease it.

In a medium bowl, put all the ingredients and, with a fork, mix until well combined.

Place half of the mixture into the preheated waffle iron and cook for about 3–5 min.

Repeat with the remaining mixture.

Serve warm.

Nutrition:
Calories 153
Total Fat: 12.3 g.
Cholesterol 96 mg.
Sodium 65 mg.
Total Carbs: 3.6 g.
Fiber 1.6 g.
Sugar 1.2 g.
Protein: 7.9 g.

113.   CINNAMON WAFFLES
Preparation time: 10 min.
Cooking time: 8 min.
Servings: 2
Ingredients:
For the waffles:
- 1 large organic egg, beaten
- 3/4 c. mozzarella cheese, shredded
- 1/2 tbsp. unsalted butter, melted
- 2 tbsp. blanched almond flour
- 2 tbsp. erythritol
- 1/2 tsp. ground cinnamon
- 1/2 tsp. Psyllium husk powder
- 1/4 tsp. organic baking powder
- 1/2 tsp. organic vanilla extract

For the topping::
- 1 tsp. powdered Erythritol
- 3/4 tsp. ground cinnamon

Directions:
Preheat a waffle iron and then grease it.

For the waffles:
In a medium bowl, put all the ingredients and, with a fork, mix until well combined.

Place half of the mixture into the preheated waffle iron and cook for about 3–5 min.

Repeat with the remaining mixture.

For the topping:
Into a small bowl, mix together the erythritol and cinnamon.

Place the waffles onto serving plates and set them aside to cool slightly.

Sprinkle with the cinnamon mixture and serve immediately.

Nutrition:
Calories 142
Total Fat: 10.6 g.
Cholesterol 106 mg.
Sodium 122 mg.
Total Carbs: 4.1 g.
Fiber 2 g.
Sugar 0.3 g.
Protein: 7.7 g.

114.   LAYERED WAFFLES
Preparation time: 5 min.
Cooking time: 10 min.
Servings: 2
Ingredients:
- 1 organic egg, beaten and divided
- 1/2 c. cheddar cheese, shredded and divided
- Pinch of salt

Directions:
Preheat a mini waffle iron and then grease it.

Place about 1/8 c. cheese in the bottom of the waffle iron and top with half of the beaten egg.

Now, place 1/8 c. cheese on top and cook for about 4–5 min.

Repeat with the remaining cheese and egg.

Serve warm.

Nutrition:
Calories 145
Total Fat: 11.6 g.
Cholesterol 112 mg.
Sodium 284 g.
Total Carbs: 0.5 g.
Fiber 0 g.
Sugar 0.3 g.
Protein: 9.8 g.

115.   BLUEBERRY CREAM CHEESE WAFFLES

Preparation time: 10 min.
Cooking time: 8 min.
Servings: 2
Ingredients:

- 1 organic egg, beaten
- 1/3 c. mozzarella cheese, shredded
- 1 tsp. cream cheese, softened
- 1 tsp. coconut flour
- 1/4 tsp. organic baking powder
- 3/4 tsp. powdered erythritol
- 1/4 tsp. ground cinnamon
- 1/4 tsp. organic vanilla extract
- Pinch of salt
- 1 tbsp. fresh blueberries

Directions:

Preheat a mini waffle iron and then grease it.
In a bowl, place all the ingredients except for blueberries and beat until well combined.
Fold in the blueberries.
Place half of the mixture into the preheated waffle iron and cook for about 4 min.
Repeat with the remaining mixture.
Serve warm.

Nutrition:

Calories 90
Total Fat: 5 g.
Cholesterol 97 mg.
Sodium 161 mg.
Total Carbs: 5.7 g.
Fiber 2.8 g.
Sugar 1.2 g.
Protein: 5.7 g.

116.   RASPBERRY WAFFLES

Preparation time: 10 min.
Cooking time: 8 min.
Servings: 2
Ingredients:

- 1 organic egg, beaten
- 1 tbsp. cream cheese, softened
- 1/2 c. mozzarella cheese, shredded
- 1 tbsp. powdered erythritol
- 1/4 tsp. organic raspberry extract
- 1/4 tsp. organic vanilla extract

Directions:

Preheat a mini waffle iron and then grease it.
In a medium bowl, put all the ingredients and, with a fork, mix until well combined.
Place half of the mixture into the preheated waffle iron and cook for about 4 min.
Repeat with the remaining mixture.
Serve warm.

Nutrition:

Calories 69
Total Fat: 5.2 g.
Cholesterol 91 mg.
Sodium 88 mg.
Total Carbs: 0.6 g.
Fiber 0 g.
Sugar 0.2 g.
Protein: 5.2 g.

117.   RED   VELVET WAFFLES

Preparation time: 10 min.
Cooking time: 8 min.
Servings: 2
Ingredients:

- 2 tbsp. cacao powder
- 2 tbsp. erythritol
- 1 organic egg, beaten
- 2 drops super red food coloring
- 1/4 tsp. organic baking powder

- 1 tbsp. heavy whipping cream

Directions:
Preheat a mini waffle iron and then grease it.

In a medium bowl, put all the ingredients and, with a fork, mix until well combined.

Place half of the mixture into the preheated waffle iron and cook for about 4 min.

Repeat with the remaining mixture.

Serve warm.

Nutrition:
Calories 70

Total Fat: 6 g.

Cholesterol 92 mg.

Sodium 34 mg.

Total Carbs: 3.2 g.

Fiber 1.5 g.

Sugar 0.2 g.

Protein: 3.9 g.

118. WALNUT PUMPKIN WAFFLES

Preparation time: 10 min.

Cooking time: 10 min.

Servings: 2

Ingredients:
- 1 organic egg, beaten
- 1/2 c. mozzarella cheese, shredded
- 2 tbsp. almond flour
- 1 tbsp. sugar-free pumpkin puree
- 1 tsp. erythritol
- 1/4 tsp. ground cinnamon
- 2 tbsp. walnuts, toasted and chopped

Directions:
Preheat a mini waffle iron and then grease it.

In a bowl, add all the ingredients except the walnuts, and beat until well combined.

Fold in the walnuts.

Place half of the mixture into the preheated waffle iron and cook for about 5 min.

Repeat with the remaining mixture.

Serve warm.

Nutrition:
Calories 148

Total Fat: 11.8 g.

Cholesterol 86 mg.

Sodium 74 mg.

Total Carbs: 3.3 g.

Fiber 1.7 g.

Sugar 0.8 g.

Protein: 6.7 g.

119. PUMPKIN CREAM CHEESE WAFFLES

Preparation time: 10 min.

Cooking time: 10 min.

Servings: 2

Ingredients:
- 1 organic egg, beaten
- 1/2 c. mozzarella cheese, shredded
- 1 1/2 tbsp. sugar-free pumpkin puree
- 2 tsp. heavy cream
- 1 tsp. cream cheese, softened
- 1 tbsp. almond flour
- 1 tbsp. erythritol
- 1/2 tsp. pumpkin pie spice
- 1/2 tsp. organic baking powder
- 1 tsp. organic vanilla extract

Directions:
Preheat a mini waffle iron and then grease it.

In a medium bowl, put all the ingredients and, with a fork, mix until well combined.

Place half of the mixture into the preheated waffle iron and cook for about 3–5 min.

Repeat with the remaining mixture.

Serve warm.

Nutrition:
Calories 110

Total Fat: 7.8 g.

Cholesterol 94 mg.

Sodium 82 mg.

Total Carbs: 3.3 g.

Fiber 0.8 g.

Sugar 1 g.

Protein: 5.2 g.

120. PUMPKIN WAFFLE

Preparation time: 5 min.
Cooking time: 5 min.
Servings: 2
Ingredients:

- 1/2 oz. cream cheese
- 1 large egg
- 1/2 c. mozzarella cheese (shredded)
- 2 tbsp. pumpkin puree
- 2 1/2 tbsp. erythritol
- 3 tsp. coconut flour
- 1/2 tbsp. pumpkin pie spice
- 1/2 tsp. vanilla essence (optional)
- 1/4 tsp. baking powder (optional)

Directions:

Preheat the waffle iron for about 5 min. until hot. If your recipe includes cream cheese, put it in a bowl first. Gently heat in a microwave (15–30 sec.) or double boiler until soft and stir.

Stir all the remaining ingredients (except toppings, if any).

Pour a sufficient amount of the waffle dough into the waffle maker and cover the surface firmly. (For a normal waffle maker, about 1/2 c., for a mini waffle maker, about 1/4 c.)

Cook for about 3–4 min. until brown and crisp. Carefully remove the waffle from the waffle maker and set it aside for a crisp noise. (Cooling is important for the texture!) If there is any dough, repeat with the remaining dough.

Nutrition:

Calories 208
Fat: 16 g.
Protein: 11 g.
Total carbs 4 g.
Pure carbs 2 g.
Fiber 2 g.
Sugar 0 g.

121. KETO BELGIAN WAFFLE

Preparation time: 2 min.
Cooking time: 4 min.
Servings: 2
Ingredients:

- large eggs
- 1/2 c. shred cheddar/jack cheese (other cheeses can be substituted)

Directions:

Preheat the waffle iron. While heating, break the eggs into small bowls, whisk and mix.

Next, add the shredded cheese and mix.

Pour the waffle dough evenly into the preheated waffle iron. Each waffle cavity can be completely filled. This fabric expands, but not as much as regular waffle fabric.

Close the waffle iron lid and cook for 4 min.

When ready, lift the lid and pierce the end of the waffle and remove it. This creates two Belgian-sized waffles.

Nutrition:

Calories 87
Total Fat: 5.7 g.
Cholesterol 104 mg.
Sodium 136.9 mg.
Total Carbohydrate 2.8 g
Sugars 1.1 g.
Protein: 6.3 g.

122. GRILLED CHEESE WAFFLE

Preparation time: 3 min.
Cooking time: 8 min.
Servings: 1
Ingredients:

- 1 egg
- 1/4 tsp. garlic powder
- 1/2 c. shred cheddar
- 2 American cheese or 1/4 c. shredded cheese
- 1 tbsp. butter

Directions:

In a small bowl, mix the bacon, garlic powder, and shredded cheddar cheese.

After heating the mini waffle maker, add half the mixture of the scramble. Cook and cook for 4 min.

Add to the mini waffle maker the remainder of the scramble mixture and cook for 4 min.

Steam the stove pan over moderate heat when both waffles are finished.

Attach 1 spoonful of butter and dissolve. Place one waffle in the pan once the butter has melted. Place your favorite cheese on top of the waffle and finish with a second waffle.

Cook the waffle for 1 min. on the first side, turn it over and cook for another 1–2 min. on the other side to finish the cheese melting.

Cut the bread when the cheese melts and eat it!

Nutrition:

Calories 549

Carbohydrates 3 g.

Protein: 27 g.

Fats 48 g

Cholesterol 295 mg.

Sodium 1216 mg.

Potassium 172 mg.

Sugar 1 g.

123.   GARLIC   PARMESAN WAFFLE

Preparation time: 7 min.
Cooking time: 7 min.
Servings: 2
Ingredients:

* 1/2 c. mozzarella cheese (shredded)
* 1/3 c. grated parmesan cheese
* 1 large egg
* 1 piece of garlic (chopped or used 1/2 to reduce the flavor of garlic)
* 1/2 tsp. Italian seasoning
* 1/4 tsp. baking powder (optional)

Directions:

Preheat the waffle iron for about 5 min. until hot. If your recipe includes cream cheese, put it in a bowl first. Gently heat in a microwave (15–30 sec.) or double boiler until soft and stir.

Stir all the remaining ingredients (except toppings, if any).

Pour a sufficient amount of the waffle dough into the waffle maker and cover the surface firmly. (For a normal waffle maker, about 1/2 c., for a mini waffle maker, about 1/4 c.)

Cook for about 3–4 min. until brown and crisp. Carefully remove the waffle from the waffle maker and set it aside for a crisp noise. (Cooling is important for the texture!) If there is any dough, repeat with the remaining dough.

Nutrition:

Calories 208

Fat: 16 g.

Protein: 11 g.

Total carbs 4 g.

Pure carbohydrates 2 g.

Fiber 2 g.

Sugar 0 g.

124.   TRADITIONAL   KETO LOW-CARB WAFFLE

Preparation time: 5 min.
Cooking time: 8 min.
Servings: 1
Ingredients:

* 1 egg
* 1/2 c. shredded cheddar cheese

Directions:

Turn on or plug in the waffle maker, heat, and grease both sides.

After breaking the eggs into a small bowl, add 1/2 c. cheddar cheese and mix.

Pour half of the dough into the waffle maker and close the top.

Cook for 3–4 min. or until the desired degree of baking is achieved.

Carefully remove from the waffle maker and leave for 2–3 min. to give time to crisp.

Follow the directions again to make a second waffle.

Nutrition:
Calories 291
Carbohydrates 1 g.
Protein: 20 g.
Fat: 23 g.
Saturated Fat: 13 g.
Cholesterol 223 mg.
Sodium 413 mg.
Potassium 116 mg.
Sugar 1 g.

125. WAFFLE BREAKFAST SANDWICH

Preparation time: 2 min.
Cooking time: 7 min.
Servings: 1
Ingredients:
For the waffle:
- 1 egg
- 1/2 c. mozzarella cheese
- 2 tbsp. almond flour

For the sandwiches:
- 1 egg
- 1 slice of the cheese
- 2 slices of bacon

Directions:
Preheat your waffle iron.

When preheating the waffle iron, bring together in a bowl the milk, egg, and almond flour.

Using cooking spray, spray the waffle iron and pour the batter over the waffle iron. Open it and let it steam.

Fry the bacon in a pan while the waffle is frying. Make any kind of egg you want. Microwave the bacon.

Assemble your sandwich and eat it!

Nutrition:
Calories 493

Sugar 2 g.
Fat: 32 g.
Saturated Fat: 11 g.
Carbohydrate 6 g.
Fiber 3 g.
Protein: 46 g.

126. SPICY JALAPENO POPPER WAFFLE

Preparation time: 5 min.
Cooking time: 5 min.
Servings: 2
Ingredients:
- 1 oz. cream cheese
- 1 large egg
- 1 c. cheddar cheese (shredded)
- 2 tbsp. bacon bit
- 1/2 tbsp. jalapeno
- 1/4 tsp. baking powder (optional)
- Healthy yam keto sweetener

Directions:
Preheat the waffle iron for about 5 min. until hot. If your recipe includes cream cheese, put it in a bowl first. Gently heat in a microwave (15–30 sec.) or double boiler until soft and stir.

Stir all the remaining ingredients (except toppings, if any).

Pour a sufficient amount of the waffle dough into the waffle maker and cover the surface firmly. (For a normal waffle maker, about 1/2 c., for a mini waffle maker, about 1/4 c.)

Cook for about 3–4 min. until brown and crisp. Carefully remove the waffle from the waffle maker and set it aside for a crisp noise. (Cooling is important for the texture!) If there is any dough, repeat with the remaining dough.

Nutrition:
Calories 243
Fat: 19 g.
Protein: 11 g.
Total carbs 5 g.
Pure carbohydrates 2 g.

Fiber 2 g.
Sugar 0 g.

127. ZUCCHINI WAFFLES

Preparation time: 10 min.
Cooking time: 5 min.
Servings: 2
Ingredients:

- 1/2 c. mozzarella cheese, finely shredded
- 1 egg
- 4 tbsp. parmesan cheese, finely shredded
- 1 c. zucchini, grated
- 1/4 tsp. garlic powder
- 1/4 tsp. black pepper, ground
- 1/2 tsp. Italian seasoning
- 1/4 tsp. salt

Directions:

Sprinkle the zucchini with a pinch of salt, and set it aside for a few minutes. Squeeze out the excess water.

Warm-up your mini waffle maker.

Mix all the ingredients into a small bowl.

For a crispy crust, add 1 tsp. shredded cheese to the waffle maker and cook for 30 sec.

Then, pour the mixture into the waffle maker and cook for 5 min. or until crispy.

Carefully remove.

Enjoy!

Nutrition:

Calories: 190
Fats 13 g.
Carbs: 4 g.
Protein: 16 g.

128. GOAT CHEESE WAFFLE BITES

Preparation time: 10 min.
Cooking time: 14 min.
Servings: 2
Ingredients:

- 1 egg, beaten
- 1/4 c. crumbled goat cheese

- 1/2 c. grated cheddar cheese
- 1 tsp. xylitol

Directions:

Preheat the waffle iron.

Next, add and mix all the ingredients into a bowl. Spoon half of the batter into the waffle iron, cover, and cook for 6–7 min. or until crispy.

Lastly, dish the waffle, make another, and serve warm.

Nutrition:

Calories: 65
Fats 4.82 g.
Carbs: 0.51 g.
Protein: 4.48 g.

129. FLUFFY KETO WAFFLE

Preparation time: 3 min.
Cooking time: 4 min.
Servings: 1
Ingredients:

- 1 egg
- 1/2 c. cheddar cheese, shredded

Directions:

Switch on the waffle maker according to the manufacturer's instructions

Crack the egg and combine with cheddar cheese into a small bowl

Place half batter on the waffle maker and spread evenly.

Cook for 4 min. or as desired

Gently remove from the waffle maker and set aside for 2 min. so it cools down and become crispy

Repeat for the remaining batter

Serve with the desired toppings

Nutrition:

Calories: 130
Fats 9.64 g.
Carbs: 1.02 g.
Protein: 8.97 g.

130. TRADITIONAL WAFFLE

Preparation time: 5 min.
Cooking time: 4 min.
Servings: 2 mini waffles
Ingredients:

- 1 large egg
- 1/2 c. finely shredded mozzarella

Directions:

Switch on the mini waffle maker according to the manufacturer's instructions

Spray the waffle iron with non-stick spray

Crack the egg and combine with mozzarella cheese into a small bowl

Place half batter on the waffle maker and spread evenly.

Cook for 4 min. or as desired

Gently remove from the waffle maker and set it aside for 2 min. so it cools down and become crispy

Repeat with the remaining batter.

Serve warm with the desired toppings (optional)—butter, strawberries, and sugar-free syrup

Nutrition:

Calories: 151

Fats 10.75 g.

Carbs: 0.99 g.

Protein: 12.12 g.

131. FLUFFY SANDWICH BREAKFAST WAFFLE

Preparation time: 5 min.
Cooking time: 3 min.
Servings: 2
Ingredients:

- 1/2 tsp. psyllium husk powder (optional)
- 1 tbsp almond flour
- 1/4 tsp. baking powder (optional)
- 1 large Egg
- 1/2 c. Mozzarella cheese, shredded

- 1 tbsp. vanilla or
- Dash of cinnamon

Directions:

Switch on the waffle maker according to the manufacturer's instructions

Crack the egg and combine with cheddar cheese into a small bowl

Add remaining ingredients and combine thoroughly.

Place half batter on the waffle maker and spread evenly.

Cook for 4 min. or as desired

Gently remove from the waffle maker and set aside for 2 min. so it cools down and become crispy

Repeat for the remaining batter

Serve with keto ice cream topping

Nutrition:

Calories: 90

Fats 2.56 g.

Carbs: 2.55 g.

Protein: 10.44 g.

132. KETO PLAIN PREPPED WAFFLES

Preparation time: 3 min.
Cooking time: 6 min.
Servings: 1
Ingredients:

- 2 small eggs
- 1/2 c. shredded cheddar cheese

Directions:

Reheat the mini waffle maker until hot

Whisk the egg in a bowl, add the cheese, then mix well

Stir in the remaining ingredients (except toppings, if any).

Grease the waffle maker and scoop 1/2 of the batter onto the waffle maker, spread across evenly

Cook until a bit browned and crispy, about 4 min.

Gently remove from the waffle maker and let it cool

Repeat with the remaining batter.

Store in the fridge for 3–5 days.

Nutrition:

Calories: 54,

Fats 3.61 g.

Carbs: 0.27 g.

Protein: 4.77 g.

133. VANILLA KETO WAFFLE

Preparation time: 3 min.

Cooking time: 4 min.

Servings: 1

Ingredients:

- 1 egg
- 1/2 c. cheddar cheese, shredded
- 1/2 tsp. vanilla extract

Directions:

Switch on the waffle maker according to the manufacturer's instructions

Crack the egg and combine with cheddar cheese into a small bowl

Add vanilla extract and combine thoroughly.

Place half batter on the waffle maker and spread evenly.

Cook for 4 min. or as desired

Gently remove from the waffle maker and set aside for 2 min. so it cools down and become crispy

Repeat for the remaining batter

Nutrition:

Calories: 136

Fats 9.64 g.

Carbs: 1.28 g.

Protein: 8.97 g.

134. CRISPY SANDWICH WAFFLE

Preparation time: 3 min.

Cooking time: 4 min.

Servings: 1

Ingredients:

- 1 egg
- 1/2 c. cheddar cheese, shredded
- 1 tbsp. coconut flour

Directions:

Using a mini waffle maker, preheat according to the maker's instructions.

Combine egg and cheddar cheese in a mixing bowl. Stir thoroughly

Add coconut flour for added texture if so desired

Place half batter on the waffle maker and spread evenly.

Cook for 4 min. or as desired

Gently remove from the waffle maker and set aside for 2 min. so it cools down and become crispy

Repeat for the remaining batter

Stuff 2 waffles with the desired sandwich

Nutrition:

Calories: 200

Fats: 12 g.

Carbs: 2,7 g.

Protein: 7,2 g

135. FLAKY DELIGHT WAFFLE

Preparation time: 3 min.

Cooking time: 4 min.

Servings: 1

Ingredients:

- 1 egg
- 1/2 c. cheddar cheese, shredded
- 1/2 c. coconut flakes

Directions:

Switch on the waffle maker according to the manufacturer's instructions

Crack the egg and combine with cheddar cheese into a small bowl

Place half batter on the waffle maker and spread evenly.

Sprinkle coconut flakes and cook for 4 min. or as desired

Gently remove from the waffle maker and set aside for 2 min. so it cools down and become crispy

Repeat for the remaining batter

Serve with the desired toppings

Nutrition:

Calories 291

Net carbs 1 g.

Fat 23 g.

Protein 20 g.

136.   KETO MINTY BASE WAFFLE

Preparation time: 3 min.

Cooking time: 4 min.

Servings: 1

Ingredients:

- 1 egg
- 1/2 c. cheddar cheese, shredded
- 1 tbsp. mint extract (low-carb)

Directions:

Using a mini waffle maker, preheat according to the maker's instructions.

Combine egg and cheddar cheese in a mixing bowl. Stir thoroughly

Add mint extract and place half batter on the waffle maker; spread evenly.

Cook for 4 min. or as desired

Gently remove from the waffle maker and set aside for 2 min. so it cools down and become crispy

Repeat for the remaining batter

Garnish with the desired toppings

Nutrition:

Calories 170

Net carbs 2 g.

Fat 14 g.

Protein 10 g.

137.   OKONOMIYAKI WAFFLE

Preparation time: 22 min.

Cooking time: 11 min.

Servings: 2

Ingredients:

For the waffle:

- 1/2 c. mozzarella cheese
- 1/2 tsp. baking powder
- 2 egg
- 2 onions (chopped)
- 1/4 c. cabbage (shredded)

For the sauce:

- 4 tsp. soy sauce
- 2 tbsp. swerve/monk fruit
- 4 tbsp. ketchup (sugar-free)
- 4 tsp. Worcestershire sauce

For the toppings:

- 2 tbsp. kewpie mayo
- 2 tbsp. b beni shoga
- 1 green onion stalk
- 4 tbsp. bonito flakes
- 2 tbsp. dried seaweed powder

Directions:

Prepare a mix of chopped onions and finely cut cabbage and set it aside.

Using a mixing bowl, prepare another mix for the sauce containing all the ingredients for the sauce and also set it aside.

Quickly, preheat a mini-sized waffle and grease it. In another mixing bowl, prepare a mix of shredded mozzarella cheese with cabbage, beaten eggs, and baking powder.

Combine the mixture and pour it into the lower side of the waffle maker.

With the lid closed, cook for 5 min. to a crunch. Once timed out, take out the waffles and serve on a plate.

Repeat the process for the remaining waffle mixture.

Garnish the waffles with beni shoga, bonito flakes, chopped onions, and dried seaweed powder. Pour the prepared sauce with Kewpie mayo.

Serve and enjoy.

Nutrition:
Calories 298

Net carbs 14.63 g.

Fat 17.1 g.

Protein 23.2 g.

138. RICH AND CREAMY MINI WAFFLE

Preparation time: 12 min.
Cooking time: 6 min.
Servings: 2
Ingredients:
- 3/4 tbsp. baking powder
- 2 eggs
- 2 tbsp. cream cheese
- 2 tbsp. almond flour
- 2 tbsp. water (optional)
- 1 c. shredded mozzarella

Directions:
Preheat and grease the waffle maker.

Prepare a mix of all the ingredients in a mixing bowl.

Pour the mixture into a large-sized waffle maker and spread evenly.

Heat the mixtures to a crunchy form for 5 min.

Repeat the process for the remaining mixture.

Serve hot and enjoy the crispy taste.

Nutrition:
Calories 266

Net carbs 6.43 g.

Fat 14.55 g.

Protein 28.2 g.

139. JALAPENO BACON SWISS WAFFLE

Preparation time: 18 min.
Cooking time: 12 min.
Servings: 2
Ingredients:
- 1/2 c. shredded swiss cheese
- 1 tbsp. fresh jalapenos (diced)
- 2 tbsp. bacon piece
- 1 egg

Directions:
First, preheat and grease the waffle maker.

Using a pan, cook the bacon pieces, put off the heat and shred the cheese and egg.

Add in the diced fresh jalapenos and mix evenly.

Heat the waffle maker to get the mixture into a crispy form.

Repeat the process for the remaining mixture.

Serve the dish to enjoy.

Nutrition:
Calories 218

Net carbs 2.85 g.

Fat 16.65 g.

Protein 14.33 g.

140. SAVORY CAULIFLOWER WAFFLES WITH CREAM CHEESE FROSTING

Preparation time: 30 min.
Cooking time: 15 min.
Servings: 4
Ingredients:
- 2 tbsp. cream cheese or a mixture of 1 tbsp. cream cheese and 1 1/2 tbsp. shredded mozzarella cheese
- 1/2 tbsp. unsalted butter, melted
- 1 tbsp. finely shredded and chopped carrot
- 1 tbsp. sweetener of your choice
- 1 tbsp. almond flour

- 1 tsp. pumpkin pie spice
- 1/2 tsp. keto-friendly flavor of choice
- 1/2 tsp. baking powder
- I pinch of salt
- 1 egg

For the cream cheese frosting:
- 1 tbsp. cream cheese
- 1 tbsp. unsalted butter
- 1 tsp. sweetener of choice

Directions:
For the cream cheese frosting:
Heat the butter and cream cheese for the frosting
Mix until smooth and add the sweetener.

For the waffles:
Heat up the waffle maker.
Melt the cheese cream, mozzarella, and butter for 15 sec. in a low heat
Mix flour, sweetener, flavor, salt
Mix the melted butter content with the dry ingredients
Whisk the egg thoroughly
Gently whisk the egg into the existing batter thoroughly
Add the carrot and the pumpkin pie spice. Mix thoroughly
Grease the waffle maker
Add the batter to the waffle maker
Repeat the baking procedures till the batter is finished
Drizzle the frosting over the waffle as desired.

Nutrition:
Calories 116
Net carbs 6.17 g.
Fat 8.77 g.
Protein 3.4 g.

141. CHOCOLATE WAFFLES WITH RASPBERRIES

Preparation time: 5 min.
Cooking time: 5 min.
Servings: 4
Ingredients:
- 2 c. almond/coconut flour
- 1 tbsp. mozzarella cheese
- 2 tsps. baking powder
- Pinch of salt
- oz. unsweetened chocolate, coarsely chopped
- 1 3/4 c. Lekanto sugar-free maple syrup
- 2 large eggs
- 2 tbsps. unsalted butter, melted
- 1/2 pint fresh raspberries

For the berry syrup:
- 3 fresh berries
- 1/2 c. water
- 1 tsp. grated lemon zest
- 1/2 c. sweetener
- 1 tbsp. lemon juice

Directions:
For the berry syrup:
Mix the berries and water in a large saucepan and boil over medium-high heat.
Crush the berries with a spoon or masher. Lower the heat and cook the mixture for 10 min.
Place a fine-mesh sieve over a bowl or cup.
Pour the berries into the sieve, pressing lightly to release the juices.
Pour the juice into a small size saucepan and gently stir in the lemon zest, sugar, and lemon juice. Boil over medium heat, stirring continuously to dissolve the sugar. Leave to simmer for about 8–10 min. until the syrup has thickened slightly.
Serve warm or refrigerate for about 1 week

For the waffles:

Heat up a waffle iron.

In a large bowl, mix the flour, sweetener, baking powder, and salt.

Stir in the chocolate.

Whisk the cheese, eggs, and butter together in a separate medium bowl.

Gently mix the egg mixture into the dry ingredients.

Lightly grease the waffle iron.

Ladle the batter into the waffle iron.

Bake until crispy and golden brown, according to the manufacturer's directions.

Repeat the baking procedure until all batter is baked.

Sprinkle with raspberries to serve.

Serve with maple syrup

Enjoy!

Nutrition:

Calories 161

Net carbs 31.2 g.

Fat 2.71 g.

Protein 2.85 g.

142.   YEAST-RISEN OVERNIGHT WAFFLES

Preparation time: 10 min.

Cooking time: 10 min.

Servings: 4

Ingredients:

- 2 c. almond flour
- 1 tbsp. sweetener
- 1/2 tsp. salt
- 1/2 tsp. instant yeast
- 2 c. cheese, slightly warmed
- 1/2 c. unsalted butter, melt down and cooled to room temperature
- 1 tsp. pure vanilla extract
- 2 large eggs, separated the next day

Note:

Warming the cheese gives the yeast a head start. Do not make it too hot or the yeast will die and the batter won't bubble.

Some versions of overnight waffles require the mixture to stay on the counter at room temperature.

Directions:

Mix the flour, sweetener, salt, and yeast in a large bowl.

In a medium-size bowl, mix the cheese, butter, and vanilla together.

Gently mix the wet ingredients with the dry ingredients.

Stir the mixture thoroughly.

Close up the mix with plastic wrap or a tight-fitting lid and leave for an hour at room temperature before refrigerating overnight.

The next morning, the batter will bubble a bit.

Preheat the waffle iron on medium. Gently grease the waffle iron.

Stir the egg yolks into the batter.

Place the egg whites in a medium-size bowl, and beat them thoroughly.

Gently mix the dry and wet ingredients together until smooth.

Ladle the batter in the waffle iron and bake for about 3–5 min. until light golden brown.

Serve with butter and maple syrup.

Nutrition:

Calories 432

Net carbs 3.8 g.

Fat 37.99 g.

Protein 18.74 g.

143. WHITE MUSHROOM WAFFLES WITH SALTED CARAMEL SAUCE

Preparation time: 15 min.
Cooking time: 15 min.
Servings: 4–6
Ingredients:

* 4 white mushrooms (washed and shredded)
* 3/4 c. whole cheese
* 3 large eggs
* 4 tbsps. unsalted butter, melted
* 2 c. almond flour
* 2 tbsps. sweetener
* 1 1/2 tbsps. baking powder
* 1/2 tsp. salt

For 1 c. salted caramel sauce:

* 1/4 c. sweetener
* 4 tbsps. unsalted butter, melted
* 1 tsp. vanilla
* 3/4 c. cheese cream
* 1 tsp. salt

Directions:

Heat a waffle iron beforehand according to the manufacturer's instructions.

In a bowl (medium size), whisk the white mushroom, cheese, eggs, and butter.

In a bowl (large size), mix the flour, sweetener, baking powder, and salt together.

Gently mix the butter mixture into the dry ingredients until thoroughly mixed.

Lightly grease the waffle iron.

Ladle the batter in the preheated waffle iron.

Bake until golden brown.

Repeat the baking procedure until all the batter is baked.

Drizzle with the warm salted caramel to serve.

Nutrition:

Calories 217
Net carbs 12.81 g.
Fat 15.21 g.
Protein 7.9 g.

144. LEMON–POPPYSEED WAFFLES

Preparation time: 10 min.
Cooking time: 20 min.
Servings: 6
Ingredients:

* 2 large eggs
* 1 1/2 c. cream cheese
* 1/2 c. (4 oz/125 g.) no salt butter, melted
* 2 tbsp. finely grated lemon zest
* 2 tbsp. fresh lemon juice
* 1 tsp. French vanilla flavor
* 1 1/2 c. (7 1/2 oz/235 g) almond flour
* 1/3 c. (3 oz/90 g) monk fruit or any keto-friendly sweetener of choice
* 1 1/2 tsp. baking powder
* 1 tsp. baking soda
* 1/4 tsp. salt
* 2 tbsp. poppy seeds

Directions:
For the waffle:

Heat a waffle maker beforehand

In a bowl (medium), whisk together the eggs, cheese, butter, lemon zest, lemon juice, and vanilla.

In a bowl (large), combine the flour, sweetener, baking powder, baking soda, and salt. Stir in the poppy seeds.

Create a hole in the center of the bowl containing the dry ingredients. Pour in the egg mixture.

Whisk thoroughly until mostly smooth.

Grease the waffle maker

Ladle the batter in the waffle maker, using 1/2–3/4 c. batter per batch.

Bake for about 3–4 min. until the waffles are crisp and golden brown.

Remove the waffles from the waffle maker.

Either you serve immediately or leave to cool before serving.

Top with any keto-friendly sauce and dust with cheese.

Nutrition:

Calories 736

Net Carbs 21.66 g.

Fat 66.36 g.

Protein 17.48 g.

145. GINGERBREAD WAFFLES WITH SUGAR-FREE MAPLE SYRUP

Preparation time: 15 min.

Cooking time: 15 min.

Servings: 6

Ingredients:

For the maple butter:

- 6 tbsp. (3 oz./90 g.) unsalted butter, softened
- 1 1/2 tbsp. pure maple syrup
- Pinch of salt
- Pinch of cinnamon

For the waffles:

- 2 large eggs
- 1 1/2 c. any keto cheese
- 1/2 c. (4 oz/125 g) no salt butter, melted,
- 1 tsp. keto-friendly flavor of choice
- 1 1/2 c. (7 1/2 oz./235 g.) almond/coconut flour
- 3 tbsp. Lekanto sugar-free maple syrup
- 1 tbsp. baking powder
- 1 1/2 tsp.s ground ginger
- 1 tsp. cinnamon
- 1/4 tsp. ground cloves
- Pinch of salt

Directions:

For the maple butter:

To prepare the maple butter, in a bowl (small size), whisk together the butter, maple syrup, cinnamon, and salt. Scoop into a ramekin or other serving dish. Place it in the freezer for 5 min. or in the refrigerator for 15 min. to firm up before serving.

For the waffles:

Preheat a waffle maker

Whisk together the eggs, cheese, butter, and flavor in a medium bowl.

Mix the flour, maple syrup, baking powder, ginger, cinnamon, cloves, and salt together in a large bowl.

Carefully pour the egg mixture into the dry ingredients.

Whisk thoroughly till smooth.

Grease the waffle maker

Ladle the batter into the waffle maker.

Cook for about 3–4 min. till the waffles are crisp and browned.

Remove the waffles from the waffle maker and serve right away, or allow cooling before serving.

Top with pats of maple butter and/or drizzle with maple syrup

Nutrition:

Calories 520

Net carbs 26.42 g.

Fat 36.4 g.

Protein 23.42 g.

146. PEANUT BUTTER AND JAM WAFFLE

Preparation time: 15 min.

Cooking time: 15 min.

Servings: 6

Ingredients:

For the maple butter:

- 1 c. jam or preserves of your choice, such as raspberry, strawberry, or blackberry
- 2 large eggs
- 1 1/2 c. cheese of your choice
- 1/2 c. natural peanut butter
- 1/4 c. unsalted butter, melted,
- 1 1/2 c. almond flour
- 3 tbsp. keto-friendly sweetener

- 1 tbsp. baking powder
- 1/2 tsp. salt

Directions:
For the jam:
Place the jam in a small saucepan.

Heat for about 1–3 min. until just gently warmed and loose enough to pour; stir continuously.

Stir and place in a serving bowl or pitcher.

For the waffles:
Preheat a waffle maker

Whip the eggs, cheese, 1/2 c. peanut butter, and butter on medium speed for about 2 min. in the bowl until smooth.

In a bowl (medium), mix together the flour, sweetener, baking powder, and salt.

Add the dry ingredients to the peanut butter mixture until well mixed. Ladle the batter into the waffle maker.

Cook for about 3–4 min. until the waffles are crisp and browned.

Remove the waffles from the waffle maker.

Repeat the procedure until all the batter is finished.

Cut the waffles into half or quarters.

Place a waffle piece on a plate; spread some peanut butter on top.

Pour some of the warmed jam on top, then top with another piece of the waffle, or leave open-faced, if desired.

Repeat with the remaining waffles and serve right away or allow cooling.

Note:
For best results, use salted but unsweetened peanut butter.

Nutrition:
Calories 571

Net carbs 23.31 g.

Fat 42.08 g.

Protein 28.08 g.

147. CREAM CAKE WAFFLE
Preparation time: 7 min.
Cooking time: 12 min.
Servings: 4
Ingredients:
For the waffle:
- 4 oz. cream cheese, softened
- 4 eggs
- 4 tbsp. coconut flour
- 1 tbsp. almond flour
- 1 1/2 tsp. baking powder
- 1 tbsp. butter, softened
- 1 tsp. vanilla extract
- 1/2 tsp. cinnamon
- 1 tbsp. sweetener
- 1 tbsp. shredded coconut, colored and unsweetened
- 1 tbsp. walnuts, chopped

For the Italian cream frosting:
- 2 oz. cream cheese, softened
- 2 tbsp. butter, room temperature
- 2 tbsp. sweetener
- 1/2 tsp. vanilla

Directions:
Add the almond flour, coconut flour, eggs, cream cheese, softened butter, vanilla, cinnamon, sweetener, and baking powder in a blender and blend until smooth.

Add the walnuts and shredded coconut to the mixture.

Blend the ingredients on the high setting until you have a creamy mixture.

Preheat your waffle maker and add 1/4 of the ingredients.

Cook for 3 min. and repeat the process until you have 4 waffles.

Remove and set aside.

In the meantime, start making your frosting by mixing all the ingredients.

Stir until you have a smooth and creamy mixture.

Cool, frost the cake, and enjoy.

Nutrition:

Calories: 127

Fats: 10 g.

Carbs: 5.5 g.

Protein: 7 g.

148.   TURNIP HASH BROWN WAFFLES

Preparation time: 10 min.

Cooking time: 20 min.

Servings: 6

Ingredients:

- 1 large turnip, peeled and shredded
- 1/2 medium white onion, minced
- 2 garlic cloves, pressed
- 1 c. grated Swiss cheese
- 2 eggs, beaten
- Salt and black pepper to taste

Directions:

Pour the turnips into a medium safe microwave bowl, sprinkle with 1 tbsp. water, and steam in the microwave for 1–2 min. or until softened.

Remove the bowl and mix in the remaining ingredients except for 1/4 c. Swiss cheese.

Preheat the waffle iron.

Once heated, sprinkle half of the Swiss cheese on the bottom of the waffle iron and add half of the turnip mixture. Close and cook for 8–9 min. or until the waffle is crispy.

Plate the waffle and make the second one in the same manner.

Nutrition:

Calories: 133

Fats 13 g.

Carbs: 3 g.

Protein: 5 g

149.   SOUTH-WESTERN WAFFLES

Preparation time: 5 min.

Cooking time: 6 min.

Servings: 2

Ingredients:

- 1 large organic egg, beaten
- 1/2 c. Colby Jack cheese, shredded finely
- 1/8 tsp. organic vanilla extract

Directions:

Preheat a mini waffle iron and then grease it.

In a small bowl, add the egg, vanilla extract, and cheese and stir to combine.

Place half of the mixture into the preheated waffle iron and cook for about 3 min. or until golden brown.

Repeat with the remaining mixture.

Serve warm.

Nutrition:

Calories: 147

Carbohydrates: 1.2 g.

Protein: 9.2 g.

Fat: 11.5 g.

Sugar: 0.2 g.

Sodium: 215 mg.

Fiber: 0 g.

150.   UNIQUE WAFFLES

Preparation time: 5 min.

Cooking time: 8 min.

Servings: 1

Ingredients:

- 2 oz. Colby Jack cheese, sliced thinly in triangles
- 1 large organic egg, beaten

Directions:

Preheat a waffle iron and then grease it.

Arrange 1 thin layer of the cheese slices in the bottom of the preheated waffle iron.

Place the beaten egg on top of the cheese.

Now, arrange another layer of the cheese slice on top to cover it evenly.

Cook for about 5–8 min. or until golden brown.

Serve warm.

Nutrition:
Calories: 292
Carbohydrates: 2.4 g.
Protein: 18.3 g.
Fat: 23 g.
Sugar: 0.4 g.
Sodium: 431 mg.
Fiber: 0 g.

151.   FLUFFIER WAFFLES

Preparation time: 5 min.
Cooking time: 10 min.
Servings: 2
Ingredients:

- 1 large organic egg, beaten
- 1/2 c. cheddar cheese, shredded
- 2 tbsp. almond flour

Directions:
Preheat a mini waffle iron and then grease it.

In a bowl, add the egg, cheddar cheese, and almond flour and beat until well combined.

Place half of the mixture into the preheated waffle iron and cook for about 3–5 min. or until golden brown.

Repeat with the remaining mixture.

Serve warm.

Nutrition:
Calories: 195
Carbohydrates: 1.8 g.
Protein: 10.2 g.
Fat: 15.6 g.
Sugar: 0.6 g.
Sodium: 210 mg.
Fiber: 0.8 g.

152.   EASIEST WAFFLES

Preparation time: 5 min.
Cooking time: 10 min.
Servings: 1
Ingredients:

- 1 organic egg, beaten
- 2 tbsp. almond flour
- 1/2 tsp. organic baking powder
- 1/2 c. Mozzarella cheese, shredded

Directions:
Preheat a mini waffle iron and then grease it.

In a bowl, add all the ingredients and beat until well combined.

Place half of the mixture into the preheated waffle iron and cook for about 3–5 min. or until golden brown.

Repeat with the remaining mixture.

Serve warm.

Nutrition:
Calories: 98
Carbohydrates: 2.3 g.
Protein: 4.8 g.
Fat: 7.2 g.
Sugar: 0.4 g.
Sodium: 74 mg.
Fiber: 0.8 g.

153.   LIGHTER WAFFLES

Preparation time: 10 min.
Cooking time: 5 min.
Servings: 1
Ingredients:

- 1 organic egg, beaten
- 1/3 c. Cheddar cheese, shredded
- 1/2 tsp. ground flaxseed
- 1/4 tsp. organic baking powder
- 2 tbsp. Parmesan cheese, shredded

Directions:
Preheat a mini waffle iron and then grease it.

In a bowl, add all the ingredients except Parmesan and beat until well combined.

Place half of the Parmesan cheese in the bottom of the preheated waffle iron.

Place the egg mixture over the cheese and top with the remaining Parmesan cheese.

Cook for about 3–5 min. or until golden brown.

Serve warm.

Nutrition:

Calories: 264

Carbohydrates: 2.1 g.

Protein: 18.9 g.

Fat: 20 g.

Sugar: 0.6 g.

Sodium: 467 mg.

Fiber: 0.4 g.

154.   EXTRA   SOFT WAFFLES

Preparation time: 10 min.

Cooking time: 16 min.

Servings: 4

Ingredients:

- 2 tbsp. butter, melted and cooled
- 2 large organic eggs
- 2 oz. cream cheese, softened
- 1/4 c. powdered erythritol
- 1 1/2 tsp. organic vanilla extract
- Pinch of salt
- 1/4 c. almond flour
- 2 tbsp. coconut flour
- 1 tsp. organic baking powder

Directions:

Preheat a mini waffle iron and then grease it.

In a bowl, add the butter and eggs and beat until creamy.

Add the cream cheese, Erythritol, vanilla extract, and salt and beat until well combined.

Add the flour and baking powder and beat until well combined.

Place 1/4 of the mixture into the preheated waffle iron and cook for about 4 min. or until golden brown.

Repeat with the remaining mixture.

Serve warm.

Nutrition:

Calories: 217

Carbohydrates: 6.6 g.

Protein: 5.3 g.

Fat: 18 g.

Sugar: 1.2 g.

Sodium: 173 mg.

Fiber: 3.3 g.

155.   ULTIMATE BREAKFAST WAFFLES

Preparation time: 10 min.

Cooking time: 12 min.

Servings: 2

Ingredients:

- 1 organic egg, beaten
- 1 tsp. organic vanilla extract
- 1 tbsp. almond flour
- 1 tsp. organic baking powder
- Pinch of ground cinnamon
- 1 c. Mozzarella cheese, shredded

Directions:

Preheat a mini waffle iron and then grease it.

In a bowl, add the egg and vanilla extract and beat until well combined.

Add the flour, baking powder, and cinnamon and mix well.

Add the Mozzarella cheese and stir to combine.

Place half of the mixture into the preheated waffle iron and cook for about 5–6 min. or until golden brown.

Repeat with the remaining mixture.

Serve warm.

Nutrition:

Calories: 103

Carbohydrates: 2.8 g.

Protein: 6.8 g.

Fat: 6.6 g.

Sugar: 0.6 g.

Sodium: 118 mg.

Fiber: 0.5 g.

156. BIOLOGICAL WAFFLES

Preparation time: 5 min.
Cooking time: 8 min.
Servings: 2
Ingredients:
- 1/2 c. Mozzarella cheese, shredded
- 1 large organic egg, beaten
- 2 tbsp. blanched almond flour
- 1/2 tsp. Psyllium husk powder
- 1/4 tsp. organic baking powder

Directions:
Preheat a mini waffle iron and then grease it.
In a bowl, add all the ingredients and beat until well combined.
Place half of the mixture into the preheated waffle iron and cook for about 3–4 min. or until golden brown.
Repeat with the remaining mixture.
Serve warm.

Nutrition:
Calories: 101
Carbohydrates: 2.9 g.
Protein: 6.7 g.
Fat: 7.1 g.
Sugar: 0.2 g.
Sodium: 81 mg.
Fiber: 1.3 g.

157. WHITE BREAD WAFFLES

Preparation time: 5 min.
Cooking time: 10 min.
Servings: 2
Ingredients:
- 1 large organic egg, beaten
- 1 tbsp. mayonnaise
- 2 tbsp. almond flour
- 1/8 tsp. organic baking powder
- 1 tsp. water

Directions:
Preheat a mini waffle iron and then grease it.
In a bowl, add all the ingredients and beat until well combined.
Place half of the mixture into the preheated waffle iron and cook for about 4–5 min. or until golden brown.
Repeat with the remaining mixture.
Serve warm.

Nutrition:
Calories: 145
Carbohydrates: 2.4 g.
Protein: 2.8 g.
Fat: 12.8 g.
Sugar: 0.5 g.
Sodium: 76 mg.
Fiber: 1.1 g.

158. PROTEIN-RICH WAFFLES

Preparation time: 5 min.
Cooking time: 20 min.
Servings: 4
Ingredients:
- 1/2 scoop unsweetened protein powder
- 2 large organic eggs
- 1/2 c. mozzarella cheese, shredded
- 1 tbsp. erythritol
- 1/4 tsp. organic vanilla extract

Directions:
Preheat a mini waffle iron and then grease it.
In a bowl, add all the ingredients and beat until well combined.
Place 1/4 of the mixture into the preheated waffle iron and cook for about 4–5 min. or until golden brown.
Repeat with the remaining mixture.
Serve warm.

Nutrition:
Calories: 61
Carbohydrates: 0.4 g.
Protein: 7.3 g.

Fat: 3.3 g.
Sugar: 0.2 g.
Sodium: 89 mg.
Fiber: 0 g.

159. NUT BUTTER WAFFLES

Preparation time: 5 min.
Cooking time: 10 min.
Servings: 2
Ingredients:

- 1 large organic egg, beaten
- 1/3 c. mozzarella cheese, shredded
- 1 tbsp. monk fruit sweetener
- 2 tbsp. almond butter
- 1 tsp. organic vanilla extract

Directions:
Preheat a mini waffle iron and then grease it.
In a bowl, add all the ingredients and beat until well combined.
Place half of the mixture into the preheated waffle iron and cook for about 3–5 min. or until golden brown.
Repeat with the remaining mixture.
Serve warm.
Nutrition:
Calories: 149
Carbohydrates: 3.6 g.
Protein: 7.5 g.
Fat: 12 g.
Sugar: 1.1 g.
Sodium: 60 mg.
Fiber: 1.6 g.

160. SATURDAY MORNING WAFFLES

Preparation time: 5 min.
Cooking time: 8 min.
Servings: 2
Ingredients:

- 1 organic egg, beaten
- 1/2 c. mozzarella cheese, shredded

- 3 tbsp. granulated Erythritol
- 2 tbsp. peanut butter

Directions:
Preheat a mini waffle iron and then grease it.
In a bowl, add all the ingredients and beat until well combined.
Place half of the mixture into the preheated waffle iron and cook for about 4 min. or until golden brown.
Repeat with the remaining mixture.
Serve warm.
Nutrition:
Calories: 145
Carbohydrates: 3.6 g.
Protein: 8.8 g.
Fat: 11.5 g.
Sugar: 1.7 g.
Sodium: 147 mg.
Fiber: 1 g.

161. VERSATILE WAFFLES

Preparation time: 10 min.
Cooking time: 6 min.
Servings: 2
Ingredients:
For the waffles:

- 1 organic egg, beaten
- 1 tbsp. heavy whipping cream
- 2 tbsp. sugar-free peanut butter powder
- 2 tbsp. monk fruit sweetener
- 1/4 tsp. organic baking powder
- 1/4 tsp. peanut butter extract

For the frosting:

- 2 tbsp. monk fruit sweetener
- 1 tbsp. butter, softened
- 1 tbsp. natural peanut butter
- 2 tbsp. cream cheese, softened
- 1/4 tsp. organic vanilla extract

Directions:
Preheat a mini waffle iron and then grease it.

For the waffles:

In a bowl, add all the ingredients and beat until well combined.

Place half of the mixture into the preheated waffle iron and cook for about 3 min.

Repeat with the remaining mixture.

For the frosting

In a bowl, add all the ingredients, and with a hand mixer, beat until well combined.

Place the waffles onto serving plates.

Spread frosting over each waffle and serve.

Nutrition:

Calories: 221

Carbohydrates: 4.3 g.

Protein: 9.2 g.

Fat: 19 g.

Sugar: 0.8 g.

Sodium: 107 mg.

Fiber: 1.5 g.

162. ZINGY WAFFLES

Preparation time: 10 min.

Cooking time: 10 min.

Servings: 2

Ingredients:

For the waffles:

- 1 organic egg, beaten
- 1 oz. cream cheese, softened
- 2 tbsp. almond flour
- 1 tbsp. fresh lemon juice
- 2 tsp. monk fruit sweetener
- 1/2 tsp. fresh lemon zest, grated
- 1/4 tsp. organic baking powder
- Pinch of salt

For the frosting:

- 4 tsp. heavy cream
- 2 tbsp. powdered Erythritol
- 1 tsp. fresh lemon juice
- Pinch of fresh lemon zest, grated

Directions:

Preheat a mini waffle iron and then grease it.

For the waffles:

In a bowl, add all the ingredients and beat until well combined.

Place half of the mixture into the preheated waffle iron and cook for about 3–5 min.

Repeat with the remaining mixture.

For the frosting:

In a bowl, add all the ingredients and, with a hand mixer, beat until well combined.

Place the waffles onto serving plates.

Spread frosting over each waffle and serve.

Nutrition:

Calories: 163

Carbohydrates: 2.6 g.

Protein: 4.1 g.

Fat: 14.6 g.

Sugar: 0.7 g.

Sodium: 156 mg.

Fiber: 0.8 g.

163. CINNAMON CHURRO WAFFLES

Preparation time: 10 min.

Cooking time: 8 min.

Servings: 2

Ingredients:

- 1 large organic egg, beaten
- 3/4 c. mozzarella cheese, shredded
- 1/2 tbsp. unsalted butter, melted
- 2 tbsp. blanched almond flour
- 2 tbsp. erythritol
- 1/2 tsp. ground cinnamon
- 1/2 tsp. psyllium husk powder
- 1/4 tsp. organic baking powder
- 1/2 tsp. organic vanilla extract

For the topping::

- 1/4 c. erythritol
- 3/4 tsp. ground cinnamon

- 1 tbsp. unsalted butter, melted

Directions:

Preheat a waffle iron and then grease it.

For the waffles:

In a bowl, add all the ingredients and beat until well combined.

Place half the mixture into the preheated waffle iron and cook for about 3–5 min. or until golden brown.

Repeat with the remaining mixture.

For the topping:

Into a small bowl, mix together the erythritol and cinnamon.

Place the waffles onto serving plates and set them aside to cool slightly.

Brush the waffles with melted butter and then sprinkle with the cinnamon mixture.

Serve immediately.

Nutrition:

Calories: 193
Carbohydrates: 4.1 g.
Protein: 7.8 g.
Fat: 16.4 g.
Sugar: 0.4 g.
Sodium: 163 mg.
Fiber: 2 g.

164. VANILLA CHEESECAKE WAFFLES

Preparation time: 10 min.
Cooking time: 8 min.
Servings: 2
Ingredients:

- 2 tsp. coconut flour
- 4 tsp. erythritol
- 1/4 tsp. organic baking powder
- 1 organic egg, beaten
- 1 oz. cream cheese, softened
- 1/2 tsp. organic vanilla extract

Directions:

Preheat a mini waffle iron and then grease it.

In a bowl, add flour, erythritol, and baking powder and mix well.

Add the egg, cream cheese, and vanilla extract and beat until well combined.

Place half of the mixture into the preheated waffle iron and cook for about 3–4 min. or until golden brown.

Repeat with the remaining mixture.

Serve warm.

Nutrition:

Calories: 145
Carbohydrates: 8 g.
Protein: 5.8 g.
Fat: 9.1 g.
Sugar: 1.3 g.
Sodium: 103 mg.
Fiber: 5 g.

165. AMERICAN BLUEBERRY WAFFLES

Preparation time: 10 min.
Cooking time: 25 min.
Servings: 5
Ingredients:

- 1 c. Mozzarella cheese, shredded
- 2 tbsp. almond flour
- 1 tsp. organic baking powder
- 2 organic eggs
- 1 tsp. ground cinnamon
- 2 tsp. Erythritol
- 3 tbsp. fresh blueberries

Directions:

Preheat a mini waffle iron and then grease it.

In a bowl, add all the ingredients except the blueberries and beat until well combined.

Fold in the blueberries.

Divide the mixture into 5 portions.

Place 1 portion of the mixture into the preheated waffle iron and cook for about 3–5 min. or until golden brown.

Repeat with the remaining mixture.

Serve warm.

Nutrition:
Calories: 64
Carbohydrates: 2.5 g.
Protein: 3.9 g.
Fat: 4.3 g.
Sugar: 0.8 g.
Sodium: 60 mg.
Fiber: 0.7 g.

166. WONDERFUL BLUEBERRY WAFFLES

Preparation time: 10 min.
Cooking time: 8 min.
Servings: 2
Ingredients:

- 1 organic egg, beaten
- 1 tbsp. cream cheese, softened
- 3 tbsp. almond flour
- 1/4 tsp. organic baking powder
- 1 tsp. organic blueberry extract
- 5–6 fresh blueberries

Directions:
Preheat a mini waffle iron and then grease it.
In a bowl, add all the ingredients except the blueberries and beat until well combined.
Fold in the blueberries.
Divide the mixture into 5 portions.
Place 1 portion of the mixture into the preheated waffle iron and cook for about 3–4 min. or until golden brown.
Repeat with the remaining mixture.
Serve warm.

Nutrition:
Calories: 131
Carbohydrates: 4.7 g.
Protein: 3.3 g.
Fat: 9.6 g.
Sugar: 2.2 g.
Sodium: 46 mg.
Fiber: 1.5 g.

167. CRUNCHY WAFFLES

Preparation Time: 10 minutes
Cooking Time: 10 minutes
Serving: 2
Ingredients:

- 1 organic egg, beaten
- 1 tsp. organic vanilla extract
- 1 tbsp. almond flour
- 1 tsp. organic baking powder
- Pinch of ground cinnamon
- 1 C. Mozzarella cheese, shredded

Direction:
1. Preheat a mini waffle iron and then grease it.
2. In a bowl, add the egg and vanilla extract and mix well.
3. Add the flour, baking powder and cinnamon and mix until well combined.
4. Add the Mozzarella cheese and stir to combine.
5. Place half of the mixture into preheated waffle iron and cook for about 4-5 minutes or until golden brown.
6. Repeat with the remaining mixture.
7. Serve warm.
Nutrition:
Calories per serving: 103;
Carbohydrates: 2.9g;
Protein: 6.8g;
Fat: 6.6g;
Sugar: 0.6g;
Sodium: 118mg;
Fiber: 0.5g

168. MOUTHWATERING WAFFLES

Preparation time: 10 min.
Cooking time: 8 min.
Servings: 2
Ingredients:

- 1 organic egg, beaten

- 1/3 c. mozzarella cheese, shredded
- 1 tsp. cream cheese, softened
- 1 tsp. coconut flour
- 1/4 tsp. organic baking powder
- 3/4 tsp. powdered Erythritol
- 1/4 tsp. ground cinnamon
- 1/4 tsp. organic vanilla extract
- Pinch of salt
- 1 tbsp. fresh blueberries

Directions:

Preheat a mini waffle iron and then grease it.

In a bowl, add all the ingredients except blueberries and beat until well combined.

Fold in the blueberries.

Place half of the mixture into the preheated waffle iron and cook for about 4 min. or until golden brown.

Repeat with the remaining mixture.

Serve warm.

Nutrition:

Calories: 86

Carbohydrates: 5.6 g.

Protein: 5.3 g.

Fat: 4.6 g.

Sugar: 1.2 g.

Sodium: 157 mg.

Fiber: 2.8 g.

CHAPTER 7. VEGETARIAN WAFFLE RECIPES

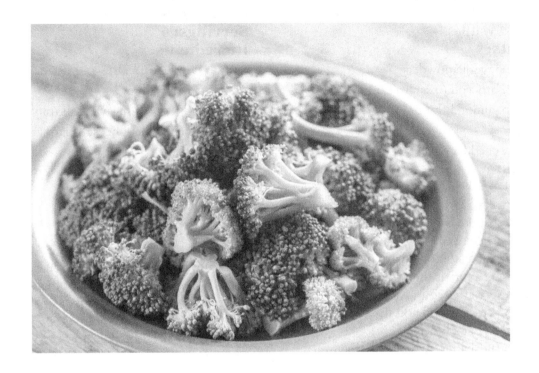

169. BROCCOLI AND CHEESE WAFFLE

Preparation time: 10 min.
Cooking time: 10 min.
Servings: 2 waffles
Ingredients:

- 1/4 tsp. garlic powder
- 1/4 c. broccoli (freshly chopped)
- 1 tbsp. almond flour
- 1 egg
- 1/2 c. cheddar cheese

Directions:

Take a bowl of the size you prefer and add almond flour, egg, 1/4 tsp. garlic powder, and cheddar cheese one after the other or in any order and mix them well. You may use a fork to mix the ingredients. You may prefer other mixers, but using a fork is the easiest way I know. Add the cheese waffle you just made with half the amount of broccoli and add the mixture to a mini waffle maker at a time.

Leave the waffle batter to cook in the waffle maker for about 4 min. The best way to know if the waffle is cooked is when you cannot see the waffle emit any steam.

Give about 1–2 min. for each waffle so that it sits on a plate in an associated manner.

Enjoy the waffle alone or by bathing in sour cream (or ranch dressing).

Nutrition:

Calories: 170
Carb: 2 g.
Protein: 11 g.
Fat: 13 g.
Fiber: 1 g.

170. CHEDDAR JALAPENO WAFFLE

Preparation time: 5 min.
Cooking time: 10 min.
Servings: 6
Ingredients:

- 8 oz. cream cheese
- 3 eggs (large)
- 1/4 tsp. Himalayan salt (pink)
- 1 c. cheddar cheese (sharp and shredded)
- 4 slices of bacon
- 1 tsp. baking powder
- 2–3 jalapeno peppers
- 3 tbsp. coconut flour

Directions:

Take jalapeno peppers and wash them properly, dry, and remove the seeds. Take one of the peppers and dice it. Chop the others.

Light a stove and place a pan on it. Cook the bacon before crispy and brown.

Use a small-sized mixing bowl to whisk baking powder, flour, and salt until they are mixed properly.

Use a mixing bowl, batter the cream cheese until it is light and creamy.

Preheat the waffle maker and drizzle handsomely with non-stick spray (low-carb).

Take another large-sized mixing bowl to add the egg into it and batter before fluffy.

Add 1/2 c. cream and another 1/2 c. shredded cheese. Mix them well until mixed properly.

Add the remaining ingredients (dry) to the egg mixture and mix until well combined.

Fold in the jalapeno (diced).

Take a waffle maker and put it on medium temperature settings. Pour the batter into the waffle maker and heat the batter for a longer time. Cook the batter for about 5 min. until it starts to brown from the outer side.

Let the waffle cool down to some extent. Top the waffle (or waffles) with the remaining cream cheese.

Serve with jalapeno slices, crumbled bacon pieces, and enjoy.

Nutrition:
Calories: 119
Carb: 2 g.
Protein: 10 g.
Fat: 8 g.
Fiber: 0 g.

171. SPINACH PROTEIN WAFFLES

Preparation time: 3 min.
Cooking time: 3 min.
Servings: 1 waffle
Ingredients:

- 1/3 c. oats
- 1/3 c. plain Greek yogurt (or non-dairy yogurt)
- 1 handful of spinach
- 1 egg (large)
- Cheddar cheese
- A dash of stevia

Directions:
Plug in your waffle iron and allow it to heat up.

Whisk the egg and add the oats, yogurt, cheddar cheese, spinach, and stevia into it and blend everything together to get a smooth batter.

When the waffle iron turns hot, pour the entire batter into it.

Close the lid of the waffle maker and let it cook for about 5 min. until it's no longer steaming.

Your waffle will be slightly golden brown around the edges.

Take it out carefully with the help of a spatula and place it on a platter.

Top it with your favorite topping, and your spinach protein waffle is ready to serve.

Nutrition:
Calories: 217

Protein: 18 g.
Fat: 7 g.
Carbs: 22 g.
Fiber: 3 g.

172. CAULIFLOWER HASH BROWN WAFFLES

Preparation time: 5 min.
Cooking time: 10 min.
Servings: 2
Ingredients:

- 2 eggs (large)
- Half a cup of low-fat cheddar cheese (shredded)
- 2 green onions, chopped
- 1 package or 12 oz. cauliflower rice
- Half 1 tsp. garlic powder

1/4 tsp. each of:

- Salt
- Pepper

Directions:
Heat your waffle maker and spray it with a non-stick cooking spray.

Steam the cauliflower rice as per the directions given on the package.

Let it cool down and then transfer it onto a clean dish towel and ring to eliminate any excess water.

Add the cauliflower rice into a large bowl along with the eggs, cheddar cheese, garlic powder, chopped green onions, salt, and pepper, and mix everything together to form a batter.

Add the batter into the waffle iron and let it cook for about 3–4 min.

When the waffle turns brown and crisp around the edges, remove it from the waffle maker and transfer it to a plate. Cut into four pieces and serve.

Nutrition:
Calories: 208
Protein: 16 g.
Fat: 11 g.
Carbs: 13 g.

Fiber: 4 g.

173. SPINACH, POTATO, AND FETA WAFFLE

Preparation time: 10 min.
Cooking time: 10 min.
Servings: 3–4
Ingredients:

- 1 potato like Maris Piper (large), cooked and cubed
- 4 eggs (large)
- 80 g. or 2.8 oz. crumbled feta cheese
- 100 g. or 3.5 oz. baby spinach, finely chopped
- 2 tbsp. olive oil
- 1/4 c. or 40 g. all-purpose flour
- 1 tbsp. flat-leaf parsley, finely chopped
- 3 spring onions, finely chopped
- 1/2 tsp. baking powder
- 1 tsp. dill, finely chopped (optional)
- 1/4 tsp. salt
- Cooking spray for the waffle maker

For the tzatziki:

- 150 g. or 5.3 oz. cucumber with the seeds eliminated (almost half large cucumber)
- 1 garlic clove (large), minced
- 300 g. or 10.5 oz. Greek yogurt
- 1 tsp. salt
- 1/2 tsp. dried oregano or mint
- 1 tbsp. lemon juice
- 1 tbsp. olive oil (to drizzle)

Directions:

Coarsely grate the cucumber into a bowl and season it with salt. Allow it to rest for about 5 min. and then squeeze out most of the moisture with the help of your hands.

Add the Greek yogurt, minced garlic, chopped oregano, and lemon juice into the grated cucumber and mix well.

Drizzle it with olive oil and keep it covered in the fridge until needed.

Boil the potato until it gets soft. Let it cool and then peel and cut it into small cubes. Keep them aside.

Preheat your waffle iron and spray it with a non-stick cooking spray.

Whisk the eggs, salt, and oil in a large bowl and add the flour and baking powder into it. Mix everything together to get a smooth batter.

Add the boiled potatoes, feta cheese, chopped spinach, spring onions, and herbs into the batter and fold them in.

Pour some batter into the waffle maker so that about half of the surface is covered.

Cook your waffle for about 5 min. until they turn golden and firm. Transfer the waffle carefully to a warm plate.

Repeat the process with the rest of the batter, and you will end up with 3–4 large waffle frittatas depending on the size and depth of your waffle iron.

You can serve the waffles either hot or cold and have the tzatziki as a side dip.

Nutrition:

Calories: 201
Protein: 12 g.
Fat: 15 g.
Carbs: 4 g.
Fiber: 1 g.

174. PARMESAN WAFFLE WITH ROASTED VEGGIES

Preparation time: 10 min.
Cooking time: 25 min.
Servings: 4
Ingredients:

- 1 egg
- 1 c. all-purpose baking mix
- 1 c. milk
- 2 tbsp. olive oil (extra-virgin)
- 1 orange or yellow bell pepper, chopped
- 1 zucchini, diced
- 1 pint of cherry tomatoes, halved

- 1 eggplant (small), peeled (optional), and diced
- 1 clove of garlic, chopped
- 1/2 red onion, thinly sliced
- 1–2 teaspoons of balsamic vinegar
- 1/2 c. grated parmesan cheese and some more for serving
- 2–3 tbsp. Italian parsley, fresh basil, or both, finely chopped
- Kosher salt

Directions:

Preheat your oven to 425 °F.

On a large rimmed baking sheet, toss the diced onion, bell pepper, eggplant, tomatoes, and zucchini along with some olive oil and 1 tsp. salt. Roast them for about 25 min. until they turn tender and golden around the edges.

Add in the vinegar, chopped garlic, and herbs and stir to mix them together.

Preheat your waffle maker.

Whisk the egg in a bowl along with the grated cheese, baking mix, and milk until you get a smooth batter.

Pour the batter into the hot waffle maker and bake for 3–4 min. until it turns golden brown.

Top the waffles with some grated parmesan cheese and vegetables and serve them right away.

Nutrition:

Calories: 606
Protein: 14 g.
Fat: 28
Carbs: 78 g.
Fiber: 6 g.

175. VEGAN WAFFLE

Preparation time: 5 min.
Cooking time: 25 min.
Servings: 2
Ingredients:

- 1 tbsp. flaxseed meal
- 2 1/2 tbsp. water
- 1/4 c. low-carb vegan cheese
- 2 tbsp. coconut flour
- 1 tbsp. low-carb vegan cream cheese, softened
- Pinch of salt

Directions:

Turn on the waffle maker to heat and oil it with cooking spray.

Mix the flaxseed and water in a container. Leave for 5 min., until thickened and gooey.

Whisk the remaining ingredients for the waffle.

Pour 1 1/2 of the batter into the center of the waffle maker. Close and cook for 3–5 min.

Remove the waffle and serve.

Nutrition:

Carbs: 33 g.
Fat: 25 g.
Protein: 25 g.
Calories: 450

176. LEMONY FRESH HERBS WAFFLES

Preparation time: 15 min.
Cooking time: 24 min.
Servings: 6
Ingredients:

- 1/2 c. ground flaxseed
- 2 organic eggs
- 1/2 c. goat cheddar cheese, grated
- 2–4 tbsp. plain Greek yogurt
- 1 tbsp. avocado oil
- 1/2 tsp. baking soda
- 1 tsp. fresh lemon juice
- 2 tbsp. fresh chives, minced
- 1 tbsp. fresh basil, minced
- 1/2 tbsp. fresh mint, minced
- 1/4 tbsp. fresh thyme, minced
- 1/4 tbsp. fresh oregano, minced
- Salt and pepper, to taste

Directions:

Preheat a waffle iron and then grease it.

In a container, add all the ingredients and, with a fork, mix until well combined.

Divide the mixture into 6 portions.

Add 1 portion of the mixture into the preheated waffle iron and cook for 4–5 min. or until golden brown.

Repeat with the remaining mixture.

Serve warm.

Nutrition:
Calories: 11
Carb: 0.9 g.
Fat: 7.9 g.
Saturated Fat: 3 g.
Carbohydrates: 3.7 g.
Dietary Fiber: 2.8 g.
Sugar: 0.7 g.
Protein: 6.4 g.

177.   BASIL WAFFLES
Preparation time: 10 min.
Cooking time: 16 min.
Servings: 2
Ingredients:
- 2 organic eggs, beaten
- 1/2 c. Mozzarella cheese, shredded
- 1 tbsp. Parmesan cheese, grated
- 1 tsp. dried basil, crushed
- Pinch of salt

Directions:
Preheat a mini waffle iron and then grease it.

In a container, add all the ingredients and mix until well combined.

Add 1/of the mixture into the preheated waffle iron and cook for about 3–4 min. or until golden brown.

Repeat with the remaining mixture.

Serve warm.

Nutrition:
Net Carb: 0.4 g.
Fat: 4.2 g.
Saturated Fat: 1.6 g.
Carbohydrates: 0.4 g.
Dietary Fiber: 0 g.
Sugar: 0.2 g.
Protein: 5.7 g.

178.   BACON WAFFLES
Preparation time: 6 min.
Cooking time: 5 min.
Servings: 2
Ingredients:
- 2 eggs
- 1/2 c. cheddar cheese
- 1/2 c. mozzarella cheese
- 1/4 tsp. baking powder
- 1/2 tbsp. almond flour
- 1 tbsp. butter, for the waffle maker

For the filling:
- 1/4 c. bacon, chopped
- 2 tbsp. green onions, chopped

Directions:
Turn on the waffle maker to heat and oil it with cooking spray.

Add the eggs, mozzarella, cheddar, butter, almond flour, and baking powder to a blender and pulse 10 times, so the cheese is still chunky.

Add bacon and green onions. Pulse 2-times to combine.

Add 1/2 of the batter to the waffle maker and cook for 3 min., until golden brown.

Repeat with the remaining batter.

Add your toppings and serve hot.

Nutrition:
Carbs: 3 g.
Fat: 38 g.
Protein: 23 g.
Calories: 446

179.   HERB WAFFLES
Preparation time: 10 min.
Cooking time: 12 min.
Servings: 2
Ingredients:
- 4 tbsp. almond flour
- 1 tbsp. coconut flour

- 1 tsp. mixed dried herbs
- 1/2 tsp. organic baking powder
- 1/4 tsp. garlic powder
- 1/4 tsp. onion powder
- Salt and ground black pepper, to taste
- 1/4 c. cream cheese, softened
- 3 large organic eggs
- 1/2 c. cheddar cheese, grated
- 1/3 c. Parmesan cheese, grated

Directions:

Preheat a waffle iron and then grease it.

In a container, mix together the flour, dried herbs, baking powder, and seasoning, and mix well.

In a container, put the cream cheese and eggs and beat until well combined.

Add the flour mixture, cheddar, and Parmesan cheese, and mix until well combined.

Add the desired amount of the mixture into the preheated waffle iron and cook for about 2–3 min.

Repeat with the remaining mixture.

Serve warm.

Nutrition:

Calories 240
Net Carb: g
Total Fat: 19 g.
Saturated Fat: 5 g.
Cholesterol 176 mg.
Sodium 280 mg.
Total Carbs: 4 g.
Fiber 1.6 g.
Sugar 0.7 g.
Protein: 12.3 g.

180.   SCALLION WAFFLES

Preparation time: 6 min.
Cooking time: 8 min.
Servings: 2
Ingredients:

- 1 organic egg, beaten
- 1/2 c. mozzarella cheese, shredded
- 1 tbsp. scallion, chopped
- 1/2 tsp. Italian seasoning

Directions:

Preheat a mini waffle iron and then grease it.

In a container, add all the ingredients and with a fork, mix until well combined.

Add half of the mixture into the preheated waffle iron and cook for about 4 min. or until golden brown.

Repeat with the remaining mixture.

Serve warm.

Nutrition:

Calories: 5
Carb: 0.7 g.
Fat: 3.8 g.
Saturated Fat: 1.5 g.
Carbohydrates: 0.8 g.
Dietary Fiber: 0.g
Sugar: 0.3 g.
Protein: 4.8 g.

181.   CRISPY   BAGEL WAFFLES

Preparation time: 5 min.
Cooking time: 30 min.
Servings: 2
Ingredients:

- 2 eggs
- 1/2 c. parmesan cheese
- 1 tsp. bagel seasoning
- 1/2 c. mozzarella cheese
- 2 tsp. almond flour

Directions:

Turn on the waffle maker to heat and oil it with cooking spray.

Evenly sprinkle half of the cheeses into a griddle and let them melt. Then toast for 30 sec. and leave them to wait for the batter.

Whisk the eggs, the other half of the cheeses, almond flour, and bagel seasoning in a container. Pour the batter into the waffle maker. Cook for 4–5 min.

Let cool for 2–3 min. before serving.

Nutrition:
Fat: 20 g.
Protein: 21 g.
Calories: 287

182. SAUSAGE AND VEGGIES WAFFLES

Preparation time: 10 min.
Cooking time: 20 min.
Servings: 2
Ingredients:

- 1/3 c. unsweetened almond milk
- 4 organic eggs
- 2 tbsp. gluten-free breakfast sausage, cut into slices
- 2 tbsp. broccoli florets, chopped
- 2 tbsp. bell peppers, seeded and chopped
- 2 tbsp. Mozzarella cheese, shredded

Directions:
Preheat a waffle iron and then grease it.
In a container, add the almond milk and eggs and beat well.
Add the remaining ingredients and stir to combine well.
Add 1/4 of the mixture into the preheated waffle iron and cook for about 5 min. or until golden brown.
Repeat with the remaining mixture.
Serve warm.

Nutrition:
Calories: 132
Net Carb: 1.2 g.
Fat: 9.2 g.
Saturated Fat: 3.5 g.
Carbohydrates: 1.4 g.
Dietary Fiber: 0.2 g.
Sugar: 0.5 g.
Protein: 11.1 g.

183. BROCCOLI AND ALMOND FLOUR WAFFLES

Preparation time: 6 min.
Cooking time: 8 min.
Servings: 2
Ingredients:

- 1 organic egg, beaten
- 1/2 c. cheddar cheese, shredded
- 1/4 c. fresh broccoli, chopped
- 1 tbsp. almond flour
- 1/4 tsp. garlic powder

Directions:
Preheat a mini waffle iron and then grease it.
In a container, add all the ingredients and mix until well combined.
Add half of the mixture into the preheated waffle iron and cook for about 4 min. or until golden brown.
Repeat with the remaining mixture.
Serve warm.

Nutrition:
Calories: 173
Net Carb: 1.5 g.
Fat: 13.5 g.
Saturated Fat: 8 g.
Carbohydrates: 2.2 g.
Dietary Fiber: 0.7 g.
Sugar: 0.7 g.
Protein: 10.2 g.

184. SPINACH AND CAULIFLOWER WAFFLES

Preparation time: 6 min.
Cooking time: 10 min.
Servings: 2
Ingredients:

- 1/2 c. frozen chopped spinach, thawed and squeezed
- 1/2 c. cauliflower, chopped finely
- 1/2 c. Cheddar cheese, shredded
- 1/2 c. Mozzarella cheese, shredded

- 1/3 c. Parmesan cheese, shredded
- 2 organic eggs
- 1 tbsp. butter, melted
- 1 tsp. garlic powder
- 1 tsp. onion powder
- Salt and pepper, to taste

Directions:

Preheat a waffle iron and then grease it.

In a container, add all the ingredients and mix until well combined.

Add half of the mixture into the preheated waffle iron and cook for about 4–5 min. or until golden brown.

Repeat with the remaining mixture.

Serve warm.

Nutrition:

Calories: 320
Net Carb: 4 g.
Fat: 24.5 g.
Saturated Fat: 14 g.
Carbohydrates: 5 g.
Dietary Fiber: 1 g.
Sugar: 1.9 g.
Protein: 20.8 g.

185.   ROSEMARY WAFFLES

Preparation time: 6 min.
Cooking time: 8 min.
Servings: 2
Ingredients:

- 1 organic egg, beaten
- 1/2 c. Cheddar cheese, shredded
- 1 tbsp. almond flour
- 1 tbsp. fresh rosemary, chopped
- Salt and black pepper

Directions:

Preheat a mini waffle iron and then grease it.

For the waffles:

In a container, add all the ingredients and, with a fork, mix until well combined.

Add half of the mixture into the preheated waffle iron and cook for about 4 min. or until golden brown.

Repeat with the remaining mixture.

Serve warm.

Nutrition:

Calories: 173
Net Carb: 1.1 g.
Fat: 13.7 g.
Saturated Fat: 9 g.
Carbohydrates: 2.2 g.
Dietary Fiber: 1.1 g.
Sugar: 0.4 g.
Protein: 9.9 g.

186.   ZUCCHINI WAFFLES WITH PEANUT BUTTER

Preparation time: 10 min.
Cooking time: 5 min.
Servings: 2
Ingredients:

- 1 c. zucchini grated
- 1 egg beaten
- 1/2 c. shredded parmesan cheese
- 1/4 c. shredded mozzarella cheese
- 1 tsp. dried basil
- 1/2 tsp. salt
- 1/2 tsp. black pepper
- 2 tbsps. peanut butter for topping

Directions:

Sprinkle salt over the zucchini and let it sit for 4–5 min.

Squeeze out water from the zucchini.

Beat the egg with zucchini, basil. Salt mozzarella cheese, and pepper.

Sprinkle 1/2 of the parmesan cheese over the preheated waffle maker and pour the zucchini batter over it.

Sprinkle the remaining cheese over it.

Close the lid.

Cook the zucchini waffles for about 4–8 min. Utes.

Remove the waffle from the maker and repeat with the remaining batter.

Serve with peanut butter on top and enjoy!

Nutrition:

Protein: 52% 88

Fat: 41% 69

Carbohydrates: 7% 12

187.   3-CHEESE BROCCOLI WAFFLES

Preparation time: 10 min.

Cooking time: 16 min.

Servings: 2

Ingredients:

- 1/2 c. cooked broccoli, chopped finely
- 2 organic eggs, beaten
- 1/2 c. Cheddar cheese, shredded
- 1/2 c. Mozzarella cheese, shredded
- 2 tbsp. Parmesan cheese, grated
- 1/2 tsp. onion powder

Directions:

Preheat a waffle iron and then grease it.

In a container, add all the ingredients and mix until well combined.

Add half of the mixture into the preheated waffle iron and cook for about 4 min. or until golden brown.

Repeat with the remaining mixture.

Serve warm.

Nutrition:

Calories: 112

Net Carb: 1.2 g.

Fat: 8.1 g.

Saturated Fat: 4.3 g.

Carbohydrates: 1.5 g.

Dietary Fiber: 0.3 g.

Sugar: 0.5 g.

Protein: 8.

188.   GARLIC MOZZARELLA WAFFLE STICKS

Preparation time: 10 min.

Cooking time: 14 min.

Servings: 2

Ingredients:

- 1/2 tsp. garlic powder
- 1 tsp. Italian seasoning
- 1 egg, beaten
- 1/2 c. grated mozzarella cheese
- 1 tsp. chive-flavored cream cheese
- Tomato sauce dip for serving

Directions:

Preheat the waffle iron.

Next, combine all the ingredients into a medium bowl until well-mixed. Add the batter to the waffle iron, close, and cook for 6–7 min. or until crispy.

Lastly, remove the waffle onto a plate and make a second one. Cut the waffles into bite-size sticks and serve warm with a tomato sauce dip.

Nutrition:

Calories: 119

Net Carb: 1.2 g.

Fat: 5.54 g.

Protein: 13.81 g.

Carbohydrates: 3.01 g.

Dietary Fiber: 0.8 g.

Sugar: 1.01 g.

189.   BACON AND VEGGIES WAFFLES

Preparation time: 15 min.

Cooking time: 24 min.

Servings: 6

Ingredients:

- 2 cooked bacon slices, crumbled
- 1/2 c. frozen chopped spinach, thawed and squeezed
- 1/2 c. cauliflower rice

- 2 organic eggs
- 1/2 c. cheddar cheese, shredded
- 1/2 c. mozzarella cheese, shredded
- 1/4 c. parmesan cheese, grated
- 1 tbsp. butter, melted
- 1 tsp. garlic powder
- 1 tsp. onion powder

Directions:
Preheat a mini waffle iron and then grease it.
In a container, add all the ingredients except the blueberries and beat until well combined.
Fold in the blueberries.
Divide the mixture into 6 portions.
Add 1 portion of the mixture into the preheated waffle iron and cook for about 3–4 min. or until golden brown.
Repeat with the remaining mixture.
Serve warm.

Nutrition:
Calories: 10
Carb: 1.2 g.
Fat: 8.4 g.
Saturated Fat: 4.6 g.
Carbohydrates: 1.5 g.
Dietary Fiber: 0.3 g.
Sugar: 0.6 g.
Protein: 7.1 g.

190. GARLIC AND ONION POWDER WAFFLES

Preparation time: 5 min.
Cooking time: 5 min.
Servings: 2
Ingredients:
- 1 organic egg, beaten
- 1/4 c. Cheddar cheese, shredded
- 2 tbsp. almond flour
- 1/2 tsp. organic baking powder
- 1/4 tsp. garlic powder
- 1/4 tsp. onion powder
- Pinch of salt

Directions:
Preheat a waffle iron and then grease it.
In a container, add all the ingredients and beat until well combined.
Add the mixture into the preheated waffle iron and cook for about 5 min. or until golden brown.
Serve warm.

Nutrition:
Calories: 274
Net Carb: 3.3 g.
Fat: 21.3 g.
Saturated Fat: 7.8 g.
Dietary Fiber: 1.7 g.
Sugar: 1.4 g.
Protein: 12.8 g.

191. SAVORY BAGEL SEASONING WAFFLES

Preparation time: 10 min.
Cooking time: 5 min.
Servings: 4
Ingredients:
- 2 tbsps. everything bagel seasoning
- 2 eggs
- 1 c. mozzarella cheese
- 1/2 c. grated parmesan

Directions:
Preheat the square waffle maker and grease it with cooking spray.
Mix together eggs, mozzarella cheese, and grated cheese in a container.
Pour 1/4 of the batter into the waffle maker.
Sprinkle 1 tbsp. of the everything bagel seasoning over the batter.
Close the lid.
Cook the waffles for about 3–4 min. Utes.
Repeat with the remaining batter.
Serve hot and enjoy!

Nutrition:
Protein: 34% 71
Fat: 60% 125
Carbohydrates: 6% 13

192. DRIED HERBS WAFFLES

Preparation time: 6 min.
Cooking time: 8 min.
Servings: 2
Ingredients:

- 1 organic egg, beaten
- 1/2 c. Cheddar cheese, shredded
- 1 tbsp. almond flour
- Pinch of dried thyme, crushed
- Pinch of dried rosemary, crushed

Directions:

Preheat a mini waffle iron and then grease it.

In a container, add all the ingredients and beat until well combined.

Add half of the mixture into the preheated waffle iron and cook for about 4 min. or until golden brown.

Repeat with the remaining mixture.

Serve warm.

Nutrition:

Calories: 1
Carb: 0.9 g.
Fat: 13.4 g.
Saturated Fat: 6.8 g.
Carbohydrates: 1.3 g.
Dietary Fiber: 0.4 g.
Sugar: 0.4 g.
Protein: 9.8 g.

193. ZUCCHINI AND BASIL WAFFLES

Preparation time: 6 min.
Cooking time: 10 min.
Servings: 2
Ingredients:

- 1 organic egg, beaten
- 1/4 c. Mozzarella cheese, shredded
- 2 tbsp. Parmesan cheese, grated
- 1/2 of zucchini, grated and squeezed
- 1/4 tsp. dried basil, crushed
- Freshly ground black pepper, as required

Directions:

Preheat a mini waffle iron and then grease it.

In a container, add all fixing and mix until well combined.

Add half of the mixture into the preheated waffle iron and cook for about 4–5 min. or until golden brown.

Repeat with the remaining mixture.

Serve warm.

Nutrition:

Net Carb: 1 g.
Fat: 4.1 g.
Saturated Fat: 1.7 g.
Carbohydrates: 1.3 g.
Dietary Fiber: 0.3 g.
Sugar: 0.7 g.
Protein: 6.1 g.

194. HASH BROWN WAFFLE

Preparation time: 6 min.
Cooking time: 10 min.
Servings: 2
Ingredients:

- 1 large jicama root, peeled and shredded
- 1/2 onion, minced
- 2 garlic cloves, pressed
- 1 c. cheddar shredded cheese
- 2 eggs
- Salt and pepper, to taste

Directions:

Add the jicama in a colander, sprinkle with 2 tsp. salt, and let it drain.

Squeeze out all the excess liquid.

Microwave the jicama for 5–8 min.

Mix 3/4 of the cheese and all the other ingredients in a container.

Sprinkle 1–2 tsp. cheese on the waffle maker, add 3 tbsp. of the mixture, and top with 1–2 tsp. cheese.

Cook for 5-minutes, or until done.

Remove and repeat for the remaining batter. Serve while hot with the preferred toppings.

Nutrition:
Carbs: 1 g.
Fat: 6 g.
Protein: 4 g.
Calories: 194

195. GARLIC MAYO VEGAN WAFFLES

Preparation time: 8 min.
Cooking time: 5 min.
Servings: 2
Ingredients:
- 1 tbsp. chia seeds
- 2 1/2 tbsps. water
- 1/4 c. low-carb vegan cheese
- 2 tbsps. coconut flour
- 1 c. low-carb vegan cream cheese, softened
- 1 tsp. garlic powder
- Pinch of salt
- Pinch of pepper
- 2 tbsps. vegan garlic mayo for topping

Directions:
Preheat your square waffle maker.
In a container, mix the chia seeds and water, let it stand for 5 min. Utes.
Add all the ingredients to the chia seeds mixture and mix well.
Pour the vegan waffle batter into a greased waffle maker
Once the waffles are cooked, remove them from the maker.
Top with garlic mayo and pepper.
Enjoy!

Nutrition:
Protein: 32% 42
Fat: 63% 82
Carbohydrates: 5% 6

196. BROCCOLI WAFFLE

Preparation time: 10 min.
Cooking time: 15 min.
Servings: 4
Ingredients:
For the batter:
- 4 eggs
- 2 c. grated mozzarella cheese
- 1 c. steamed broccoli, chopped
- Salt and pepper to taste
- 1 clove garlic, minced
- 1 tsp. chili flakes
- 2 tbsp. almond flour
- 2 tsp. baking powder

Other:
- 2 tbsp. cooking spray to brush the waffle maker
- 1/4 c. mascarpone cheese for serving

Directions:
Preheat the waffle maker.
Add the eggs, grated mozzarella, chopped broccoli, salt, pepper, minced garlic, chili flakes, almond flour, and baking powder to a container. Mix with a fork.
Brush the heated waffle maker with cooking spray and add a few tablespoons of the batter.
Close the lid and cook for about 7 min. depending on your waffle maker.
Serve each waffle with mascarpone cheese.

Nutrition:
Calories 229
Fat 15 g.
Carbs 6 g.
Sugar 1.1 g.
Protein: 13.1 g.
Sodium 194 mg.

197. CELERY AND COTTAGE CHEESE WAFFLE

Preparation time: 9 min.
Cooking time: 15 min.
Servings: 4
Ingredients:
For the batter:

- 4 eggs
- 2 c. grated cheddar cheese
- 1 c. fresh celery, chopped
- Salt and pepper to taste
- 2 tbsp. chopped almonds
- 2 tsp. baking powder

Other:

- 2 tbsp. cooking spray to brush the waffle maker
- 1/4 c. cottage cheese for serving

Directions:
Preheat the waffle maker.
Add the eggs, grated cheddar cheese, chopped celery, salt and pepper, chopped almonds, and baking powder to a container.
Mix with a fork.
Brush the heated waffle maker with cooking spray and add a few tablespoons of the batter.
Close the lid and cook for about 7 min. depending on your waffle maker.
Serve each waffle with cottage cheese on top.

Nutrition:
Calories 385
Fat 31.6 g.
Carbs 4 g.
Sugar 1.5 g.
Protein: 22.2 g.
Sodium 492 mg.

198. LETTUCE WAFFLE SANDWICH

Preparation time: 9 min.
Cooking time: 5 min.
Servings: 2
Ingredients:

- 1 large egg
- 1 tbsp. almond flour
- 1 tbsp. full-fat Greek yogurt
- 1/8 tsp. baking powder
- 1/4 c. shredded Swiss cheese
- 4 lettuce leaves

Directions:
Switch on your mini waffle maker.
Grease it with cooking spray.
Mix together egg, almond flour, yogurt, baking powder, and cheese in the mixing container.
Pour 1/2 c. of the batter into the center of your waffle iron and close the lid.
Cook the waffles for about 2–3 min. Utes until cooked through.
Repeat with the remaining batter
Once cooked, carefully transfer to a plate. Serve the lettuce leaves between 2 waffles.
Enjoy!

Nutrition:
Protein: 22% 40
Fat: 66% 120
Carbohydrates: 12% 22

199. COCOA WAFFLES WITH COCONUT CREAM

Preparation time: 9 min.
Cooking time: 5 min.
Servings: 2
Ingredients:

- 1 egg
- 1/2 c. mozzarella cheese
- 1 tsp. stevia
- 1 tsp. vanilla
- 2 tbsps. almond flour

- 1 tbsp. sugar-free chocolate chips
- 2 tbsps. cocoa powder

For the topping:
- 1 scoop coconut cream
- 1 tbsp. coconut flour

Directions:

Mix together the waffle ingredients in a container and mix well.

Preheat your mini waffle maker. Spray the waffle maker with cooking spray.

Pour 1/2 batter into the mini waffle maker and close the lid.

Cook the waffles for about 2 min. and remove them from the maker.

Make the waffles from the rest of the batter.

Serve with a scoop of coconut cream between two waffles.

Drizzle coconut flour on top.

Enjoy with afternoon coffee!

Nutrition:

Protein: 26% 60

Fat: 65% 152

Carbohydrates: 21

200. SHRIMP AVOCADO WAFFLE SANDWICH

Preparation time: 8 min.
Cooking time: 32 min.
Servings: 2
Ingredients:
- 2 c. shredded mozzarella cheese
- 4 large eggs
- 1/2 tsp. curry powder
- 1/2 tsp. oregano

For the shrimp sandwich filling:
- 1-lb. raw shrimp (peeled and deveined)
- 1 large avocado (diced)
- 4 slices cooked bacon
- 2 tbsp. sour cream
- 1/2 tsp. paprika
- 1 tsp. Cajun seasoning
- 1 tbsp. olive oil
- 1/4 c. onion (finely chopped)
- 1 red bell pepper (diced)

Directions:

Plug the waffle maker to preheat it and spray it with a non-stick cooking spray.

Break the eggs into a mixing container and beat. Add the cheese, oregano, and curry. Mix until the ingredients are well combined.

Pour an appropriate amount of the batter into the waffle maker and spread out the batter to the edges to cover all the holes on the waffle maker. This should make 8 mini waffles.

Cook for 4–5 min. or according to your waffle maker's settings.

After the cooking cycle, use a silicone or plastic utensil to remove the waffle from the waffle maker.

Repeat steps 3–5 until you have cooked all the batter into the waffles.

Heat up the olive oil in a large skillet over to high heat.

Add the shrimp and cook until the shrimp is pink and tender.

Remove the skillet from the heat and use a slotted spoon to transfer the shrimp to a paper towel-lined plate to drain for a few minutes.

Put the shrimp in a mixing container. Add paprika and Cajun seasoning. Toss until the shrimps are all coated with seasoning.

To assemble the sandwich, add one waffle on a flat surface and spread some sour cream over it. Layer some shrimp, onion, avocado, diced pepper, and one slice of bacon over it. Cover with another waffle.

Repeat step 11 until you have assembled all the ingredients into sandwiches.

Serve and enjoy.

Nutrition:

Fat: 32.1 g. 41%

Carbohydrate 10.8 g. 4%

Sugars 2.5 g.
Protein: 44.8 g.

201. BANANA WAFFLE

Preparation time: 8 min.
Cooking time: 16 min.
Servings: 2
Ingredients:

- 1/2 tsp. banana flavoring
- 1/8 tsp. salt
- 2 tbsp. almond flour
- 1/2 shredded mozzarella cheese
- 2 eggs (beaten)
- 1/2 tsp. baking powder
- 1/2 tsp. cinnamon
- 2 tbsp. swerve sweetener

Directions:

Plug the waffle maker to preheat it and spray it with a non-stick spray.

In a mixing container, combine the baking powder, cinnamon, swerve, salt, almond flour, and cheese. Add the egg and banana flavor. Mix until the ingredients are well combined.

Pour 1/4 of the batter into your waffle maker and spread out the batter to cover all the holes on the waffle maker.

Cook for 4–5 min. or according to your waffle maker's settings.

After the cooking cycle, use a silicone or plastic utensil to remove the waffle from the waffle maker.

Repeat steps 3–5 until you have cooked all the batter into the waffles.

Serve warm and enjoy.

Nutrition:

Fat: 12.5 g. 16%
Carbohydrate 11 g. 7%
Sugars 0.7 g.
Protein: 8.8 g

202. CINNAMON ROLL WAFFLE

Preparation time: 10 min.
Cooking time: 9 min.
Servings: 2
Ingredients:

- 1 egg (beaten)
- 1/2 c. shredded mozzarella cheese
- 1 tsp. cinnamon
- 1 tsp. sugar-free maple syrup
- 1/4 tsp. baking powder
- 1 tbsp. almond flour
- 1/2 tsp. vanilla extract

For the topping:

- 2 tsp. granulated swerve
- 1 tbsp. heavy cream
- 4 tbsp. cream cheese

Directions:

Plug the waffle maker to preheat it and spray it with a non-stick spray.

In a container, whisk together the egg, maple syrup, and vanilla extract.

In another mixing container, combine the cinnamon, almond flour, baking powder, and mozzarella cheese.

Pour the egg mixture into the flour mixture and mix until the ingredients are well combined.

Pour an appropriate amount of the batter into the waffle maker and spread out the batter to the edges to cover all the holes on the waffle maker.

Close the waffle maker and bake for about 3 min. or according to your waffle maker's settings.

After the cooking cycle, use a silicone or plastic utensil to remove the waffle from the waffle maker.

Repeat steps 5–7 until you have cooked all the batter into the waffles.

For the topping, combine the cream cheese, swerve, and heavy cream in a microwave-safe dish.

Add the dish into a microwave and microwave on high until the mixture is melted and smooth. Stir every 15 sec.

Top the waffles with the cream mixture and enjoy.

Nutrition:
Fat: 9.9 g. 13%

Carbohydrate 3.8 g. 1%

Sugars 0.3 g.

Protein: 4.8 g.

203. GARLIC CAULIFLOWER WAFFLE

Preparation time: 10 min.

Cooking time: 8 min.

Servings: 2

Ingredients:

- 1 egg, beaten
- 1 c. cauliflower rice
- 1/2 c. cheddar cheese, shredded
- 1 tsp. garlic powder

Directions:
Plug in your waffle maker.

Mix all the ingredients in a container.

Transfer half of the mixture to the waffle maker.

Close the device and cook for 4–5 min.

Put the waffle on a plate to cool for 2 min.

Repeat the procedure to make the next waffle.

Nutrition:
Calories 1

Total Fat: 12.5 g.

Saturated Fat: 7 g.

Cholesterol 112 mg.

Sodium 267 mg.

Total Carbohydrate 4.9 g.

Dietary Fiber 0.1 g.

Total Sugars 2.7 g.

Protein: 12 g.

Potassium 73 mg.

204. CHEESE GARLIC WAFFLE

Preparation time: 10 min.

Cooking time: 8 min.

Servings: 2

Ingredients:

For the waffle:

- 1 egg
- 1 tsp. cream cheese
- 1/2 c. mozzarella cheese, shredded
- 1/2 tsp. garlic powder
- 1 tsp. Italian seasoning

For the topping:

- 1 tbsp. butter
- 1/2 tsp. garlic powder
- 1/2 tsp. Italian seasoning
- 2 tbsp. mozzarella cheese, shredded

Directions:
Plug in your waffle maker to preheat.

Preheat your oven to 350 °F.

In a container, combine all the waffle ingredients.

Cook in the waffle maker for 4–5 min. per waffle.

Transfer to a baking pan.

Spread butter on top of each waffle.

Sprinkle garlic powder and Italian seasoning on top.

Top with mozzarella cheese.

Bake until the cheese has melted.

Nutrition:
Calories: 141

Total Fat: 13 g.

Saturated Fat: 8 g.

Cholesterol 115.8 mg.

Sodium 255.8 mg.

Potassium 350 mg.

Total Carbohydrate 2.6 g.

Dietary Fiber 0.7 g.

205. CINNAMON CREAM CHEESE WAFFLE

Preparation time: 10 min.
Cooking time: 15 min.
Servings: 2
Ingredients:

- 2 eggs, lightly beaten
- 1 tsp. collagen
- 1/4 tsp. baking powder, gluten-free
- 1 tsp. monk fruit sweetener
- 1/2 tsp. cinnamon
- 1/4 c. cream cheese, softened
- Pinch of salt

Directions:

Preheat your waffle maker.

Add all the ingredients into the container and beat using a hand mixer until well combined.

Spray the waffle maker with cooking spray.

Pour 1/2 batter into the hot waffle maker and cook for 3 min. or until golden brown. Repeat with the remaining batter.

Serve and enjoy.

Nutrition:

Calories 179
Fat: 14.5 g.
Carbohydrates 1.9 g.
Sugar 0.4 g.
Protein 10.8 g.
Cholesterol 19 mg.

206. APPLE CINNAMON WAFFLES

Preparation time: 6 min.
Cooking time: 20 min.
Servings: 2
Ingredients:

- 3 eggs, lightly beaten
- 1 c. mozzarella cheese, shredded
- 1/4 c. apple, chopped
- 1/2 tsp. monk fruit sweetener
- 1 1/2 tsp. cinnamon
- 1/4 tsp. baking powder, gluten-free
- 2 tbsp. coconut flour

Directions:

Preheat your waffle maker.

Add remaining ingredients and stir until well combined.

Spray the waffle maker with cooking spray.

Pour 1/3 of the batter into the hot waffle maker and cook for 4–5 min. or until golden brown. Repeat with the remaining batter.

Serve and enjoy.

Nutrition:

Calories 142
Fat: 7.4 g.
Carbohydrates 9.7 g.
Sugar 3 g.
Protein 9 g.
Cholesterol 169 mg.

207. BLUEBERRY WAFFLES

Preparation time: 8 min.
Cooking time: 15 min.
Servings: 2
Ingredients:

- 2 eggs
- 1/2 c. blueberries
- 1/2 tsp. baking powder
- 1/2 tsp. vanilla
- 2 tsp. Swerve
- 3 tbsp. almond flour
- 1 c. mozzarella cheese, shredded

Directions:

Preheat your waffle maker.

In a container, mix eggs, baking powder vanilla, Swerve, almond flour, and cheese.

Add blueberries and stir well. ,

Spray the waffle maker with cooking spray.

Pour 1/4 batter into the hot waffle maker and cook for 8 min. or until golden brown. Repeat with the remaining batter.

Serve and enjoy.

Nutrition:
Calories 96
Fat: 6.1 g.
Carbohydrates 5 g.
Sugar 2.2 g.
Protein 6.1 g.
Cholesterol 86 mg.

208. PUMPKIN CHEESECAKE WAFFLE

Preparation time: 10 min.
Cooking time: 15 min.
Servings: 2
Ingredients:
For the waffle:
- 1 egg
- 1/2 tsp. vanilla
- 1/2 tsp. baking powder, gluten-free
- 1/4 tsp. pumpkin spice
- 1 tsp. cream cheese, softened
- 2 tsp. heavy cream
- 1 tbsp. Swerve
- 1 tbsp. almond flour
- 2 tsp. pumpkin puree
- 1/2 c. mozzarella cheese, shredded

For the filling:
- 1/4 tsp. vanilla
- 1 tbsp. Swerve
- 2 tbsp. cream cheese

Directions:
Preheat your mini waffle maker.
In a container, mix all the waffle ingredients.
Spray the waffle maker with cooking spray.
Pour half batter into the hot waffle maker and cook for 3–5 min. Repeat with the remaining batter.
In a container, combine all the filling ingredients.
Spread the filling mixture between two waffles and put in the fridge for 10 min.
Serve and enjoy.

Nutrition:
Calories 107
Fat: 7.2 g.
Carbohydrates 5 g.
Sugar 0.7 g.
Protein 6.7 g.
Cholesterol 93 mg.

209. OKRA FRITTER WAFFLE

Preparation time: 10 min.
Cooking time: 10 min.
Servings: 2
Ingredients:
- 1 egg:
- 1/4 c. mozzarella cheese
- 1/2 tbsp. onion powder
- 2 tbsp. heavy cream
- 1 tbsp. mayo
- 2 garlic cloves (finely chopped)
- 1/4 c. almond flour
- 1 c. okra
- 1/4 tsp. salt, or as per your taste
- 1/4 tsp. black pepper, or as per your taste

Directions:
Combine egg, mayo, and heavy cream and whisk
When mixed, add almond flour and make a uniform batter
Leave it for 5–10 min.
Now add okra and the rest of the ingredients and mix well
Preheat a mini waffle maker if needed and grease it
Pour the mixture into the lower plate of the waffle maker and spread it evenly to cover the plate properly
Close the lid
Cook for at least 4 min. to get the desired crunch
Remove the waffle from the heat

Make as many waffles as your mixture and waffle maker allow

Serve hot and enjoy!

Nutrition:
Calories: 192
Fat: 13.05 g.
Carbohydrates 8.73 g.
Sugar: 2.45 g.
Protein: 10.8 g.
Cholesterol: 335 mg.

210.   SPINACH ZUCCHINI WAFFLE

Preparation time: 10 min.
Cooking time: 5 min.
Servings: 2
Ingredients:

- 1 zucchini (small)
- 1 egg
- 1/2 c. shredded mozzarella
- 1 tbsp. parmesan
- Pepper, as per your taste
- 1 tsp. basil
- 1/2 c. spinach

Directions:
Preheat your waffle iron
Grate the zucchini finely
Boil spinach for 5 min. and strain water
Add all the ingredients to zucchini in a bowl and mix well
Now add the spinach
Grease your waffle iron lightly
Pour the mixture into a full-size waffle maker and spread evenly
Cook till it turns crispy
Make as many waffles as your mixture and waffle maker allow
Serve crispy and with your favorite keto sauce

Nutrition:
Calories: 120
Fat: 5.85 g.

Carbohydrates 9.3 g.
Sugar: 4.44 g.
Protein: 7.81 g.
Cholesterol: 313 mg.

211.   OKRA CAULI WAFFLE

Preparation time: 10 min.
Cooking time: 15 min.
Servings: 2
Ingredients:

- 1/2 c. cauliflower
- 1/2 c. okra
- 2 egg
- 1 c. mozzarella cheese (shredded)
- 1 tbsp. butter
- 2 tbsp. almond flour
- 1/4 tsp. turmeric
- 1/4 tsp. baking powder
- A pinch of onion powder
- A pinch of garlic powder
- A pinch of salt

Directions:
In a deep saucepan, boil okra and cauliflower for 5 min. or till it tenders, strain, and set aside
Mix all the remaining ingredients well together
Pour a thin layer on a preheated waffle iron
Remove any excess water from the vegetables and add a layer to the mixture
Add more mixture over the top
Cook the waffle for around 5 min.
Serve hot with your favorite keto sauce

Nutrition:
Calories: 269
Fat: 14.23 g.
Carbohydrates: 7.02 g.
Sugar: 2.43 g.
Protein: 28.4 g.
Cholesterol: 636 mg.

212. CRISPY CAULI WAFFLE

Preparation time: 5 min.
Cooking time: 5 min.
Servings: 2
Ingredients:

- 1 c. cauliflower rice
- 1 egg
- 1/2 c. parmesan cheese (shredded)
- 1/2 c. mozzarella cheese (shredded)
- 1/4 tsp. salt, or as per your taste
- 1/4 tsp. black pepper, or as per your taste
- 1/2 tsp. Italian seasoning:
- 1/2 tsp. garlic powder

Directions:
Preheat a mini waffle maker if needed and grease it
Add all the ingredients, except for the parmesan cheese, into a blender
Mix them all well
Spread 1/8 c. shredded parmesan cheese to the lower plate of the waffle maker
Pour the cauliflower mixture above the cheese
Sprinkle 1/8 c. shredded parmesan cheese on top of the mixture
Close the lid
Cook for at least 5 min. to get the desired crunch
Remove the waffle from the heat
Serve hot and enjoy!

Nutrition:
Calories: 230
Fat: 14.23 g.
Carbohydrates 7.02 g.
Sugar: 2.17 g.
Protein: 21.85 g.
Cholesterol: 336 mg.

213. JICAMA LOADED WAFFLE

Preparation time: 5 min.
Cooking time: 5 min.
Servings: 2
Ingredients:

- 2 egg
- 1 c. cheddar cheese
- 1/2 medium onion minced
- 1 large jicama root
- 2 garlic cloves
- 1/4 tsp. salt, or as per your taste
- 1/4 tsp. black pepper, or as per your taste

Directions:
With a peeler or knife, peel the jicama and blend it in a food processor
Put this in a large colander with a pinch of salt and let it drain
Make it dry as much as possible
Microwave it for around 7 min.
Now add the remaining ingredients to the blended jicama and mix well
Preheat a mini waffle maker if needed and grease it
Pour the mixture into the lower plate of the waffle maker and spread it evenly to cover the plate properly
Close the lid
Cook for at least 4 min. to get the desired crunch
Remove the waffle from the heat
Make as many waffles as your mixture and waffle maker allow
Serve hot and enjoy!

Nutrition:
Calories: 416
Fat: 13.26 g.
Carbohydrates 58.03 g.
Sugar: 12.94 g.
Protein: 17.09 g.
Cholesterol: 630 mg.

214. SPINACH GARLIC BUTTER WAFFLE

Preparation time: 15 min.
Cooking time: 5 min.
Servings: 2
Ingredients:
For the waffle:

- 2 egg
- 1 c. mozzarella cheese (shredded)
- 1/2 tsp. garlic powder
- 1 tsp. Italian seasoning
- 1 tsp. cream cheese
- 1/2 c. spinach

For the garlic butter topping::

- 1/2 tsp. garlic powder
- 1/2 tsp. Italian seasoning
- 1 tbsp. butter

Directions:

In a small saucepan, add 1/4 c. water with spinach and simmer for 5 min.

Drain the excess water from the spinach and set it aside

Preheat a mini waffle maker if needed and grease it

In a mixing bowl, add all the ingredients of the waffle along with the prepared spinach and mix well

Pour the mixture to the lower plate of the waffle maker and spread it evenly to cover the plate properly and close the lid

Cook for at least 4 min. to get the desired crunch

In the meanwhile, melt the butter and add the garlic butter ingredients

Remove the waffle from the heat and apply the garlic butter immediately

Make as many waffles as your mixture and waffle maker allow

Nutrition:

Calories: 266
Fat: 14.25 g.
Carbohydrates 5.76 g.
Sugar: 1.88 g.
Protein: 27.86 g.
Cholesterol: 639 mg.

215. ALL GREEN WAFFLE

Preparation time: 10 min.
Cooking time: 5 min.
Servings: 4
Ingredients:
For the waffle:

- 1/2 c. cabbage
- 1/2 c. broccoli
- 1/2 c. zucchini
- 2 egg
- 1 c. mozzarella cheese (shredded)
- 1 tbsp. butter
- 2 tbsp. almond flour
- 1/4 tsp. baking powder
- A pinch of onion powder
- A pinch of garlic powder
- A pinch of salt

For the filling:

- 1/2 c. cucumber diced
- 4 lettuce leave

Directions:

In a deep saucepan, boil cabbage, broccoli, and zucchini for 5 min. or till it tenders, strain and blend

Mix all the remaining ingredients well together

Pour a thin layer on a preheated waffle iron

Add a layer of the blended vegetables to the mixture

Add more mixture over the top

Cook the waffle for around 5 min.

Remove from the heat, fold, and add lettuce and cucumber

Serve with your favorite sauce

Nutrition:

Calories: 153

Fat: 8.64 g.
Carbohydrates 3.1 g.
Sugar: 1.42 g.
Protein: 15.72 g.
Cholesterol: 324 mg.

216. BROCCOLI CAULI CABBAGE WAFFLE

Preparation time: 10 min.
Cooking time: 5 min.
Servings: 4
Ingredients:

- 1/2 c. cauliflower
- 1/2 c. cabbage
- 1/2 c. broccoli
- 2 egg
- 1 c. mozzarella cheese (shredded)
- 1 tbsp. butter
- 2 tbsp. almond flour
- 1/4 tsp. turmeric
- 1/4 tsp. baking powder
- A pinch of onion powder
- A pinch of garlic powder
- A pinch of salt

Directions:
In a deep saucepan, boil cabbage, broccoli, and cauliflower for 5 min. or till it tenders, strain, and set aside
Mix all the remaining ingredients well together
Pour a thin layer on a preheated waffle iron
Remove any excess water from the vegetables and add a layer to the mixture
Add more mixture over the top
Cook the waffle for around 5 min.
Serve hot with your favorite keto sauce

Nutrition:
Calories: 135
Fat: 7.14 g.
Carbohydrates 3.54 g.
Sugar: 1.48 g.

Protein: 14.28 g.
Cholesterol: 318 mg.

217. PEPPERMINT MOCHA WAFFLE

Preparation time: 10 min.
Cooking time: 10 min.
Servings: 2
Ingredients:
For the waffle:

- 1 egg
- 2 tbsp. powdered sweetener
- 2 tbsp. cream cheese
- 2 tbsp. butter (melted)
- 2 tsp. coconut flour
- 1 tsp. almond flour
- 1/4 tsp. baking powder
- 1/4 tsp. vanilla extract
- 1 tbsp. cocoa powder (unsweetened)
- A pinch of salt

For the filling:

- 1/2 c. heavy cream
- 2 tbsp. powdered sweetener
- 2 tbsp. butter
- 1/4 tsp. vanilla extract
- 1/8 tsp. peppermint extract
- Starlight mints, for garnishing

Directions:
Preheat a mini waffle maker if needed and grease it
In a mixing bowl, add all the waffle ingredients
Mix them all well
Pour the mixture to the lower plate of the waffle maker and spread it evenly to cover the plate properly and close the lid
Cook for at least 4 min. to get the desired crunch
Remove the waffle from the heat and keep aside for around 1 min.

Make as many waffles as your mixture and waffle maker allow

For the filling, add all the filling ingredients and beat at high speed using the hand blender

On each waffle spread the filling and top with starlight mint

Nutrition:
Calories: 454
Fat: 36.43 g.
Carbohydrates 24.91 g.
Sugar: 20.74 g.
Protein: 7.77 g.
Cholesterol: 394 mg.

218. EASY BROCCOLI WAFFLE

Preparation time: 5 min.
Cooking time: 5 min.
Servings: 2
Ingredients:

- 1 c. broccoli
- 2 egg
- 1 c. mozzarella cheese (shredded)
- 1 tbsp. butter
- 2 tbsp. almond flour
- 1/4 tsp. turmeric
- 1/4 tsp. baking powder
- A pinch of onion powder
- A pinch of garlic powder
- A pinch of salt

Directions:
In a deep saucepan, boil broccoli for 5 min. or till it tenders, strain, and set aside
Mix all the remaining ingredients well together
Pour a thin layer on a preheated waffle iron
Remove any excess water from the broccoli and add 1 tbsp. broccoli to the mixture
Add more mixture over the top
Cook the waffle for around 5 min.

Serve hot with your favorite keto sauce
Nutrition:
Calories: 258
Fat: 14.21 g.
Carbohydrates 4.39 g.
Sugar: 1.63 g.
Protein: 28.04 g.
Cholesterol: 636 mg

219. SPINACH AND CABBAGE WAFFLE

Preparation time: 10 min.
Cooking time: 5 min.
Servings: 2
Ingredients:
For the waffle:

- 2 egg
- 1 c. mozzarella cheese (shredded)
- 1 tbsp. butter
- 2 tbsp. almond flour
- 1/4 tsp. turmeric
- 1/4 tsp. baking powder
- A pinch of onion powder
- A pinch of garlic powder
- A pinch of salt
- 1/4 tsp. black pepper, or as per your taste
- 1/2 c. spinach
- 1/2 c. cabbage

Directions:
Boil the spinach and cabbage in water for around 10 min. and drain the remaining water
In a mixing bowl, add all the above-mentioned ingredients
Mix well and add the boiled spinach and cabbage

Pour the mixture into the lower plate of the waffle maker and spread it evenly to cover the plate properly

Cook for at least 4 min. to get the desired crunch

Remove the waffle from the heat

Make as many waffles as your mixture and waffle maker allow

Serve hot and enjoy!

Nutrition:
Calories: 265
Fat: 14.19 g.
Carbohydrates 6.27 g.
Sugar: 2.72 g.
Protein: 28.05 g.
Cholesterol: 636 mg.

220. GARLIC BROCCOLI WAFFLE

Preparation time: 15 min.
Cooking time: 5 min.
Servings: 2
Ingredients:
For the waffle:

- 2 egg
- 1 c. mozzarella cheese (shredded)
- 1/2 tsp. garlic powder
- 1 tsp. Italian seasoning
- 1 tsp. cream cheese

For the garlic butter topping::
1/2 tsp. garlic powder
1/2 tsp. Italian seasoning
1 tbsp. butter

For the broccoli:
1/2 c. broccoli
1/4 tsp. salt, or as per your taste
1/4 tsp. black pepper, or as per your taste

Directions:
In a small saucepan, add broccoli and water and boil for 10 min.

When it tenders, remove it from water and blend with a hand mixer and add salt and pepper

Preheat a mini waffle maker if needed and grease it

In a mixing bowl, add all the ingredients of the waffle and mix well

Pour the thin layer of the mixture into the lower plate of the waffle maker and spread it evenly to cover the plate properly

Add 1/2 tbsp. the broccoli paste over the mixture

Add a thin layer of the waffle mixture again on the broccoli paste

Cook for at least 4 min. to get the desired crunch

In the meanwhile, melt the butter and add the garlic butter ingredients

Remove the waffle from the heat and apply the garlic butter immediately and serve hot

Nutrition:
Calories: 269
Fat: 14.28 g.
Carbohydrates 6.31 g.
Sugar: 2.17 g.
Protein: 28.08 g.
Cholesterol: 639 mg.

221. JALAPENO ZUCCHINI WAFFLE

Preparation time: 10 min.
Cooking time: 5 min.
Servings: 2
Ingredients:

- 1 small zucchini
- 1/8 tsp. onion powder
- 1/8 tsp. garlic powder
- 1 egg
- 1/4 c. cheddar cheese
- 1 jalapeno, diced
- 1 cream cheese, tbsp.
- 1/8 tbsp. parmesan cheese

Directions:
Preheat a mini waffle maker if needed and grease it
In a mixing bowl, beat the eggs and add all the ingredients
Mix them all well
Pour the mixture into the lower plate of the waffle maker and spread it evenly to cover the plate properly
Close the lid
Cook for at least 4 min. to get the desired crunch
Remove the waffle from the heat and keep aside for around 1 min.
Make as many waffles as your mixture and waffle maker allow
Serve hot and enjoy!
Nutrition:
Calories: 91
Fat: 7.09 g.
Carbohydrates: 1.25 g.
Sugar: 0.6 g.
Protein: 5.31 g.
Cholesterol: 316 mg.

222. CRISPY BROCCOLI AND ARTICHOKE WAFFLE

Preparation time: 10 min.
Cooking time: 10 min.
Servings: 2
Ingredients:
- 1/2 c. artichokes, chopped
- 1/2 c. broccoli, chopped and boiled
- 1 egg
- 1/2 c. mozzarella cheese (shredded)
- 1 oz. cream cheese
- Salt, as per your taste
- Pepper, as per your taste
- 1/4 tsp. garlic powder

Directions:
Preheat a mini waffle maker if needed and grease it

In a mixing bowl, add all the ingredients
Mix them all well
Pour the mixture into the lower plate of the waffle maker and spread it evenly to cover the plate properly
Close the lid
Cook for at least 4 min. to get the desired crunch
Remove the waffle from the heat and keep aside for around 1 min.
Make as many waffles as your mixture and waffle maker allow
Serve hot with your favorite keto sauce
Nutrition:
Calories: 180
Fat: 9.27 g.
Carbohydrates 8.98 g.
Sugar: 2.86 g.
Protein: 16.66 g.
Cholesterol: 328 mg.

223. OLIVE AND SPINACH WAFFLES

Preparation time: 10 min.
Cooking time: 15 min.
Servings: 2
Ingredients:
For the waffle:
- 2 egg
- 1 c. mozzarella cheese (shredded)
- 1 tbsp. butter
- 2 tbsp. almond flour
- 1/4 tsp. turmeric
- 1/4 tsp. baking powder
- A pinch of onion powder
- A pinch of garlic powder
- A pinch of salt
- 1/4 tsp. black pepper, or as per your taste
- 1/2 c. spinach
- 5–10 olives

Directions:

Boil the spinach in water for around 10 min. and drain the remaining water

In a mixing bowl, add all the above-mentioned ingredients except for olives

Mix well and add the boiled spinach

Pour the mixture into the lower plate of the waffle maker and spread it evenly to cover the plate properly

Sprinkle the sliced olives as per choice over the mixture and close the lid

Cook for at least 4 min. to get the desired crunch

Remove the waffle from the heat

Make as many waffles as your mixture and waffle maker allow

Serve hot and enjoy!

Nutrition:

Calories: 272

Fat: 15.71 g.

Carbohydrates 5.02 g.

Sugar: 1.93 g.

Protein: 27.83 g.

Cholesterol: 636 mg.

224. SIMPLE CABBAGE WAFFLES

Preparation time: 10 min.

Cooking time: 15 min.

Servings: 2

Ingredients:

- 2 egg
- 1 c. mozzarella cheese, (shredded)
- 2 tbsp. butter
- 2 tbsp. almond flour
- 1/4 tsp. turmeric
- 1/4 tsp. baking powder
- A pinch of onion powder
- A pinch of garlic powder
- Salt, as per your taste
- 1 c. cabbage, shredded

Directions:

Take a frying pan and melt 1 tbsp. butter

Add the shredded cabbage and sauté for 4 min. and set aside

In a mixing bowl, add all the ingredients and mix well

Pour a thin layer on a preheated waffle iron

Add the cabbage on top of the mixture

Add more mixture over the top

Cook the waffle for around 5 min.

Serve hot with your favorite keto sauce

Nutrition:

Calories: 303

Fat: 18.04 g.

Carbohydrates 7.1 g.

Sugar: 3.26 g.

Protein: 28.27 g.

Cholesterol: 644 mg.

225. CABBAGE AND ARTICHOKE WAFFLE

Preparation time: 10 min.

Cooking time: 20 min.

Servings: 2

Ingredients:

- 1/2 c. artichokes, chopped
- 1/2 c. cabbage
- 1/2 tbsp. black pepper
- 1 egg
- 1/2 c. mozzarella cheese (shredded)
- 1 oz. cream cheese
- Salt, as per your taste
- 1/4 tsp. garlic powder
- 1/4 tsp. turmeric
- 1/4 tsp. baking powder

Directions:

Take a frying pan and melt 1 tbsp. butter

Add the shredded cabbage and sauté for 4 min. and set aside

In a mixing bowl, add all the ingredients and mix well

Pour a thin layer on a preheated waffle iron
Add cabbage on top of the mixture
Add more mixture over the top
Cook the waffle for around 5 min.
Serve hot with your favorite keto sauce
Nutrition:
Calories: 182
Fat: 9.28 g.
Carbohydrates 9.9 g.
Sugar: 2.56 g.
Protein: 16.43 g.
Cholesterol: 328 mg.

226. ZUCCHINI BBQ WAFFLE

Preparation time: 10 min.
Cooking time: 20 min.
Servings: 2
Ingredients:
- 1/2 c. zucchini
- 1 tbsp. BBQ sauce (sugar-free)
- 2 tbsp. almond flour
- 1 egg
- 1/2 c. cheddar cheese

Directions:
Finely grate the zucchini
Preheat your waffle iron
In the mixing bowl, add all the waffle ingredients including the zucchini, and mix well
Grease your waffle iron lightly
Pour the mixture to the bottom plate evenly; also spread it out to get better results and close the upper plate and heat
Cook for 6 min. or until the waffle is done
Make as many waffles as your mixture and waffle maker allow
Nutrition:
Calories: 75
Fat: 5.44 g.
Carbohydrates 1.46 g.
Sugar: 0.73 g.

Protein: 4.95 g.
Cholesterol: 309 mg.

227. EGGPLANT BBQ WAFFLE

Preparation time: 10 min.
Cooking time: 20 min.
Servings: 2
Ingredients:
- 1/2 c. eggplant
- 1 tbsp. BBQ sauce (sugar-free)
- 2 tbsp. almond flour
- 1 egg
- 1/2 c. cheddar cheese

Directions:
Boil the eggplant in water, and strain
Preheat your waffle iron
In the mixing bowl, add all the waffle ingredients including the zucchini, and mix well
Grease your waffle iron lightly
Pour the mixture to the bottom plate evenly; also spread it out to get better results and close the upper plate and heat
Cook for 6 min. or until the waffle is done
Make as many waffles as your mixture and waffle maker allow
Nutrition:
Calories: 79
Fat: 5.47 g.
Carbohydrates 2.58 g.
Sugar: 1.46 g.
Protein: 5.08 g.
Cholesterol: 309 mg.

228. SLICED EGGPLANT WAFFLES

Preparation time: 15 min.
Cooking time: 20 min.
Servings: 2
Ingredients:
For the waffles:
- 2 eggs

- 1/2 c. cheddar cheese
- 2 tbsp. parmesan cheese
- 1/4 tsp. Italian season

For the eggplant:
- 1 big eggplant
- 1 pinch of salt
- 1 pinch of black pepper

Directions:
Cut the eggplant in slices and boil in water and strain

Add a pinch of salt and pepper

Add all the waffle ingredients into a bowl and mix well to make a mixture

Preheat a mini waffle maker if needed and grease it

Pour the mixture into the lower plate of the waffle maker and spread it evenly to cover the plate properly

Add the eggplant over two slices on the mixture and cover the lid

Cook for at least 4 min. to get the desired crunch

Remove the waffle from the heat and keep aside for around 1 min.

Make as many waffles as your mixture and waffle maker allow

Serve hot with your favorite sauce

Nutrition:
Calories: 285
Fat: 16.34 g.
Carbohydrates 18.53 g.
Sugar: 10.69 g.
Protein: 17.57 g.
Cholesterol: 933 mg.

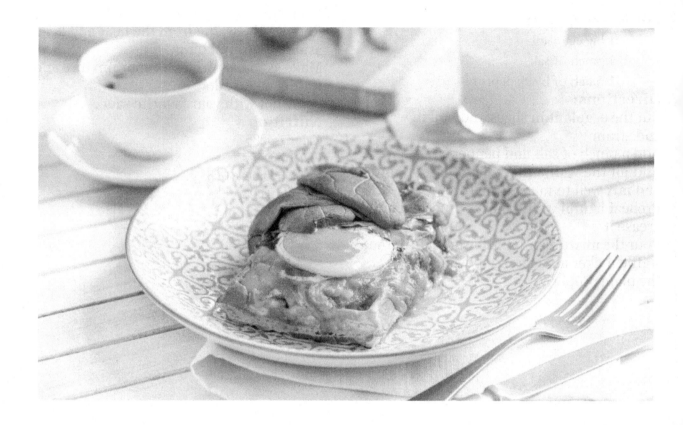

229. BBQ SAUCE PORK WAFFLE

Preparation time: 10 min.
Cooking time: 15 min.
Servings: 2
Ingredients:

- 1/2 lb. ground pork
- 3 eggs
- 1 c. grated mozzarella cheese
- Salt and pepper to taste
- 1 clove garlic, minced
- 1 tsp. dried rosemary
- 3 tbsp. sugar-free BBQ sauce

Other:

2 tbsp. butter to brush the waffle maker
1/2 lb. pork rinds for serving
1/4 c. sugar-free BBQ sauce for serving

Directions:

Preheat the waffle maker.

Add the ground pork, eggs, mozzarella, salt and pepper, minced garlic, dried rosemary, and BBQ sauce to a bowl.

Mix until combined.

Brush the heated waffle maker with butter and add a few tablespoons of the batter.

Close the lid and cook for about 7–8 min. depending on your waffle maker.

Serve each waffle with some pork rinds and a tablespoon of BBQ sauce.

Nutrition:

Calories 350
Fat 21.1 g.
Carbs 2 g.
Sugar 0.3 g.
Protein: 36.9 g.
Sodium 801 mg.

230. BEEF AND TOMATO WAFFLE

Preparation time: 10 min.
Cooking time: 15 min.
Servings: 2
Ingredients:
For the batter:

- 4 eggs
- 1/4 c. cream cheese
- 1 c. grated mozzarella cheese
- Salt and pepper to taste
- 1/4 c. almond flour
- 1 tsp. freshly chopped dill

For the beef:

- 1-lb. beef loin
- Salt and pepper to taste
- 1 tbsp. balsamic vinegar
- 2 tbsp. olive oil
- 1 tsp. freshly chopped rosemary

Other:

- 2 tbsp. cooking spray to brush the waffle maker
- 4 tomato slices for serving

Directions:

Preheat the waffle maker.

Add the eggs, cream cheese, grated mozzarella cheese, salt and pepper, almond flour, and freshly chopped dill to a bowl.

Mix until combined and the batter forms.

Brush the heated waffle maker with cooking spray and add a few tablespoons of the batter.

Close the lid and cook for about 8–10 min. depending on your waffle maker.

Meanwhile, heat the olive oil in a nonstick frying pan and season the beef loin with salt and pepper and freshly chopped rosemary.

Cook the beef on each side for about 5 min. and drizzle with some balsamic vinegar.

Serve each waffle with a slice of tomato and cooked beef loin slices.

Nutrition:
Calories 4
Fat 35.8 g.
Carbs 3.3 g.
Sugar 0.8 g.
Protein: 40.3 g.
Sodium 200 mg.

231. BEEF WAFFLE SANDWICH

Preparation time: 10 min.
Cooking time: 15 min.
Servings: 2
Ingredients:
For the batter:

- 3 eggs
- 2 c. grated mozzarella cheese
- 1/4 c. cream cheese
- Salt and pepper to taste
- 1 tsp. Italian seasoning

For the beef:

- 2 tbsp. butter
- 1-lb. beef tenderloin
- Salt and pepper to taste
- 2 tsp. Dijon mustard
- 1 tsp. dried paprika

Other:

- 2 tbsp. cooking spray to brush the waffle maker
- 4 lettuce leaves for serving
- 4 tomato slices for serving
- 4 leaves fresh basil

Directions:
Preheat the waffle maker.
Add the eggs, grated mozzarella, cream cheese, salt and pepper, and Italian seasoning to a bowl. Mix until combined and batter forms.
Brush the heated waffle maker with cooking spray and add a few tablespoons of the batter.
Close the lid and cook for about 7 min. depending on your waffle maker.

Meanwhile, melt and heat the butter in a nonstick frying pan.
Season the beef loin with salt and pepper, brush it with Dijon mustard, and sprinkle some dried paprika on top.
Cook the beef on each side for about 5 min.
Thinly slice the beef and assemble the waffle sandwiches.
Cut each waffle in half and on one-half place a lettuce leaf, tomato slice, basil leaf, and some sliced beef.
Cover with the other waffle half and serve.

Nutrition:
Calories 477
Fat 32.8 g.
Carbs 2.3 g.
Sugar 0.9 g.
Protein: 42.2 g.
Sodium 299 mg.

232. BEEF WAFFLE TACO

Preparation time: 10 min.
Cooking time: 15 min.
Servings: 2
Ingredients:
For the batter:

- 4 eggs
- 2 c. grated cheddar cheese
- 1/4 c. heavy cream
- Salt and pepper to taste
- 1/4 c. almond flour
- 2 tsp. baking powder

For the beef:

- 2 tbsp. butter
- 1/2 onion, diced
- 1-lb. ground beef
- Salt and pepper to taste
- 1 tsp. dried oregano
- 1 tbsp. sugar-free ketchup

Other:
- 2 tbsp. cooking spray to brush the waffle maker
- 2 tbsp. freshly chopped parsley

Directions:
Preheat the waffle maker.

Add the eggs, grated cheddar cheese, heavy cream, salt and pepper, almond flour, and baking powder to a bowl.

Brush the heated waffle maker with cooking spray and add a few tablespoons of the batter.

Close the lid and cook for about 5–7 min. depending on your waffle maker.

Once the waffle is ready, place it in a napkin holder to harden into the shape of a taco as it cools.

Meanwhile, melt and heat the butter in a nonstick frying pan and start cooking the diced onion.

Once the onion is tender, add the ground beef. Season with salt and pepper and dried oregano and stir in the sugar-free ketchup.

Cook for about 7 min.

Serve the cooked ground meat in each taco waffle sprinkled with some freshly chopped parsley.

Nutrition:
Calories 719
Fat 51.7 g.
Carbs 7.3 g.
Sugar 1.3 g.
Protein: 56.1 g.
Sodium 573 mg.

233. BEEF WAFFLE TOWER

Preparation time: 10 min.
Cooking time: 15 min.
Servings: 2
Ingredients:
For the batter:
- 4 eggs
- 2 c. grated mozzarella cheese
- Salt and pepper to taste
- 2 tbsp. almond flour
- 1 tsp. Italian seasoning

For the beef:
- 2 tbsp. butter
- 1-lb. beef tenderloin
- Salt and pepper to taste
- 1 tsp. chili flakes

Other:
- 2 tbsp. cooking spray to brush the waffle maker

Directions:
Preheat the waffle maker.

Add the eggs, grated mozzarella cheese, salt and pepper, almond flour, and Italian seasoning to a bowl.

Mix until everything is fully combined.

Brush the heated waffle maker with cooking spray and add a few tablespoons of the batter.

Close the lid and cook for about 7 min. depending on your waffle maker.

Meanwhile, heat the butter in a nonstick frying pan and season the beef tenderloin with salt and pepper and chili flakes.

Cook the beef tenderloin for about 5 minutes on each side.

When serving, assemble the waffle tower by placing one waffle on a plate, a layer of diced beef tenderloin, another waffle, another layer of beef, and so on until you finish with the waffles and beef.

Serve and enjoy.

Nutrition:
Calories 412
Fat 25 g.
Carbs 1.8 g.
Sugar 0.5 g.
Protein: 43.2 g.
Sodium 256 mg.

234.   BEEF MEATBALLS ON A WAFFLE

Preparation time: 10 min.
Cooking time: 20 min.
Servings: 2
Ingredients:
For the batter:

- 4 eggs
- 2 1/2 c. grated gouda cheese
- 1/4 c. heavy cream
- Salt and pepper to taste
- 1 spring onion, finely chopped

For the beef meatballs:

- 1-lb. ground beef
- Salt and pepper to taste
- 2 tsp. Dijon mustard
- 1 spring onion, finely chopped
- 5 tbsp. almond flour
- 2 tbsp. butter

Other:

- 2 tbsp. cooking spray to brush the waffle maker
- 2 tbsp. freshly chopped parsley

Directions:
Preheat the waffle maker.
Add the eggs, grated Gouda cheese, heavy cream, salt and pepper, and finely chopped spring onion to a bowl.
Mix until combined and batter forms.
Brush the heated waffle maker with cooking spray and add a few tablespoons of the batter.
Close the lid and cook for about 7 min. depending on your waffle maker.
Meanwhile, mix the ground beef meat, salt and pepper, Dijon mustard, chopped spring onion, and almond flour in a large bowl.
Form small meatballs with your hands.
Heat the butter in a nonstick frying pan and cook the beef meatballs for about 3–4 min. on each side.

Serve each waffle with a couple of meatballs and some freshly chopped parsley on top.
Nutrition:
Calories 670
Fat 47.4 g.,
Carbs 4.6 g.
Sugar 1.7 g.
Protein: 54.9 g.
Sodium 622 mg.

235.   BEEF MEATS WAFFLE

Preparation time: 10 min.
Cooking time: 15 min.
Servings: 2
Ingredients:
For the meatza waffle batter:

- 1/2 lb. ground beef
- 4 eggs
- 2 c. grated cheddar cheese
- Salt and pepper to taste
- 1 tsp. Italian seasoning
- 2 tbsp. tomato sauce

Other:

- 2 tbsp. cooking spray to brush the waffle maker
- 1/4 c. tomato sauce for serving
- 2 tbsp. freshly chopped basil for serving

Directions:
Preheat the waffle maker.
Add the ground beef, eggs, grated cheddar cheese, salt and pepper, Italian seasoning, and tomato sauce to a bowl.
Mix until everything is fully combined.
Brush the heated waffle maker with cooking spray and add a few tablespoons of the batter.
Close the lid and cook for about 7–10 min. depending on your waffle maker.
Serve with tomato sauce and freshly chopped basil on top.
Nutrition:
Calories 4
Fat 34.6 g.

Carbs 2.5 g.
Sugar 1.7 g.
Protein: 36.5 g.
Sodium 581 mg.

236. CHICKEN JALAPENO WAFFLE

Preparation time: 10 min.
Cooking time: 8–10 min.
Servings: 2
Ingredients:
For the batter:

- 1/2 lb. ground chicken
- 4 eggs
- 1 c. grated mozzarella cheese
- 2 tbsp. sour cream
- 1 green jalapeno, chopped
- Salt and pepper to taste
- 1 tsp. dried oregano
- 1/2 tsp. dried garlic

Other:
2 tbsp. butter to brush the waffle maker
1/4 c. sour cream to garnish
1 green jalapeno, diced, to garnish

Directions:
Preheat the waffle maker.
Add the ground chicken, eggs, mozzarella cheese, sour cream, chopped jalapeno, salt and pepper, dried oregano, and dried garlic to a bowl.
Mix everything until the batter forms.
Brush the heated waffle maker with butter and add a few tablespoons of the batter.
Close the lid and cook for about 8–10 min. depending on your waffle maker.
Serve with a tablespoon of sour cream and sliced jalapeno on top.

Nutrition:
Calories 284
Fat 19.4 g.
Carbs 2.2 g.
Sugar 0.6 g.
Protein: 24 g.

Sodium 204 mg.

237. CHICKEN TACO WAFFLE

Preparation time: 10 min.
Cooking time: 15 min.
Servings: 2
Ingredients:
For the batter:

- 4 eggs
- 2 c. grated provolone cheese
- 6 tbsp. almond flour
- 2 1/2 tsp.s baking powder
- Salt and pepper to taste

For the chicken topping:
2 tbsp. olive oil
1/2 lb. ground chicken
Salt and pepper to taste
1 garlic clove, minced
2 tsp. dried oregano

Other:
2 tbsp. butter to brush the waffle maker
2 tbsp. freshly chopped spring onion for garnishing

Directions:
Preheat the waffle maker.
Add the eggs, grated provolone cheese, almond flour, baking powder, and salt and pepper to a bowl.
Mix until just combined.
Brush the heated waffle maker with cooking spray and add a few tablespoons of the batter.
Close the lid and cook for about 7–9 min. depending on your waffle maker.
Meanwhile, heat the olive oil in a nonstick pan over medium heat and start cooking the ground chicken.
Season with salt and pepper and stir in the minced garlic and dried oregano. Cook for 10 min.

Add some of the cooked ground chicken to each waffle and serve with freshly chopped spring onion.

Nutrition:
Calories 584
Fat 44 g.
Carbs 6.4 g.
Sugar 0.8 g.
Protein: 41.3 g.
Sodium 737 mg.

238. CLASSIC GROUND PORK WAFFLE

Preparation time: 10 min.
Cooking time: 15 min.
Servings: 2
Ingredients:

- 1/2 lb. ground pork
- 3 eggs
- 1/2 c. grated mozzarella cheese
- Salt and pepper to taste
- 1 clove garlic, minced
- 1 tsp. dried oregano

Other:

- 2 tbsp. butter to brush the waffle maker
- 2 tbsp. freshly chopped parsley for garnish

Directions:
Preheat the waffle maker.
Add the ground pork, eggs, mozzarella cheese, salt and pepper, minced garlic, and dried oregano to a bowl.
Mix until combined.
Brush the heated waffle maker with butter and add a few tablespoons of the batter.
Close the lid and cook for about 7–8 min. depending on your waffle maker.
Serve with freshly chopped parsley.

Nutrition:
Calories 192
Fat 11 g.
Carbs 1 g.

Sugar 0.3 g.
Protein: 20.2 g.
Sodium 142 mg.

239. CREAMY BACON SALAD ON A WAFFLE

Preparation time: 10 min.
Cooking time: 15 min.
Servings: 2
Ingredients:

- 4 eggs
- 1 1/2 c. grated mozzarella cheese
- 1/2 c. parmesan cheese
- Salt and pepper to taste
- 1 tsp. dried oregano
- 1/4 c. almond flour
- 2 tsp. baking powder

For the bacon salad:

- 1/2 lb. cooked bacon
- 1 c. cream cheese
- 1 tsp. dried oregano
- 1 tsp. dried basil
- 1 tsp. dried rosemary
- 2 tbsp. lemon juice

Other:

- 2 tbsp. butter to brush the waffle maker
- 2 spring onions, finely chopped, for serving

Directions:
Preheat the waffle maker.
Add the eggs, mozzarella cheese, parmesan cheese, salt and pepper, dried oregano, almond flour, and baking powder to a bowl.
Mix until combined.
Brush the heated waffle maker with butter and add a few tablespoons of the batter.
Close the lid and cook for about 7 min. depending on your waffle maker.
Meanwhile, chop the cooked bacon into smaller pieces and place them in a bowl with the cream

cheese. Season with dried oregano, dried basil, dried rosemary, and lemon juice.

Mix until combined and spread each waffle with the creamy bacon salad.

To serve, sprinkle some freshly chopped spring onion on top.

Nutrition:

Calories 750

Fat 62.5 g.

Carbs 7.7 g.

Sugar 0.8 g.

Protein: 40.3 g.

Sodium 1785 mg.

240. GARLIC CHICKEN WAFFLE

Preparation time: 10 min.

Cooking time: 15 min.

Servings: 2

Ingredients:

For the batter:

- 4 eggs
- 2 c. grated mozzarella cheese
- 1/4 c. almond flour
- 2 tbsp. coconut flour
- 2 1/2 tsp.s baking powder
- Salt and pepper to taste

For the topping:

- 1-lb. diced chicken
- Salt and pepper to taste
- 1 tsp. dried oregano
- 2 garlic cloves, minced
- 3 tbsp. butter

Other:

- 2 tbsp. cooking spray for greasing the waffle maker
- 2 tbsp. freshly chopped parsley

Directions:

Preheat the waffle maker.

Add the eggs, grated mozzarella cheese, almond flour, coconut flour, and baking powder to a bowl and season with salt and pepper.

Mix until just combined.

Spray the waffle maker with cooking spray to prevent the waffles from sticking. Add a few tablespoons of the batter to the heated and greased waffle maker.

Close the lid and cook for about 7 min. depending on your waffle maker.

Repeat with the rest of the batter.

Meanwhile, melt the butter in a nonstick pan over medium heat.

Season the chicken with salt and pepper and dried oregano and mix in the minced garlic.

Cook the chicken for about 10 min., stirring constantly.

Serve each waffle with a topping of the garlic chicken mixture and sprinkle some freshly chopped parsley on top.

Nutrition:

Calories 475

Fat 29.5 g.

Carbs 7.2 g.

Sugar 0.4 g.

Protein: 44.7 g.

Sodium 286 mg.

241. GROUND CHICKEN WAFFLE

Preparation time: 10 min.

Cooking time: 8–10 min.

Servings: 2

Ingredients:

For the batter:

- 1/2 lb. ground chicken
- 4 eggs
- 3 tbsp. tomato sauce
- Salt and pepper to taste
- 1 c. grated mozzarella cheese
- 1 tsp. dried oregano

Other:

- tbsp. butter to brush the waffle maker

Directions:

Preheat the waffle maker.

Add the ground chicken, eggs, and tomato sauce to a bowl and season with salt and pepper.

Mix everything with a fork and stir in the mozzarella cheese and dried oregano.

Mix again until fully combined.

Brush the heated waffle maker with butter and add a few tablespoons of the batter.

Close the lid and cook for about 8–10 min. depending on your waffle maker.

Serve and enjoy.

Nutrition:

Calories 246
Fat 15.6 g.
Carbs 1.5 g.
Sugar 0.9 g.
Protein: 24.2 g.
Sodium 254 mg.

242. ITALIAN CHICKEN AND BASIL WAFFLE

Preparation time: 10 min.
Cooking time: 7–9 min.
Servings: 2
Ingredients:
For the batter:

- 1/2 lb. ground chicken
- 4 eggs
- 3 tbsp. tomato sauce
- Salt and pepper to taste
- 1 c. grated mozzarella cheese
- 1 tsp. dried oregano
- 3 tbsp. freshly chopped basil leaves
- 1/2 tsp. dried garlic

Other:

- 2 tbsp. butter to brush the waffle maker
- 1/4 c. tomato sauce for serving
- 1 tbsp. freshly chopped basil for serving

Directions:

Preheat the waffle maker.

Add the ground chicken, eggs, and tomato sauce to a bowl and season with salt and pepper.

Add the mozzarella cheese and season with dried oregano, freshly chopped basil, and dried garlic.

Mix until fully combined and batter forms.

Brush the heated waffle maker with butter and add a few tablespoons of the waffle batter.

Close the lid and cook for about 7–9 min. depending on your waffle maker.

Repeat with the rest of the batter.

Serve with tomato sauce and freshly chopped basil on top.

Nutrition:

Calories 250
Fat 15.7 g.
Carbs 2.5 g.
Sugar 1.5 g.
Protein: 24.5 g.
Sodium 334 mg.

243. LAMB CHOPS ON WAFFLE

Preparation time: 10 min.
Cooking time: 15 min.
Servings: 2
Ingredients:

- 4 eggs
- 2 c. grated mozzarella cheese
- Salt and pepper to taste
- 1 tsp. garlic powder
- 1/4 c. heavy cream
- 6 tbsp. almond flour
- 2 tsp. baking powder

For the lamb chops:

- 2 tbsp. herbed butter
- 1-lb. lamb chops
- Salt and pepper to taste
- 1 tsp. freshly chopped rosemary

Other:
- 2 tbsp. butter to brush the waffle maker
- 2 tbsp. freshly chopped parsley for garnish

Directions:
Preheat the waffle maker.

Add the eggs, mozzarella cheese, salt and pepper, garlic powder, heavy cream, almond flour, and baking powder to a bowl.

Mix until combined.

Brush the heated waffle maker with butter and add a few tablespoons of the batter.

Close the lid and cook for about 7 min. depending on your waffle maker.

Meanwhile, heat a nonstick frying pan and rub the lamb chops with herbed butter, salt and pepper, and freshly chopped rosemary.

Cook the lamb chops for about 3–4 min. on each side.

Serve each waffle with a few lamb chops and sprinkle on some freshly chopped parsley for a nice presentation.

Nutrition:
Calories 537
Fat 37.3 g.
Carbs 5.5 g.
Sugar 0.6 g.
Protein: 44.3 g.
Sodium 328 mg.

244. LEFTOVER TURKEY WAFFLE

Preparation time: 10 min.
Cooking time: 7–9 min.
Servings: 2
Ingredients:
For the batter:
- 1/2 lb. shredded leftover turkey meat
- 4 eggs
- 1 c. grated provolone cheese
- Salt and pepper to taste
- 1 tsp. dried basil

- 1/2 tsp. dried garlic
- 3 tbsp. sour cream
- 2 tbsp. coconut flour

Other:
- 2 tbsp. cooking spray for greasing the waffle maker
- 1/4 c. cream cheese for serving the waffles

Directions:
Preheat the waffle maker.

Add the leftover turkey, eggs, and provolone cheese to a bowl and season with salt and pepper, dried basil, and dried garlic.

Add the sour cream and coconut flour and mix until the batter forms.

Brush the heated waffle maker with cooking spray and add a few tablespoons of the waffle batter.

Close the lid and cook for about 7–9 min. depending on your waffle maker.

Repeat with the rest of the batter.

Serve with cream cheese on top of each waffle.

Nutrition:
Calories 372
Fat 27 g.
Carbs 5.4 g.
Sugar 0.6 g.
Protein: 25 g.
Sodium 795 mg.

245. MEDITERRANEAN LAMB KEBABS ON WAFFLE

Preparation time: 10 min.
Cooking time: 15 min.
Servings: 2
Ingredients:
- 4 eggs
- 2 c. grated mozzarella cheese
- Salt and pepper to taste
- 1 tsp. garlic powder
- 1/4 c. Greek yogurt
- 1/2 c. coconut flour

- 2 tsp. baking powder

For the lamb kebabs:
- 1-lb. ground lamb meat
- Salt and pepper to taste
- 1 egg
- 2 tbsp. almond flour
- 1 spring onion, finely chopped
- 1/2 tsp. dried garlic
- 2 tbsp. olive oil

Other:
2 tbsp. butter to brush the waffle maker
1/4 c. sour cream for serving
4 sprigs of fresh dill for garnish

Directions:
Preheat the waffle maker.

Add the eggs, mozzarella cheese, salt and pepper, garlic powder, Greek yogurt, coconut flour, and baking powder to a bowl.

Mix until combined.

Brush the heated waffle maker with butter and add a few tablespoons of the batter.

Close the lid and cook for about 7 min. depending on your waffle maker.

Meanwhile, add the ground lamb, salt and pepper, egg, almond flour, chopped spring onion, and dried garlic to a bowl. Mix and form medium-sized kebabs.

Impale each kebab on a skewer. Heat the olive oil in a frying pan.

Cook the lamb kebabs for about 3 min. on each side.

Serve each waffle with a tablespoon of sour cream and 1–2 lamb kebabs. Decorate with fresh dill.

Nutrition:
Calories 679
Fat 49.9 g.
Carbs 15.8 g.
Sugar 0.8 g.
Protein: 42.6 g.
Sodium 302 mg.

246.   HUMMUS   BEEF WAFFLES

Preparation time: 15 min.
Cooking time: 32 min.
Servings: 4
Ingredients:
- 2 eggs
- 1 c. + 1/4 c. finely grated cheddar cheese, divided
- 2 chopped fresh scallions
- Salt and freshly ground black pepper to taste
- 2 chicken breasts, cooked and diced
- 1/4 c. buffalo sauce
- 3 tbsp. low-carb hummus
- 2 celery stalks, chopped
- 1/4 c. crumbled blue cheese for topping

Directions:
Preheat the waffle iron.

In a medium bowl, mix the eggs, 1 c. of the cheddar cheese, scallions, salt, and black pepper, Open the iron and add 1/4 of the mixture. Close and cook until crispy, 7 min.

Transfer the waffle to a plate and make 3 more waffles in the same manner.

Preheat the oven to 400°F and line a baking sheet with parchment paper. Set aside.

Cut the waffles into quarters and arrange them on the baking sheet.

In a medium bowl, mix the chicken with the buffalo sauce, hummus, and celery.

Spoon the chicken mixture onto each quarter of the waffles and top with the remaining cheddar cheese.

Place the baking sheet in the oven and bake until the cheese melts, 4 min.

Remove from the oven and top with the blue cheese.

Servings afterward.

Nutrition:
Calories 552

Fats 28.37 g.
Carbs: 6.97 g.
Net carbs 6.07 g.
Protein: 59.8 g.

247. TURKEY WAFFLE SANDWICH

Preparation time: 10 min.
Cooking time: 15 min.
Servings: 2
Ingredients:
For the batter:

- 4 eggs
- 1/4 c. cream cheese
- 1 c. grated mozzarella cheese
- Salt and pepper to taste
- 1 tsp. dried dill
- 1/2 tsp. onion powder
- 1/2 tsp. garlic powder

For the juicy chicken:

- 2 tbsp. butter
- 1-lb. chicken breast
- Salt and pepper to taste
- 1 tsp. dried dill
- 2 tbsp. heavy cream

Other:

- 2 tbsp. butter to brush the waffle maker
- 4 lettuce leaves to garnish the sandwich
- 4 tomato slices to garnish the sandwich

Directions:
Preheat the waffle maker.
Add the eggs, cream cheese, mozzarella cheese, salt and pepper, dried dill, onion powder, and garlic powder to a bowl.
Mix everything with a fork just until the batter forms.
Brush the heated waffle maker with butter and add a few tablespoons of the batter.
Close the lid and cook for about 7 min. depending on your waffle maker.

Meanwhile, heat some butter in a nonstick pan. Season the chicken with salt and pepper and sprinkle with dried dill. Pour the heavy cream on top.
Cook the chicken slices for about 10 min. or until golden brown.
Cut each waffle in half.
On one half add a lettuce leaf, tomato slice, and chicken slice. Cover with the other waffle half to make a sandwich.
Serve and enjoy.
Nutrition:
Calories: 102
Fat: 3 g.
Protein: 9 g.
Carbohydrates: 9 g.
Fiber: 3.8 g.

248. PORK TZATZIKI WAFFLE

Preparation time: 10 min.
Cooking time: 25 min.
Servings: 2
Ingredients:

- 4 eggs
- 2 c. grated provolone cheese
- Salt and pepper to taste
- 1 tsp. dried rosemary
- 1 tsp. dried oregano

For the pork loin:

- 2 tbsp. olive oil
- 1-lb. pork tenderloin
- Salt and pepper to taste

For the tzatziki sauce:

- 1 c. sour cream
- Salt and pepper to taste
- 1 cucumber, peeled and diced
- 1 tsp. garlic powder
- 1 tsp. dried dill
- Other:
- 2 tbsp. butter to brush the waffle maker

Directions:

Preheat the waffle maker.

Add the eggs, grated provolone cheese, dried rosemary, and dried oregano to a bowl. Season with salt and pepper to taste.

Mix until combined.

Brush the heated waffle maker with butter and add a few tablespoons of the batter.

Close the lid and cook for about 7 min. depending on your waffle maker.

Meanwhile, heat the olive oil in a nonstick frying pan. Generously season the pork tenderloin with salt and pepper and cook it for about 7 min. on each side.

Mix the sour cream, salt and pepper, diced cucumber, garlic powder, and dried dill in a bowl. Serve each waffle with a few tablespoons of tzatziki sauce and slices of pork tenderloin.

Nutrition:

Calories 104

Protein: 6 g. Fat: 4 g.

Cholesterol 11 mg.

Potassium 141 mg.

Calcium 69 mg.

Fiber 2.4 g.

249.   PORK LOIN WAFFLES SANDWICH

Preparation time: 10 min.

Cooking time: 15 min.

Servings: 2

Ingredients:

- 4 eggs
- 1 c. grated mozzarella cheese
- 1 c. grated parmesan cheese
- Salt and pepper to taste
- 2 tbsp. cream cheese
- 6 tbsp. coconut flour
- 2 tsp. baking powder

For the pork loin:

- 2 tbsp. olive oil
- 1-lb. pork loin
- Salt and pepper to taste
- 2 cloves garlic, minced
- 1 tbsp. freshly chopped thyme

Other:

- 2 tbsp. cooking spray to brush the waffle maker
- 4 lettuce leaves for serving
- 4 slices of tomato for serving
- 1/4 c. sugar-free mayonnaise for serving

Directions:

Preheat the waffle maker.

Add the eggs, mozzarella cheese, parmesan cheese, salt and pepper, cream cheese, coconut flour, and baking powder to a bowl.

Mix until combined.

Brush the heated waffle maker with cooking spray and add a few tablespoons of the batter.

Close the lid and cook for about 7 min. depending on your waffle maker.

Meanwhile, heat the olive oil in a nonstick frying pan and season the pork loin with salt and pepper, minced garlic, and freshly chopped thyme.

Cook the pork loin for about 5 min. on each side. Cut each waffle in half and add some mayonnaise, lettuce leaf, tomato slice, and sliced pork loin on one half.

Cover the sandwich with the other waffle half and serve.

Nutrition:

Calories 141

Protein: 10 g.

Carbohydrates 15 g.

Fat: 0 g.

Sodium 113 mg.

Potassium 230 mg.

Phosphorus 129 mg.

250. TURKEY BBQ SAUCE WAFFLE

Preparation time: 10 min.
Cooking time: 8–10 min.
Servings: 2
Ingredients:
For the batter:
- 1/2 lb. ground turkey meat
- 3 eggs
- 1 c. grated Swiss cheese
- 1/4 c. cream cheese
- 1/4 c. BBQ sauce
- 1 tsp. dried oregano
- Salt and pepper to taste
- 2 cloves garlic, minced

Other:
- 2 tbsp. butter to brush the waffle maker
- 1/4 c. BBQ sauce for serving
- 2 tbsp. freshly chopped parsley for garnish

Directions:
Preheat the waffle maker.
Add the ground turkey, eggs, grated Swiss cheese, cream cheese, BBQ sauce, dried oregano, salt and pepper, and minced garlic to a bowl.
Mix everything until combined and batter forms.
Brush the heated waffle maker with butter and add a few tablespoons of the batter.
Close the lid and cook for about 8–10 min. depending on your waffle maker.
Serve each waffle with a tablespoon of BBQ sauce and a sprinkle of freshly chopped parsley.

Nutrition:
Calories 242
Fat: 7 g.
Carbs: 23.8 g.
Protein: 23.2 g.
Potassium (K) 263 mg.
Sodium (Na) 63 mg.
Phosphorous 30 mg.

251. PORK CHOPS ON WAFFLE

Preparation time: 15 min.
Cooking time: 15 min.
Servings: 4
Ingredients:
- 4 eggs
- 2 c. grated mozzarella cheese
- Salt and pepper to taste
- Pinch of nutmeg
- 2 tbsp. sour cream
- 6 tbsp. almond flour
- 2 tsp. baking powder

For the pork chops:
- 2 tbsp. olive oil
- 1-lb. pork chops
- Salt and pepper to taste
- 1 tsp. freshly chopped rosemary

Other:
- 2 tbsp. cooking spray to brush the waffle maker
- 2 tbsp. freshly chopped basil for decoration

Directions:
Preheat the waffle maker.
Add the eggs, mozzarella cheese, salt and pepper, nutmeg, sour cream, almond flour, and baking powder to a bowl.
Mix until combined.
Brush the heated waffle maker with cooking spray and add a few tablespoons of the batter.
Close the lid and cook for about 7 min. depending on your waffle maker.
Meanwhile, heat the butter in a nonstick grill pan and season the pork chops with salt and pepper and freshly chopped rosemary.
Cook the pork chops for about 4–5 min. on each side.
Serve each waffle with a pork chop and sprinkle some freshly chopped basil on top.

149

Nutrition:
Calories 666
Fat 55.2 g.
Carbs 4.8 g.
Sugar 0.4 g.
Protein: 37.5 g.
Sodium 235 mg.

252. CLASSIC BEEF WAFFLE

Preparation time: 20 min.
Cooking time: 10 min.
Servings: 4
Ingredients:
For the batter:

- 1/2 lb. ground beef
- 4 eggs
- 4 oz. cream cheese
- 1 c. grated mozzarella cheese
- Salt and pepper to taste
- 1 clove garlic, minced
- 1/2 tsp. freshly chopped rosemary

Other:

- 2 tbsp. butter to brush the waffle maker
- 1/4 c. sour cream
- 2 tbsp. freshly chopped parsley for garnish

Directions:
Preheat the waffle maker.
Add the ground beef, eggs, cream cheese, grated mozzarella cheese, salt and pepper, minced garlic, and freshly chopped rosemary to a bowl.
Brush the heated waffle maker with butter and add a few tablespoons of the batter.
Close the lid and cook for about 8–10 min. depending on your waffle maker.
Serve each waffle with a tablespoon of sour cream and freshly chopped parsley on top.
Serve and enjoy.

Nutrition:
Calories 368
Fat 24 g.

Carbs 2.1 g.
Sugar 0.4 g.
Protein: 27.4 g.
Sodium 291 mg.

253. SPINACH AND ARTICHOKE CHICKEN WAFFLE

Preparation time: 10 min.
Cooking time: 8 min.
Servings: 2
Ingredients:

- 1/3 c. cooked diced chicken
- 1/3 c. cooked spinach chopped
- 1/3 c. marinated artichokes chopped
- 1/3 c. shredded mozzarella cheese
- 1-oz. softened cream cheese
- 1/4 tsp. garlic powder
- 1 egg

Directions:
Heat up your mini waffle maker.
In a small bowl, mix the egg, garlic powder, cream cheese, and mozzarella cheese.
Add the spinach, artichoke, and chicken and mix well.
Add 1/3 of the batter into your mini waffle maker and cook for 4–5 min. If they are still a bit uncooked, leave it cooking for another 2 min. Then cook the rest of the batter to make a second waffle and then cook the third waffle.
After cooking, remove from the pan and let sit for 2 min.
Dip in ranch dressing, sour cream, or enjoy alone.

Nutrition:
Calories: 1
Carbohydrates: 3 g.
Protein: 11 g.
Fat: 13 g.
Saturated Fat: 6 g.
Cholesterol: 46 mg.
Sodium: 322 mg.

Potassium: 140 mg.
Fiber: 1 g.
Sugar: 1 g.

254. CHEDDAR CHICKEN AND BROCCOLI WAFFLE

Preparation time: 15 min.
Cooking time: 8 min.
Servings: 2
Ingredients:

- 1/4 c. cooked diced chicken
- 1/4 c. fresh broccoli chopped
- Shredded cheddar cheese
- 1 egg
- 1/4 tsp. garlic powder

Directions:

Heat up your Dash mini waffle maker.

In a small bowl, mix the egg, garlic powder, and cheddar cheese.

Add the broccoli and chicken and mix well.

Add 1/2 of the batter into your mini waffle maker and cook for 4–5 min. If they are still a bit uncooked, leave it cooking for another 2 min. Then cook the rest of the batter to make a second waffle and then cook the third waffle.

After cooking, remove from the pan and let sit for 2 min.

Dip in ranch dressing, sour cream, or enjoy alone.

Nutrition:

Calories: 58
Carbohydrates: 1 g.
Fat: 3 g.
Saturated Fat: 1 g.
Cholesterol: 94 mg.
Sodium: 57 mg.
Potassium: 136 mg.
Fiber: 1 g.
Sugar: 1 g.

255. BEEF AND Sour CREAM WAFFLE

Preparation time: 10 min.
Cooking time: 15 min.
Servings: 4
Ingredients:
For the batter:

- 4 eggs
- 2 c. grated mozzarella cheese
- 3 tbsp. coconut flour
- 3 tbsp. almond flour
- 2 tsp. baking powder
- Salt and pepper to taste
- 1 tbsp. freshly chopped parsley

For the seasoned beef:

- 1-lb. beef tenderloin
- Salt and pepper to taste
- 2 tbsp. olive oil
- 1 tbsp. Dijon mustard

Other:

- 2 tbsp. olive oil to brush the waffle maker
- 1/4 c. sour cream for garnish
- 2 tbsp. freshly chopped spring onion for garnish

Directions:

Preheat the waffle maker.

Add the eggs, grated mozzarella cheese, coconut flour, almond flour, baking powder, salt and pepper, and freshly chopped parsley to a bowl.

Mix until just combined and batter forms.

Brush the heated waffle maker with olive oil and add a few tablespoons of the batter.

Close the lid and cook for about 7 min. depending on your waffle maker.

Meanwhile, heat the olive oil in a nonstick pan over medium heat.

Season the beef tenderloin with salt and pepper and spread the whole piece of beef tenderloin with Dijon mustard.

Cook on each side for about 4–5 min.

Serve each waffle with sour cream and slices of the cooked beef tenderloin.

Garnish with freshly chopped spring onion.

Serve and enjoy.

Nutrition:

Calories 543

Fat 37 g.

Carbs 7.9 g.

Sugar 0.5 g.

Protein: 44.9 g.

Sodium 269 mg.

256. BEEF TERIYAKI AVOCADO WAFFLE BURGER

Preparation time: 15 min.

Cooking time: 15 min.

Servings: 2

Ingredients:

For the waffle:

- 2 egg
- 1 c. mozzarella cheese, (shredded)
- 1/2 avocado
- 2 leaves of green leaf lettuce, optional

For Patty:

- 1/2 lb. ground beef
- 1 tbsp. pork panko
- 1 egg
- 1/4 tsp. salt, or as per your taste
- 1/4 tsp. black pepper, or as per your taste

For the teriyaki sauce:

- 2 tbsp. Japanese sake
- 1 tbsp. soy sauce
- 1/8 tsp. xanthan gum
- 1 tbsp. swerve/monk fruit

Directions:

In a saucepan, add Japanese sake, soy sauce, xanthan gum, and swerve/monk fruit and bring to boil on high heat

Then lower the heat and cook the mixture for 1–2 min. and mix continuously

When xanthan gum dissolves, remove it from the heat and let it cool

Take a mixing bowl and add ground beef, pork panko, egg, salt, and pepper, and mix with your hands

When the mixture becomes smooth, turn it into a ball and press it on a plate and make it a patty

A patty should be over 1/4 in. thick and make sure to put your thumb in between the patty so that it doesn't expand upward and retains its shape

Preheat the grill to 350 °F and cook the patties from both sides on medium to low heat for 4–5 min. till the patties turn brown

You can also use a frying pan to fry the patties

Preheat a mini waffle maker if needed

In a mixing bowl, beat the eggs and add mozzarella cheese to them

Mix them all well and pour into the greasy mini waffle maker

Cook for at least 4 min. to get the desired crunch

Remove the waffle from the heat and keep it aside

Make as many waffles as your mixture and waffle maker allow

Cut the avocado into slices

Wash the green leaf lettuce and dry

Take two waffles and arrange a beef patty with the slices of avocado, green lettuce, and teriyaki sauce in between to make a burger

Serve hot and enjoy

Nutrition:

Calories 402

Fat 23.53 g.

Carbs 13.49 g.

Sugar 4.01 g.

Protein: 1299 g.

Sodium 269 mg
257.   BEEF STRIPS WAFFLE
Preparation time: 25 min.
Cooking time: 20 min.
Servings: 2
Ingredients:
For the waffle:
- 1 egg
- 1/2 c. mozzarella cheese (shredded)
- 1/4 tsp. salt, or as per your taste
- 1/4 tsp. black pepper, or as per your taste
- 1 tbsp. ginger powder

For beef strips:
- 8 pieces beef strips
- 2 tbsp. butter
- 1/4 tsp. salt, or as per your taste
- 1/4 tsp. black pepper, or as per your taste
- 1/2 tsp. red chili flakes

Directions:
In a frying pan, melt the butter and fry the beef strips on medium-low heat
Add water to make them tender and boil for 30 min.
Add the spices at the end and set them aside
Mix all the waffle ingredients well together
Pour a thin layer on a preheated waffle iron
Add beef strips and pour again more mixture over the top
Cook the waffle for around 5 min.
Make as many waffles as your mixture and waffle maker allow
Serve hot with your favorite sauce
Nutrition:
Calories 185
Fat 12.68 g.
Carbs 3.45 g.
Sugar 1.42 g.
Protein: 14.28 g.
Sodium 927 mg.

258.   BEEF BBQ WAFFLE
Preparation time: 10 min.
Cooking time: 30 min.
Servings: 2
Ingredients:
- 1/2 c. beef mince
- 1 tbsp. butter
- 1 tbsp. bbq sauce (sugar-free)
- 2 tbsp. almond flour
- 1 egg
- 1/2 c. cheddar cheese

Directions:
Cook the beef mince in the butter and 1/2 c. water on a low-medium heat for 20 min.
Then increase the flame to reduce water
Preheat your waffle iron
In the mixing bowl, add all the waffle ingredients including beef mince, and mix well
Grease your waffle iron lightly
Pour the mixture to the bottom plate evenly; also spread it out to get better results and close the upper plate and heat
Cook for 6 min. or until the waffle is done
Make as many waffles as your mixture and waffle maker allow
Nutrition:
Calories 110
Fat 9.29 g.
Carbs 1.37 g.
Sugar 0.73 g.
Protein: 5.11 g.
Sodium 146 mg.

259.   BEEF   EGGPLANT WAFFLE
Preparation time: 15 min.
Cooking time: 30 min.
Servings: 2
Ingredients:
For the waffles:
- 2 eggs

- 1/2 c. cheddar cheese
- 2 tbsp. parmesan cheese
- 1/4 tsp. Italian season
- 1 c. beef mince

For the eggplant:

1 big eggplant
1 pinch salt
1 pinch black pepper
1/2 tsp red chili flakes

Directions:

Cook the beef mince with 1/2 c. water on medium-low flame for 20 min.

Increase the flame afterward to remove excess water

Cut the eggplant in slices and boil in water and strain

Add a pinch of salt and pepper with red chili flakes

Add all the waffle ingredients into a bowl and mix well to make a mixture

Add the boiled beef

Preheat a mini waffle maker if needed and grease it

Pour the mixture into the lower plate of the waffle maker and spread it evenly to cover the plate properly

Add the eggplant about two slices on the mixture and cover the lid

Cook for at least 4 min. to get the desired crunch

Remove the waffle from the heat

Make as many waffles as your mixture and waffle maker allow

Serve hot with your favorite sauce

Nutrition:

Calories 289
Fat 12.02 g.
Carbs 34.18 g.
Sugar 20.04 g.
Protein: 15.78 g.
Sodium 234 mg.

260.   BEEF   STUFFED WAFFLES

Preparation time: 15 min.
Cooking time: 50 min.
Servings: 2
Ingredients:
For the waffle:

- 2 egg
- 1/2 c. mozzarella cheese (shredded)
- 1/4 tsp. garlic powder
- 1/4 tsp. salt, or as per your taste
- 1/4 tsp. black pepper, or as per your taste

For stuffing:

- 1 small onion, diced
- 1 c. beef mince
- 4 tbsp. butter
- 1/4 tsp. salt, or as per your taste
- 1/4 tsp. black pepper, or as per your taste

Directions:

Preheat a mini waffle maker if needed and grease it

In a mixing bowl, add all the waffle ingredients

Mix them all well

Pour the mixture to the lower plate of the waffle maker and spread it evenly to cover the plate properly and close the lid

Cook for at least 4 min. to get the desired crunch

Remove the waffle from the heat and keep it aside

Make as many waffles as your mixture and waffle maker allow

Take a small frying pan and melt the butter in it on medium-low heat

Sauté the beef mince and onion and add salt and pepper

Cook for over 20 min.

Take another bowl and tear waffles down into minute pieces

Add beef and onion to it

Take a casserole dish and add this new stuffing mixture to it

Bake it at 350 °F for around 30 min. and serve hot

Nutrition:

Calories 373

Fat 28.16 g.

Carbs 6.63 g.

Sugar 3.14 g.

Protein: 22.72 g.

Sodium 1078 mg.

261. JALAPENO BEEF WAFFLE

Preparation time: 25 min.

Cooking time: 20 min.

Servings: 2

Ingredients:

- 1/2 c. boiled beef, shredded
- 1/8 tsp. onion powder
- 1/8 tsp. garlic powder
- 1 egg
- 1/4 c. cheddar cheese
- 1 diced jalapeno
- 1 tbsp. cream cheese
- 1/8 tbsp. parmesan cheese

Directions:

Preheat a mini waffle maker if needed and grease it

In a mixing bowl, beat an egg and add all the ingredients

Mix them all well

Pour the mixture into the lower plate of the waffle maker and spread it evenly to cover the plate properly

Close the lid

Cook for at least 4 min. to get the desired crunch

Remove the waffle from the heat and keep aside for around 1 min.

Make as many waffles as your mixture and waffle maker allow

Serve hot and enjoy!

Nutrition:

Calories 90

Fat 7.06 g.

Carbs 1.08 g.

Sugar 0.6 g.

Protein: 5.16 g.

Sodium 90 mg.

262. BEEF PICKLED SANDWICH WAFFLE

Preparation time: 20 min.

Cooking time: 1 hour 10 min.

Servings: 2

Ingredients:

For the beef:

- 1 chicken breast
- 4 tbsp. parmesan cheese
- 4 tbsp. dill pickle juice
- 2 tbsp. pork rinds
- 1 tsp. flaxseed (grounded)
- 1 tsp. butter
- 1/4 tsp. salt, or as per your taste
- 1/4 tsp. black pepper, or as per your taste

For the sandwich bun:

- 1 egg
- 1 c. mozzarella cheese (shredded)
- 4 drops of stevia glycerite
- 1/4 tsp. butter extract

Directions:

Cut the beef into half-inch pieces and add in a ziplock bag with pickle juice

Keep them together for an hour to overnight

In a mixing bowl, add all the beef ingredients and mix well

Now add the beef and discard the pickle juice

Cook the beef on the frying pan for 6 min. from each side at low flame and set aside

Mix all the sandwich bun ingredients into a bowl

Put the mixture in the mini waffle maker and cook for 4 min.

Remove from the heat

Make the waffle sandwich by adding the prepared beef in between

Nutrition:

Calories 510

Fat 24.85 g.

Carbs 11.44 g.

Sugar 4.37 g.

Protein: 59.46 g.

Sodium 3232 mg.

263. GINGER BEEF WAFFLE

Preparation time: 20 min.

Cooking time: 20 min.

Servings: 2

Ingredients:

For the garlic beef:

- 1 c. beef mince
- 1/4 tsp. salt, or as per your taste
- 1/4 tsp. black pepper, or as per your taste
- 2 tbsp. butter
- 2 tbsp. garlic juvenile
- 1 tsp. garlic powder
- 1 tbsp. soy sauce
- 1/2 c. water

For the waffle:

- 2 egg
- 1 c. mozzarella cheese (shredded)
- 1 tsp. garlic powder

Directions:

In a frying pan, melt the butter and add juvenile garlic and sauté for 1 min.

Now add the beef mince and cook by adding water till it tenders

Let the water dry out, when done, add the rest of the ingredients and set aside

In a mixing bowl, beat the eggs and add mozzarella cheese to them with garlic powder

Mix them all well and pour into the greasy mini waffle maker

Cook for at least 4 min. to get the desired crunch

Remove the waffle from the heat and top with garlic beef

Make as many waffles as your mixture and waffle maker allow

Serve hot and enjoy

Nutrition:

Calories 329

Fat 18.87 g.

Carbs 10.57 g.

Sugar 3.47 g.

Protein: 29.07 g.

Sodium 1001 mg.

264. EASY BEEF BURGER WAFFLE

Preparation time: 20 min.

Cooking time: 10 min.

Servings: 2

Ingredients:

For the waffle:

- 2 egg
- 1 c. mozzarella cheese (shredded)
- 1 tbsp. butter
- 2 tbsp. almond flour
- 1/4 tsp. baking powder
- A pinch of salt

For the beef patty:

- 1 lb. ground beef
- 1/2 tbsp. onion powder
- 1/2 tbsp. garlic powder
- 1/2 tbsp. red chili flakes
- 1 c. cheddar cheese

- 1/4 tsp. salt, or as per your taste
- 1/4 tsp. black pepper, or as per your taste

For serving:s:
- 2 lettuce leaves
- 2 slices American cheese

Directions:
Mix all the beef patty ingredient in a bowl
Make equal-sized patties; either grill them or fry them on a medium-low heat
Preheat a mini waffle maker if needed and grease it
In a mixing bowl, add all the waffle ingredients and mix well
Pour the mixture to the lower plate of the waffle maker and spread it evenly to cover the plate properly and close the lid
Cook for at least 4 min. to get the desired crunch
Remove the waffle from the heat and keep aside for around 1 min.
Make as many waffles as your mixture and waffle maker allow
Serve with the beef patties, lettuce, and a cheese slice in between two waffles

Nutrition:
Calories 414
Fat 24.68 g.
Carbs 11.22 g.
Sugar 4.64 g.
Protein: 37.11 g.
Sodium 1514 mg.

265. BEEF GARLIC WAFFLE ROLL

Preparation time: 20 min.
Cooking time: 20 min.
Servings: 2
Ingredients:
- 1 c. beef mince
- 1/4 tsp. salt, or as per your taste
- 1/4 tsp. black pepper, or as per your taste
- 2 egg

- 1 tbsp. lemon juice
- 1/2 c. water
- 1 c. mozzarella cheese (shredded)
- 2 tbsp. butter
- 1 1/2 tsp. garlic powder
- 1/2 tsp. bay seasoning
- Parsley, for garnishing
- 1/2 c. cabbage

Directions:
In a frying pan, melt the butter and add the beef mince
Add 1/2 c. water for the mince to tender
When done, add salt, pepper, 1 tbsp. garlic powder, and lemon juice and set aside
In a mixing bowl, beat the eggs and add mozzarella cheese to them with 1/2 garlic powder and bay seasoning
Mix them all well and pour into the greasy mini waffle maker
Cook for at least 4 min. to get the desired crunch
Remove the waffle from the heat, add the beef mixture in between, and fold
Make as many waffles as your mixture and waffle maker allow
Top with parsley and add cabbage in between
Serve hot and enjoy!

Nutrition:
Calories 300
Fat 17.45 g.
Carbs 7.52 g.
Sugar 2.88 g.
Protein: 28.2 g.
Sodium 885 mg.

266. CAULI BEEF WAFFLE

Preparation time: 20 min.
Cooking time: 25 min.
Servings: 2
Ingredients:
- 1 c. beef fine mince

- 1 tbsp. soy sauce
- 2 cloves garlic
- 1 c. cauliflower rice
- 2 egg
- 1 c. mozzarella cheese
- Salt, as per your taste
- 1/4 tsp. black pepper, or as per your taste
- 1/4 tsp. white pepper, or as per your taste
- 1 stalk of green onion

Directions:
Melt the butter in the oven or stove and set aside

In a pot, cook the beef mince by adding 1 c. water to it with salt and bring to boil

Close the lid of the pot and cook for 15–20 min.

When done, cook on high flame till the water dries

Grate garlic finely into pieces

In a small bowl, beat the egg and mix the beef mince, garlic, cauliflower rice, soy sauce, black pepper, and white pepper

Mix all the ingredients well

Preheat the waffle maker if needed and grease it

Place around 1/8 c. shredded mozzarella cheese to the waffle maker

Pour the mixture over the cheese on the waffle maker and add 1/8 c. shredded cheese on top as well

Cook for 4–5 min. or until it is done

Repeat and make as many waffles as the batter can

Sprinkle chopped green onion on top and serve hot!

Nutrition:
Calories 256
Fat 11.3 g.
Carbs 10.04 g.
Sugar 4.89 g.
Protein: 28.95 g.

Sodium 661 mg.

267. FRIED CHICKEN PARMESAN WAFFLE

Preparation time: 15 min.
Cooking time: 20 min.
Servings: 2
Ingredients:
- 1/3 c. cheddar cheese
- 1 egg
- 1/4 tsp. baking powder
- 1 tsp. flaxseed (ground)
- 1/3 c. parmesan cheese
- 2 cm. pieces of chicken, cut boneless 1 c.
- 1 tbsp. butter
- Salt, as per your taste
- Black pepper, as per your taste

Directions:
Take a pan and heat butter

Add the chicken and sprinkle salt and pepper and fry till soften

Mix cheddar cheese, egg, baking powder, and flaxseed in a bowl

Grease your waffle iron lightly

In your mini waffle iron, shred half of the parmesan cheese

Add a small amount of the waffle mixture to your mini waffle iron

Now add a layer of chicken

Again shred the remaining parmesan cheese on top

Cook till the desired crisp is achieved

Make as many waffles as your mixture and waffle maker allow

Nutrition:
Calories 188
Fat 14.03 g.
Carbs 5.42 g.
Sugar 1.51 g.
Protein: 28.95 g.
Sodium 382 mg.

268. BOILED CHICKEN HALLOUMI WAFFLE

Preparation time: 15 min.
Cooking time: 20 min.
Servings: 2
Ingredients

- 1 c. boiled chicken, shredded
- 1/2 tsp. pepper
- A pinch of salt
- 3 oz. halloumi cheese
- 1 tbsp. oregano

Directions:

Take a bowl and add the chicken, pepper, and salt
Make 1/2 in. thick slices of Halloumi cheese and divide each further into two
Put one slice of the cheese in the unheated waffle maker and spread the chicken on it
Top with another cheese slice and sprinkle oregano
Cook the cheese for over 4–6 min. till it turns golden brown
Remove from the heat when a bit cool and serve with your favorite sauce

Nutrition:

Calories 382
Fat 31.84 g.
Carbs 4.78 g.
Sugar 0.2 g.
Protein: 18.61 g.
Sodium 729 mg.

269. SAUTÉED CHICKEN WAFFLE

Preparation time: 15 min.
Cooking time: 20 min.
Servings: 4
Ingredients:

- 1/3 c. cheddar cheese
- 1 egg
- 2 small pieces of chicken, sautéed in butter
- 1/4 tsp. baking powder
- 1/4 tsp. salt
- 2 tbsp. yogurt
- 1/3 c. mozzarella cheese

Directions:

Mix cheddar cheese, egg, yogurt, chicken, baking powder, and salt together
Preheat your waffle iron and grease it
In your mini waffle iron, shred half of the mozzarella cheese
Add the mixture to your mini waffle iron
Again shred the remaining mozzarella cheese on the mixture
Cook till the desired crisp is achieved
Make as many waffles as your mixture and waffle maker allow

Nutrition:

Calories 50
Fat 2.66 g.
Carbs 0.94 g.
Sugar 0.66 g.
Protein: 5.46 g.
Sodium 244 mg.

270. PEPPERY CHICKEN WAFFLES

Preparation time: 10 min.
Cooking time: 10 min.
Servings: 2
Ingredients:

- 1 egg:
- 1/2 c. mozzarella cheese (shredded)
- 1/2 c. boiled chicken, shredded
- 1/2 tsp. garlic powder
- 1/4 tsp. pepper
- 1/4 tsp. salt
- 1/2 tsp. dried basil

For baking:

- 1 large Red Bell Pepper, thickly sliced

159

- 1/2 c. Mozzarella cheese (shredded)
- 1/2 tsp. Oregano

Directions:
Preheat a mini waffle maker if needed and grease it
In a mixing bowl, add all the ingredients of the waffle and mix well
Pour the mixture into the waffle maker
Cook for at least 4 min. to get the desired crunch and make as many waffles as your batter allows
Preheat the oven
Spread waffles on the baking sheet and top one pepper slice
Sprinkle cheese on top and put the baking sheet into the oven
Heat for 5 min. to melt the cheese
Spread oregano on top and serve hot

Nutrition:
Calories 287
Fat 16.29 g.
Carbs 6 g.
Sugar 2.63 g.
Protein: 28.86 g.
Sodium 782 mg.

271. SAUTÉED CHICKEN LAYERED WAFFLES

Preparation time: 10 min.
Cooking time: 15 min.
Servings: 2
Ingredients:
- 1 c. chicken boneless, sautéed in butter
- 2 egg
- 1 c. mozzarella cheese (shredded)
- 1 tbsp. butter
- 1/4 tsp. turmeric
- 1/4 tsp. baking powder
- A pinch of onion powder
- A pinch of garlic powder
- A pinch of salt

Directions:
Mix all the remaining ingredients well together except the mince
Pour a thin layer on a preheated waffle iron
Add a layer of chicken mince to the mixture
Add more mixture over the top
Cook the waffle for around 5 min.
Serve hot with your favorite keto sauce

Nutrition:
Calories 1060
Fat 105.57 g.
Carbs 3.63 g.
Sugar 1.57 g.
Protein: 28.11 g.
Sodium 1284 mg.

272. CHICKEN EGGPLANT WAFFLE

Preparation time: 15 min.
Cooking time: 10 min.
Servings: 2
Ingredients:
For the waffles:
- 2 eggs
- 1/2 c. cheddar cheese
- 2 tbsp. parmesan cheese
- 1/4 tsp. Italian season
- 1 c. chicken

For the eggplant:
- 1 big eggplant
- 1 pinch of salt
- 1 pinch of black pepper

Directions:
Boil the chicken in water for 15 min. and strain
Shred the chicken into small pieces and set aside
Cut the eggplant in slices and boil in water and strain
Add a pinch of salt and pepper
Add all the waffle ingredients into a bowl and mix well to make a mixture

Add the boiled chicken as well

Preheat a mini waffle maker if needed and grease it

Pour the mixture into the lower plate of the waffle maker and spread it evenly to cover the plate properly

Add the eggplant over two slices on the mixture and cover the lid

Cook for at least 4 min. to get the desired crunch

Remove the waffle from the heat and keep aside for around 1 min.

Make as many waffles as your mixture and waffle maker allow

Serve hot with your favorite sauce

Nutrition:
Calories 818
Fat 24.9 g.
Carbs 34.14 g.
Sugar 20.04 g.
Protein: 112.75 g.
Sodium 586 mg.

273. AROMATIC CHICKEN WAFFLES

Preparation time: 10 min.
Cooking time: 30 min.
Servings: 4
Ingredients:

- 2 leg pieces of chicken
- 1 dried bay leaves
- 1 cardamom
- 4 whole black pepper
- 4 clove
- 2 c. water
- 2 eggs
- 1/4 tsp. salt
- 1 c. shredded mozzarella
- 3/4 tbsp. baking powder

Directions:
Take a large pan and boil water in it

Add in chicken, bay leaves, black pepper, cloves, and cardamom, and cover and boil for 20 min. at least

Remove the chicken and shred finely and discard the bones

Preheat your mini waffle iron if needed

Mix all the remaining above-mentioned ingredients into a bowl and add in chicken

Grease your waffle iron lightly

Cook your mixture in the mini waffle iron for at least 4 min. or till the desired crisp is achieved and serve hot

Make as many waffles as your mixture and waffle maker allow

Nutrition:
Calories 284
Fat 10.51 g.
Carbs 7.08 g.
Sugar 3.04 g.
Protein: 39.73 g.
Sodium 542 mg.

274. CHICKEN GARLIC WAFFLE ROLL

Preparation time: 10 min.
Cooking time: 30 min.
Servings: 2
Ingredients:

- 1 c. chicken mince
- 1/4 tsp. salt, or as per your taste
- 1/4 tsp. black pepper, or as per your taste
- 2 egg
- 1 tbsp. lemon juice
- 1 c. mozzarella cheese (shredded)
- 2 tbsp. butter
- 1 1/2 tsp. garlic powder
- 1/2 tsp. bay seasoning
- Parsley, for garnishing

Directions:
In a frying pan, melt the butter and add the chicken mince

When done, add salt, pepper, 1 tbsp. garlic powder, and lemon juice and set aside

In a mixing bowl, beat the eggs and add mozzarella cheese to them with 1/2 garlic powder and bay seasoning

Mix them all well and pour into the greasy mini waffle maker

Cook for at least 4 min. to get the desired crunch

Remove the waffle from the heat, add the chicken mixture in between, and fold

Make as many waffles as your mixture and waffle maker allow

Top with parsley

Serve hot and enjoy!

Nutrition:

Calories 822

Fat 30.29 g.

Carbs 5.88 g.

Sugar 2.03 g.

Protein: 124.85 g.

Sodium 1235 mg.

275. PUMPKIN CHICKEN WAFFLES

Preparation time: 10 min.
Cooking time: 10 min.
Servings: 2
Ingredients:

- 1/2 c. boiled chicken
- 1/2 c. pumpkin puree
- 1/4 tsp. pepper
- 1 egg
- 1/2 c. mozzarella cheese (shredded)
- 2 tbsp. almond flour
- A pinch of onion powder
- A pinch of garlic powder
- Salt, as per your taste

Directions:

Mix all the ingredients well together in a bowl

Pour a layer of the mixture on a preheated waffle iron

Close the lid and cook for 5 min.

Serve with your favorite sauce

Nutrition:

Calories 548

Fat 26.34 g.

Carbs 6.63 g.

Sugar 1.46 g.

Protein: 71.1 g.

Sodium 516 mg.

276. GARLICKY CHICKEN PEPPER WAFFLES

Preparation time: 5 min.
Cooking time: 5 min.
Servings: 2
Ingredients:

- 1 egg
- 1/2 c. mozzarella cheese (shredded)
- 2 garlic cloves, chopped
- 1/2 c. pepper, finely chopped
- 1/2 c. chicken, boiled and shredded
- 1 tsp. onion powder
- Salt and pepper, as per your taste

Directions:

Mix all the ingredients well together

Pour a layer on a preheated waffle iron

Cook the waffle for around 5 min.

Make as many waffles as your mixture and waffle maker allow

Nutrition:

Calories 254

Fat 16.3 g.

Carbs 6.63 g.

Sugar 2.57 g.

Protein: 20.13 g.

Sodium 283 mg.

277. SLICED CHICKEN WAFFLES

Preparation time: 10 min.
Cooking time: 25 min.
Servings: 2
Ingredients:

- 2 egg:
- 1 1/2 c. mozzarella cheese (shredded)
- 2 slices American cheese
- 2 boneless slices of chicken
- 1/4 tsp. salt
- 1/4 tsp. black pepper
- 2 tbsp.butter

Directions:

Preheat a mini waffle maker if needed and grease it

In a mixing bowl, beat the eggs and add shredded mozzarella cheese, and mix

Pour the mixture into the lower plate of the waffle maker and close the lid

Cook for at least 4 min. to get the desired crunch

Remove the waffle from the heat

Add the chicken, salt, and pepper together and mix

Fry the chicken in the butter from both sides till they turn golden

Place a cheese slice on the chicken immediately when removing from the heat

Take two waffles and put the chicken and cheese in between

Make as many waffles as your mixture and waffle maker allow

Serve hot and enjoy!

Nutrition:

Calories 420
Fat 24.58 g.
Carbs 7.17 g.
Sugar 4.4 g.
Protein: 41.91 g.
Sodium 1638 mg.

278. GINGER CHICKEN CUCUMBER WAFFLE ROLL

Preparation time: 20 min.
Cooking time: 10 min.
Servings: 2
Ingredients:
For the garlic chicken:

- 1 c. chicken mince
- 1/4 tsp. salt, or as per your taste
- 1/4 tsp. black pepper, or as per your taste
- 1 tbsp. lemon juice
- 2 tbsp. butter
- 2 tbsp. garlic juvenile
- 1 tsp. garlic powder
- 1 tbsp.soy sauce

For the waffle:

- 2 egg
- 1 c. mozzarella cheese (shredded)
- 1 tsp. garlic powder

For serving:s:

- 1/2 c. cucumber (diced)
- 1 tbsp. parsley

Directions:

In a frying pan, melt the butter and add juvenile garlic and sauté for 1 min.

Now add the chicken mince and cook till it tenders

When done, add the rest of the ingredients and set them aside

In a mixing bowl, beat the eggs and add mozzarella cheese to them with garlic powder

Mix them all well and pour into the greasy mini waffle maker

Cook for at least 4 min. to get the desired crunch

Remove the waffle from the heat, add the chicken mixture in between with cucumber, and fold

Make as many waffles as your mixture and waffle maker allow

Serve hot and top with parsley

Nutrition:
Calories 1394
Fat 44.71 g.
Carbs 11.86 g.
Sugar 4.09 g.
Protein: 223.28 g.
Sodium 1717 mg.

279. SPICED CHICKEN WAFFLES WITH SPECIAL SAUCE

Preparation time: 5 min.
Cooking time: 10 min.
Servings: 2
Ingredients:

- 1 egg:
- 1/2 c. mozzarella cheese, shredded
- 1/2 tsp. dried basil
- 1/2 tsp. smoked paprika
- 1 c. chicken, boiled and shredded
- 1 garlic, clove minced
- 1/2 tsp. salt

For the sauce:

- 1/4 c. mayonnaise
- 1 tsp. vinegar
- 3 tbsp. sweet chili sauce
- 1 tbsp. hot sauce

Directions:
Add the egg, dried basil, smoked paprika, chicken, salt, and cheese in a bowl and whisk

Preheat your mini waffle iron if needed and grease it

Cook your mixture in the mini waffle iron for at least 4 min.

Make as many waffles as you can

Combine the sauce ingredient well together

Serve the spicy waffles with the sauce

Nutrition:
Calories 490
Fat 37.32 g.
Carbs 9.02 g.
Sugar 4.14 g.
Protein: 27.63 g.
Sodium 1518 mg.

280. CHICKEN CHEESE CRISPY WAFFLES

Preparation time: 5 min.
Cooking Time: 15 min.
Servings: 2
Ingredients:

- 1 egg
- 1 1/2 c. cheddar cheese
- 1/2 c. ground chicken
- 1/2 tsp. salt
- 1/2 tsp. pepper
- 1 tsp. butter
- Cheese slices, 1 per two waffles

Directions:
Sauté ground chicken in butter and add salt and pepper

Preheat your waffle iron if needed

Mix all the egg and cheddar cheese and whisk well

Grease your waffle iron lightly

Cook in the waffle iron for about 5 min. or till the desired crisp is achieved

Make as many waffles as your mixture and waffle maker allow

Heat the pan and grease it with butter

Place one waffle on the pan and top with the cheese slice and spread the chicken on it

Close with another waffle

Grill this waffle sandwich from both sides and serve hot

Nutrition:
Calories 131

Fat 9.75 g.
Carbs 3.06 g.
Sugar 2.14 g.
Protein: 7.58 g.
Sodium 920 mg.

281. CHICKEN AND BRUSSELS SPROUT WAFFLES

Preparation time: 10 min.
Cooking time: 10 min.
Servings: 2
Ingredients:

- 1/2 c. boiled chicken
- 1/2 c. brussels sprout (shredded)
- 1/4 tsp. pepper
- 1 egg
- 1/2 c. mozzarella cheese (shredded)
- A pinch of onion powder
- A pinch of garlic powder
- Salt, as per your taste

Directions:
Mix all the ingredients well together in a bowl
Pour a layer of the mixture on a preheated waffle iron
Close the lid and cook for 5 min.
Serve with your favorite sauce
Nutrition:
Calories 381
Fat 11.34 g.
Carbs 4 g.
Sugar 1.52 g.
Protein: 62.78 g.
Sodium 446 mg.

282. CHICKEN SWISS WAFFLES WITH DIP

Preparation time: 5 min.
Cooking time: 10 min.
Servings: 2
Ingredients:
For the waffle:

- 1 egg
- 1 c. swiss cheese, shredded
- 2 garlic cloves, finely chopped
- 1 c. chicken, boiled and shredded

For the dip:

- 1/2 c. yogurt
- 1/4 c. mint
- 1/2 tsp. salt
- 1 garlic clove

Directions:
Preheat your mini waffle iron if needed and grease it
Add all the waffle ingredients and whisk
Cook your mixture in the mini waffle iron for at least 4 min.
Make as many waffles as your mixture and waffle maker allow
Blend all the dip ingredients and serve with the waffles
Nutrition:
Calories 637
Fat 48.59 g.
Carbs 12.58 g.
Sugar 7.59 g.
Protein: 36.16 g.
Sodium 744 mg.

283. CRISPY CABBAGE CHICKEN WAFFLES

Preparation time: 5 min.
Cooking time: 25 min.
Servings: 4
Ingredients:

- 2 eggs
- 1 c. mozzarella, shredded
- 2 tbsp. cream cheese

- 1 tbsp. butter
- 1/2 c. onion
- 1/2 c. tomato
- : 1 tbsp. garlic powder
- 1/4 tsp. pepper
- 1/2 tsp. basil
- 1/2 c. cabbage, finely shredded
- 1 c. chicken, boiled and shredded
- 1/4 tsp. salt

Directions:

Take a pan, heat butter and add onion and sauté for a minute

Add tomatoes and chicken and cook for 10 min.

Preheat your mini waffle iron if needed

Mix all the above-mentioned ingredients into a bowl with chicken except for the cabbage and blend using a hand blender

Add the cabbage to the mixture from the top and mix

Grease your waffle iron lightly

Cook your mixture in the mini waffle iron for at least 4 min.

Serve hot with your favorite sauce

Make as many waffles as your mixture and waffle maker allow

Nutrition:

Calories 294
Fat 20.38 g.
Carbs 6.72 g.
Sugar 2.74 g.
Protein: 20.75 g.
Sodium 479 mg.

284. OKRA CHICKEN WAFFLE

Preparation time: 10 min.
Cooking time: 10 min.
Servings: 2
Ingredients:

- 1 egg

- 1/2 c. boiled chicken shredded
- 1/2 c. mozzarella cheese
- 1/2 tbsp. onion powder
- 1 tbsp. mayo
- 2 garlic cloves (finely chopped)
- 1/4 c. almond flour
- 1/2 c. okra
- 1/4 tsp. salt, or as per your taste
- 1/4 tsp. black pepper, or as per your taste

Directions:

Combine the egg and mayo and whisk

When mixed, add almond flour and make a uniform batter

Leave it for 5–10 min.

Now add okra, chicken, and the rest of the ingredients and mix well

Preheat a mini waffle maker if needed and grease it

Pour the mixture to the lower plate of the waffle maker and cook the lid

Cook for at least 4 min. to get the desired crunch

Make as many waffles as your mixture and waffle maker allow and serve hot

Remove from the heat when a bit cool and serve with your favorite sauce

Nutrition:

Calories 139
Fat 9.42 g.
Carbs 3.47 g.
Sugar 0.93 g.
Protein: 10.09 g.
Sodium 311 mg.

285. CHICKEN ZUCCHINI WAFFLE

Preparation time: 12 min.
Cooking time: 25 min.
Servings: 2
Ingredients:

- 1 c. chicken, boneless pieces

- 1 zucchini (small)
- 2 egg
- Salt, as per your taste
- 1 c. shredded mozzarella
- 2 tbsp. parmesan
- pepper, as per your taste
- 1 tsp. basil
- 1/2 c.water

Directions:
In a small saucepan, add the chicken with a 1/2 c. water and boil till chicken tenders
Preheat your waffle iron
Grate zucchini finely
Add all the ingredients to the zucchini in a bowl and mix well
Shred the chicken finely and add it as well
Grease your waffle iron lightly
Pour the mixture into a full-size waffle maker and spread evenly
Cook till it turns crispy
Make as many waffles as your mixture and waffle maker allow
Serve crispy and hot

Nutrition:
Calories 401
Fat 13.52 g.
Carbs 7.29 g.
Sugar 2.71 g.
Protein: 60.08 g.
Sodium 644 mg.

286. GINGERY CHICKEN WAFFLE

Preparation time: 5 min.
Cooking time: 5 min.
Servings: 2
Ingredients:
- 1 egg
- 1/2 c. mozzarella cheese (shredded)
- 2 pieces of chicken, boneless shredded sautéed in butter

- 1/2 tsp. ginger: ground
- 1/2 tsp. ground cinnamon
- 1/4 tsp. ground nutmeg
- 1/8 tsp. ground cloves
- 2 tbsp. almond flour
- 1/2 tsp. baking powder

Directions:
Mix all the ingredients well together
Pour a layer on a preheated waffle iron
Cook the waffle for around 5 min.
Make as many waffles as your mixture and waffle maker allow
Serve hot

Nutrition:
Calories 117
Fat 5.56 g.
Carbs 3.34 g.
Sugar 0.83 g.
Protein: 13.78 g.
Sodium 262 mg.

287. KALE AND CHICKEN WAFFLE

Preparation time: 5 min.
Cooking time: 6 min.
Servings: 3
Ingredients:
- 2 eggs, whisked
- 1/2 c. baby kale, torn
- 1/2 c. mozzarella, shredded
- 1/4 c. cream cheese
- 1/4 c. chicken breast, skinless, cooked, and shredded
- 1/2 tsp. garlic powder
- 2 tbsp. tomato passata

Directions:
In a bowl, mix the eggs with half of the mozzarella, cream cheese, and garlic powder and stir.
Preheat the waffle iron over medium-high heat, pour 1/3 of the waffle mix, cook for 6 min. and transfer to a plate.

Repeat with the rest of the batter, spread the passata over the waffles, divide the kale and chicken and serve.

Nutrition:
Calories 302

Fat 8.3 g.
Fiber 4.2 g.
Carbs 5 g.
Protein 18 g.

CHAPTER 9. DESSERT WAFFLES

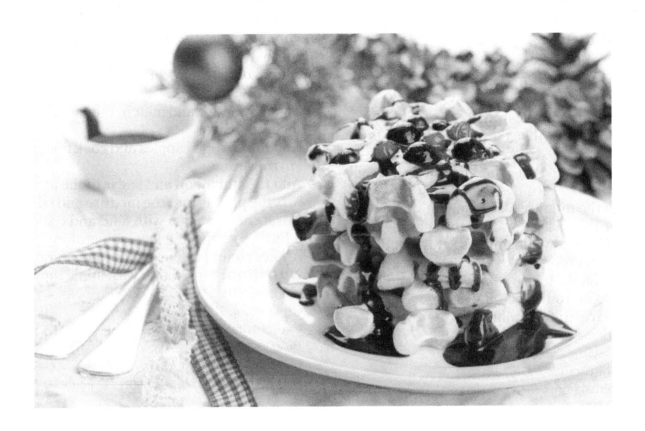

288. BELGIUM WAFFLE

Preparation time: 5 min.
Cooking time: 6 min.
Servings: 1
Ingredients:

- 1 c. grated cheddar cheese
- 2 eggs

Directions:
Preheat the waffle iron.
Beat the eggs then add the grated cheddar cheese.
Make sure that the mixture is well combined.
Cook the mixture for about 6 min.
With this classic waffle, the toppings are just about anything that is keto-friendly. It doesn't even need to be sweet toppings. Experiment to see what you like and keep an eye on your macromolecules.
Nutrition: for 1 waffle
Calories: 460
Cholesterol: 490 mg.
Carbohydrates: 2 g.
Protein: 44 g.
Fat: 33 g.

289. APPLE PIE WAFFLE

Preparation time: 45 min.
Cooking time: 15 min.
Servings: 8 mini waffles
Ingredients:

- 3 eggs
- 1 1/2 c. grated cheddar cheese

For the toppings::

- 4 Gala apples (1 1/4 lb.), chopped finely
- 1/2 tsp. ground cinnamon
- 1/4 c. sugar
- 2 tbsp. butter, melted
- 1/4 c. pecans, chopped

Directions:
For the waffle:
Preheat the waffle iron.

Combine the eggs and cheese well.
Roughly 2 tbsp. is 1 mini waffle.
Add the batter to the waffle iron and cook for about 3 min.
A total of eight waffles can be made with this batter.
Allow cooling and start on the topping.
For the topping::
Take the butter and melt in the saucepan at medium heat.
Add the chopped apples and cook for 2 min. stirring often.
Add the cinnamon and sugar to the apples.
Mix the pecans into the mixture and stir in.
Cover the saucepan with a lid and cook for a further 5 min. at a low temperature.
Apples should be cooked until tender.
Nutrition: for 1 waffle with apple topping
Calories: 250
Cholesterol: 100 mg.
Carbohydrates: 21 g.
Protein: 8 g.
Fat: 16 g.
Sugar: 16 g. (Not keto-friendly)

290. FRENCH TOAST WAFFLE

Preparation time: 5 min.
Cooking time: 10 min.
Servings: 2 mini waffles
Ingredients:

- 1 egg
- 1/2 c. grated mozzarella cheese
- 2 tbsp. almond flour
- 1 tsp. vanilla extract
- 1 tsp. cinnamon
- 1 tsp. granulated sweetener of choice
- Sugar-free cinnamon syrup

Directions:
Preheat your waffle iron.
Mix all the waffle ingredients well.

Use half of the mixture and cook the waffle for about 5 min.

Add an extra minute to the cooking if you want a crispier waffle.

Repeat until all the batter is used.

Add some sugar-free cinnamon syrup and enjoy these waffles still warm.

Nutrition: for 1 mini waffle

Calories: 180

Carbohydrates: 7 g.

Protein: 11 g.

Fat: 12 g.

291.   BANANA   NUT WAFFLE

Preparation time: 3 min.
Cooking time: 8 min.
Servings: 2 mini waffles
Ingredients:

- 1 egg
- 1/4 tsp. vanilla extract
- 1/4 tsp. banana extract
- 1 tbsp. cream cheese, room temperature, and softened
- 1/2 c. grated mozzarella cheese
- 1 tbsp. monk fruit confectioners, or confectioners sweetener of choice
- 1 tbsp. sugar-free cheesecake pudding, optional

For the toppings::

- Pecans
- Sugar-free caramel sauce. or keto-safe sauce of preference

Directions:

Preheat the waffle iron.

Beat the egg before adding the other ingredients and make sure that everything is coated in the egg mixture.

Use half of the batter and cook for about 4 min.

Remove the waffle to rest while cooking the second mini waffle.

Nutrition: for 1 mini waffle

Calories: 119

Cholesterol: 111 mg.

Carbohydrates: 2.7 g.

Protein: 8.8 g.

Fat: 7.8 g.

Sugar: 1.1 g.

292.   BANANA   FOSTER WAFFLE PANCAKES

Preparation time: 5 min.
Cooking time: 20 min.
Servings: 4 regular waffles
For the waffle:

- 4 large eggs
- 1 c. almond flour
- 1/3 c. flaxseed meal
- 1 tsp. vanilla extract
- 1/2 medium banana, slightly overripe
- 4 oz. cream cheese
- 2 tsp. baking powder
- 1/2 tsp. banana extract, optional
- Liquid stevia or sweetener of choice, optional

For the topping::

- 8 tbsp. salted butter
- 1/2 tsp. cinnamon
- 1/2 tsp. vanilla extract
- 1/2 tsp. banana extract
- 1/4 c. sugar-free maple syrup
- 1/2 c. brown sugar substitute or granulated sweetener with maple extract
- 1/2 medium banana, sliced into discs
- 1/8–1/4 tsp. xanthan gum, optional
- 2 tbsp. dark rum or bourbon, optional
- 1/4 c. pecans chopped, optional

Directions:

Preheat the waffle iron or skillet.

Add all the waffle ingredients to a blender and blend until smooth.

Add 1/4 of the batter to the waffle iron and cook for about 2–3 min., add an extra minute to cooking if the waffle isn't set. Repeat until all the batter is used.

For the topping::

At a medium temperature combine the banana extract, rum or bourbon, butter, and vanilla in a skillet.

As the mixture starts to bubble, add the sliced bananas in a single layer and allow them to cook for between 2–3 min. Do not stir.

After the time has passed, add the cinnamon, brown sugar substitute, and sugar-free maple syrup.

Stir and let the mixture simmer until all the brown sugar substitute has become melted and incorporated into the butter.

If the brown sugar substitute isn't blending with the butter, then add the xanthan gum to the simmering mixture. This will also help to thicken up the sauce.

Depending on your preference, you can either add the pecans to the simmering sauce or add it after pouring the batter on the waffles.

Add the warm sauce to the cooled waffles.

Add a scoop or two of keto-friendly ice cream to make a unique taste experience.

Or simply enjoy the waffle with no sauce.

Nutrition: for two regular waffles with 2 1/2 tbsp. of topping

Calories: 417
Cholesterol: 170 mg.
Carbohydrates: 13 g.
Protein: 10 g.
Fat: 37 g.
Sugar: 7 g.

293. CHOCOLATE CHIP WAFFLES

Preparation time: 3 min.
Cooking time: 8 min.
Servings: 2 mini waffles
Ingredients:

- 1/2 c. grated mozzarella cheese
- 1/2 tbsp. granulated Swerve, or sweetener of choice
- 1 tbsp. almond flour
- 2 tbsp. low-carb, sugar-free chocolate chips
- 1 egg
- 1/4 tsp. cinnamon

Directions:

Preheat your waffle iron.

In a bowl, mix the almond flour, egg, cinnamon, mozzarella cheese, Swerve, chocolate chips.

Place half the batter in the waffle iron and cook for 4 min.

Remove the waffle and cook the remaining batter.

Let the waffles cool before serving.

Nutrition: for 1 mini waffle

Calories: 136
Cholesterol: 104 mg.
Carbohydrates: 2 g.
Protein: 10 g.
Fat: 10 g.
Sugar: 1 g.

294. CHOCOLATE WAFFLE

Preparation time: 3 min.
Cooking time: 5 min.
Servings: 1 waffle, 2 mini waffles
Ingredients:

- 1 tsp. vanilla extract
- 1 tbsp. cocoa powder, unsweetened
- 1 egg

- 2 tbsp. almond flour
- 2 tsp. monk fruit
- 1 oz. cream cheese

Directions:
Preheat the waffle iron.
Soften the cream cheese then whisk together the other ingredients well.
Pour the batter into the center of the waffle iron and spread out.
Cook the batter for between 3–5 min.
Remove the waffle once set and serve.
Nutrition: for 1 regular waffle
Calories: 261
Carbohydrates: 4 g.
Protein: 11.5 g.
Fat: 22.2 g.

295. SWEET WAFFLES

Preparation time: 30 min. for waffle
Cooking time: 20 min. for waffle
Servings: 1 s'more, 2 mini waffles
For the waffle:
- 1 egg
- 1/2 tsp. vanilla extract
- 1/4 c. cream cheese
- 2 tbsp. almond flour
- 1 tbsp. sweetener of choice
- 1 tbsp. protein powder, unflavored
- 1/2 tsp. baking powder
- 1 tsp. ground cinnamon

For the sugar-free marshmallow:
- 100 g. (3.5 oz) xylitol, or other baking friendly sweetener
- 3 tbsp. water
- 4 gelatin sheets, or 7 g. gelatin powder

For the chocolate dip:
- 10 g. cacao butter
- 80 g. sugar-free chocolate

Directions:
For the sugar-free marshmallow:
If you do not have sugar-free marshmallow fluff, then it is suggested that you make this up to 8 hours, or even the day before, making the waffle.
Choose a container to set the marshmallow in later. This container needs to be lined with cling film.
Gelatin sheets need to be placed in water for a few minutes before use.
Melt the sugar in a cooking pot and allow it to boil for up to 3 min. before adding the gelatin sheets or powder.
Dissolve the gelatin fully.
Now that the liquid is ready, pour it into an electric mixer.
Mix the mixture until the liquid bulks up and starts to form a white marshmallow-like fluff.
Pour the marshmallow fluff into the previously prepared container and smooth the surface.
Allow the mixture to sit on a kitchen surface for no less than eight hours. For the best possible setting, allow for the fluff to rest overnight to allow it to set into the marshmallow form. Cover with cling film once cool to prevent insects from getting into the mixture.
Once fully set, the marshmallow can be cut into the desired shape.
Dust the marshmallow pieces with powdered sweetener if you want to keep it softer for longer.
For the waffle:
Preheat the waffle iron.
Beat the egg before adding the cinnamon.
Combine the remaining waffle ingredients before adding a few drops of vanilla.
Divide the batter in half and cook each portion for 3 min.

Set the waffles aside to cool.

If you want to prepare the s'mores at home, take the marshmallow fluff and spread it to the thickness of choice on one waffle before adding the second waffle on top.

Set aside the waffles to prepare the chocolate dip.

For the chocolate dip:

Make use of a double boiler or instant pot to melt the cocoa butter and sugar-free chocolate together.

Make sure the mixture is completely smooth before dipping the waffle's edges in it. Coat all the marshmallow fluff.

Put aside and allow the chocolate to harden. Whether you are making this as a snack at home or you take the individual parts with you to go camping, this waffle is something that is a must in your collection.

Nutrition: for 1 s'more sandwich with a marshmallow center, and dipped in chocolate

Calories: 368

Carbohydrates: 3 g.

Protein: 11 g.

Fat: 23 g.

296. THIN MINT COOKIE WAFFLES

Preparation time: 20 min.

Cooking time: 16 min.

Servings: 4 mini waffles

For the waffle:

- 1 c. grated mozzarella cheese
- 2 tbsp. unsweetened cocoa powder
- 2 large eggs
- 3 tbsp. Swerve confectioners, or sweetener of choice

For the filling:

- 6 oz. cream cheese, softened
- 2 tbsp. unsweetened cocoa powder
- 1/2 c. almond flour

- 1/4 c. Swerve confectioners, or sweeteners of choice
- 1 tsp. peppermint extract
- 1/2 tsp. vanilla extract

For the topping::

- 3 tbsp. sugar-free chocolate chips
- 1 tbsp. coconut oil

Directions:

For the waffle:

Preheat the waffle iron.

Mix all the waffle ingredients into a bowl and make sure everything is mixed well.

Cook 1/4 of the batter in the waffle iron for two to 4 min. The longer it is cooked, the crispier it becomes.

Continue to make waffles until the batter is finished.

For the filling and topping::

Combine all the filler ingredients and beat with a hand mixer on high.

Apply the filling to the three cooled waffles, stack, and set aside.

Heat the coconut oil and chocolate chips at 30-second intervals in a microwave until melted together.

Drizzle this over the stacked waffles and serve.

Anyone who is a fan of chocolate will not turn their nose up at this treat!

Nutrition: for 1 mini waffle

Calories: 431

Carbohydrates: 6 g. net

Protein: 16 g.

Fat: 38 g.

297. CHOCOLATE ICE CREAM SUNDAE WAFFLE

Preparation time: 5 min.

Cooking time: 20 min.

Servings: 3 mini waffles

Ingredients:

- 1 egg

- 1/2 tsp. baking powder
- 1 tsp. vanilla extract
- 1/2 c. grated mozzarella cheese
- 2 tbsp. unsweetened cocoa powder
- 3 tbsp. Swerve sweetener, or sweetener of choice

For the toppings:
- 2 c. keto-friendly vanilla ice cream
- Pecans
- Keto-friendly chocolate sauce

Directions:
Preheat the waffle iron.
Mix all the ingredients well.
Use 1/3 of the batter to make a mini waffle and cook for between five to 7 min.
Allow each cooked waffle to cool completely.
Nutrition: for 1 mini waffle only
Calories: 128
Cholesterol: 104 mg.
Carbohydrates: 3 g.
Protein: 9.5 g.
Fat: 8.7 g.
Sugar: 0.7 g.

298. FUDGY CHOCOLATE DESSERT WAFFLES

Preparation time: 5 min.
Cooking time: 20 min.
Servings: 4 mini waffles
Ingredients:
- 2 large eggs
- 2 tsp. coconut flour
- 4 tbsp. grated mozzarella cheese
- 2 tbsp. heavy whipping cream
- 1/2 tsp. baking powder
- 1/2 tsp. vanilla extract
- 1 tbsp. dark cacao (70% cocoa or higher)
- Pinch of salt
- 1/4 tsp. Stevia powder, or powdered sweetener of choice

Directions:
Preheat the waffle iron.
Beat the eggs and cream together before adding the other ingredients to the mixture.
Divide the batter into four parts and add to the waffle iron.
Cook the waffles for about three to 5 min. then remove them from the waffle iron.
Continue until all the batter is gone.
Nutrition: for 1 mini waffle
Calories: 83
Cholesterol: 102.7 mg.
Carbohydrates: 3 g.
Protein: 6.1 g.
Fat: 5.4 g.
Sugar: 0.8 g.

299. VANILLA CAKE WAFFLE

Preparation time: 3 min.
Cooking time: 12 min.
Serving size: 4 mini waffles
For the waffle:
- 2 eggs
- 2 tbsp. cream cheese room temp
- 2 tbsp. melted butter
- 1/4 c. almond flour
- 1 tsp. coconut flour
- 1/2 tsp. baking powder
- 2 tbsp. confectioners sweetener
- 1/4 tsp. Xanthan powder
- 1 tsp. cake batter extract
- 1/2 tsp. vanilla extract

For the whipped cream frosting:
- 1/2 c. heavy whipping cream
- 1/2 tsp. vanilla extract
- 2 tbsp. confectioners sweetener

Directions:
For the waffle:
Preheat the waffle iron

Use a blender to mix all the waffle ingredients. The batter may look a little watery so let it rest for a minute before use.

Add about 3 tbsp. of the batter to the waffle maker.

Cook until golden brown or about 3 min.

Remove the cooked waffle and complete until the batter is finished.

While the fourth waffle is cooking, start on the frosting.

For the frosting:

In a clean bowl, add all the frosting ingredients with a hand mixer.

The whipped cream is perfect when peaks are formed.

Once the waffles are cool, add the frosting. Waffles must be cool or frosting will melt.

Nutrition: for 1 mini waffle

Calories: 144

Cholesterol: 111 mg.

Carbohydrates: 4.7 g.

Protein: 4.7 g.

Fat: 10.2 g.

Sugar: 0.8 g.

300. PUMPKIN WAFFLES

Preparation time: 5 min.

Cooking time: 8 min.

Servings: 3 mini waffles

Ingredients:

- 2 tbsp. pumpkin puree
- 1/2 oz. cream cheese
- 2 1/2 tbsp. erythritol, or sweetener of choice
- 3 tsp. coconut flour
- 1 large egg
- 1/2 tbsp. pumpkin pie spice
- 1/2 c. grated mozzarella cheese
- 1/2 tsp. vanilla extract (optional)
- 1/4 tsp. baking powder (optional)

Directions:

Preheat your waffle pan.

Heat the cream cheese for 15–30 sec. in the microwave to soften it.

Stir all the ingredients in, use optional ingredients only if you want to.

Use half of the batter to make one regular waffle.

Cook till golden brown, about 3–4 min.

Remove from the waffle iron and allow cooling and become crispy.

Nutrition: for 1 mini waffle

Calories: 117

Carbohydrates: 3 g. net

Protein: 7 g.

Fat: 7 g.

301. PUMPKIN CHOCOLATE CHIP WAFFLES

Preparation time: 4 min.

Cooking time: 12 min.

Servings: 3 mini waffles

Ingredients:

- 1/2 c. shredded mozzarella cheese
- 1 tbsp. almond flour
- 4 tsp. pumpkin puree, make your own, or find a keto-friendly
- 2 tbsp. granulated Swerve, or sweetener of choice
- 1 egg
- 1/4 tsp. pumpkin pie spice
- 4 tsp. sugar-free chocolate chips

Directions:

Preheat the waffle iron.

Mix the egg and pumpkin very well.

To the mixture, add the almond flour, Swerve, pumpkin spice, and mozzarella.

Add the sugar-free chocolate chips.

Take half the mixture to make one mini waffle and cook for 4 min.

Once cooked, remove the waffle and cook the remaining batter.

Nutrition: for 1 mini waffle
Calories: 93
Cholesterol: 69 mg.
Carbohydrates: 2 g.
Protein: 7 g.
Fat: 7 g.
Sugar: 1 g.

302. PUMPKIN PECAN WAFFLE

Preparation time: 2 min.
Cooking time: 10 min.
Servings: 2 mini waffles
Ingredients:

- 1 egg
- 2 tbsp. almond flour
- 2 tbsp. pecans, toasted chopped
- 1/2 c. mozzarella cheese grated
- 1/2 tsp. pumpkin spice
- 1 tbsp. pumpkin puree, sugar-free
- 1 tsp. erythritol low-carb, or sweetener of choice

Directions:
Preheat the waffle iron.
First, beat the egg before adding the other ingredients. Make sure everything is coated by the egg.
Depending on the size of your waffle iron spoon in the necessary amount. Don't overfill.
Cook the batter for about 5 min. and repeat with the remaining batter if there is.
Nutrition: for 1 mini waffle
Calories: 210
Carbohydrates: 4.6 g.
Protein: 11 g.
Fat: 17 g.

303. MAPLE PECAN WAFFLES

Preparation time: 5 min.
Cooking time: 8 min.
Servings: 2 mini waffles
Ingredients:

- 1 large egg
- 1 tbsp. sweetener of choice
- 2–3 drops maple flavoring
- 1/2 c. grated mozzarella cheese
- 1 tbsp. pecans, chopped
- 1/4 c. almond flour

Directions:
Preheat the waffle iron.
Whisk the eggs before adding the chopped pecans, sweetener, maple flavoring, mozzarella cheese, almond flour. Mix well.
Take half the batter and cook for between 3–4 min.
Repeat until the batter is used up completely.
Cool each waffle completely before serving.
Nutrition: for 1 mini waffle
Calories: 162
Cholesterol: 108 mg.
Carbohydrates: 2 g.
Protein: 12 g.
Fat: 12 g.
Sugar: 0 g.

304. CHAFFLES WITH TOPPING

Preparation time: 15 minutes
Cooking Time: 10 Minutes
Servings: 3
Ingredients:

- 1 large egg
- 1 tbsp. almond flour
- 1 tbsp. full-fat Greek yogurt
- 1/8 tsp baking powder
- 1/4 cup shredded Swiss cheese
- TOPPING

- 4oz. grill prawns
- 4 oz. steamed cauliflower mash
- 1/2 zucchini sliced
- 3 lettuce leaves
- 1 tomato, sliced
- 1 tbsp. flax seeds

Directions:
Make 3 chaffles with the given chaffles ingredients.
For serving, arrange lettuce leaves on each chaffle.
Top with zucchini slice, grill prawns, cauliflower mash and a tomato slice.
Drizzle flax seeds on top.
Serve and enjoy!
Nutrition: per Servings:
Protein: 45% 71 kcal
Fat: 47% 75 kcal
Carbohydrates: 8% 12 kcal

305. MAPLE PUMPKIN WAFFLE

Preparation time: 5 min.
Cooking time: 16 min.
Servings: 4 mini waffles
Ingredients:

- 2 eggs
- 1/2 c. grated mozzarella cheese
- 3/4 tsp. baking powder
- 2 tsp. pureed pumpkin, no additives
- 3/4 tsp. pumpkin pie spice
- 1/2 tsp. vanilla
- Pinch of salt
- 4 tsp. heavy whipping cream
- 1 tsp. coconut flour

For the toppings::

- 2 tsp. sugar-free maple syrup

Directions:
Preheat the waffle iron.
Whisk together all the ingredients well.

Add 1/4 of the batter to the waffle iron and cook for 3–4 min.
Repeat until all the batter is finished.
Nutrition: for two mini waffles, excluding maple syrup
Calories: 201
Cholesterol: 200 mg.
Carbohydrates: 4 g.
Protein: 12 g.
Fat: 15 g.
Sugar: 1 g.

306. TIRAMISU WAFFLE CAKE

Preparation time: 10 min.
Cooking time: 16 min.
Servings: 4 mini waffles
For the waffle:

- 2 large eggs, room temperature
- 2 tbsp. unsalted butter, melted
- 2 tsp. instant coffee powder
- 1 oz. cream cheese, softened
- 1 tsp. vanilla extract
- 1/4 c. fine almond flour
- 2 tbsp. coconut flour
- 1 tbsp. cocoa powder, gluten-free
- 2 tbsp. powdered sweetener of choice
- 1 tsp. baking powder
- 1/8 tsp. salt

For the filling:

- 4 oz. mascarpone cheese
- 1/4 c. powdered sweetener of choice
- 1/2 tsp. vanilla extract

For the secondary filling:

- 1/2 tsp. instant coffee powder
- 1/2 tbsp. cocoa powder, gluten-free
- 1/2 tsp. hazelnut extract, optional

Directions:
Preheat the waffle iron.
Mix the melted butter and the powdered coffee.

178

With this mixture add the extracts, eggs, and cream cheese. Stir well.

Add the remaining dry ingredients together and mix well.

Pout 1/4 of the mixture into the waffle iron and cook for about 4 min.

Repeat this until all the batter is used.

While the fourth waffle is cooking, start on the cream filling.

For the secondary filling:

In a clean bowl mix the mascarpone, vanilla, and sweetener.

Divide the filling between two bowls. 1 will remain white and be the filling between the waffles.

Once the waffles are cool spread the white filling between layers. Refrigerate for about 20 min.

In the second bowl, add the instant coffee and cocoa and mix well.

Take this second filling and coat the stacked waffles.

Refrigerate the cake for another 30 min. to allow the frosting to set.

Nutrition: for 1 mini waffle

Calories: 302

Carbohydrates: 12 g.

Protein: 8 g.

Fat: 27 g.

Sugar: 6 g.

307. CHOCOLATE CHIP COOKIE WAFFLE CAKE

Preparation time: 10 min.

Cooking time: 5 min.

Servings: 2

Ingredients:

For the cake layer:

- 1 tbsp. butter melted
- 1 tbsp. Golden Monk Fruit Sweetener
- 1 egg yolk
- 1/8 tsp. vanilla essence
- 1/8 tsp. cake batter extract
- 3 tbsp. almond flour
- 1/8 tsp. baking powder
- 1 tbsp. Chocolate Chip Sugar-Free

For the frosting:

- 1 tsp. unflavored gelatin
- 4 tsp. cold water
- 1 cup HWC
- 1 tbsp. sweetener

Directions:

Mix everything and cook on a mini waffle iron for 4 min. Repeat for each layer. I decided to make three.

For the frosting:

Place the beater and mixing bowl in the freezer for about 15 min. to cool.

Sprinkle gelatin on cold water in a microwave-compatible bowl. Stir and "bloom." This takes about 5 min.

Microwave the gelatin mixture for 10 sec. It becomes liquid. Stir to make sure everything is melted.

In a chilled mixing bowl, start whipping the cream at low speed. Add the sweetener.

Do it faster and observe that peaks begin to form.

When the whipped cream has peaked, switch to low speed and squirt the melted liquid gelatin mixture slowly. Once in, switch to high speed and continue tapping until a hard peak is reached. Put it in a piping bag and pipe the cake.

Note:

This recipe uses only half of the whipped cream.

Nutrition:

Calories 84

Total Fat: 4.5 g.

Cholesterol 71.3 mg.

Sodium 122.3 mg.

Total Carbohydrate 5.3 g.

Dietary Fiber 0.9 g.

Sugars 2.1 g.
Protein: 6.1 g.

308. LIME PIE WAFFLE
Preparation time: 15 min.
Cooking time: 8 min.
Servings: 2
Ingredients:
For the waffle:
- 1 egg
- 1/4 c. almond flour
- 2 tsp. cream cheese, at room temperature
- 1 tsp. powdered sweetener swerve or monk fruit
- 1/2 tsp. lime extract or 1 tsp. fresh-squeezed lime juice
- 1/2 tsp. baking powder
- 1/2 tsp. lime zest
- Pinch of salt to bring out the flavors

For the frosting:
- 4 oz. cream cheese softened
- 4 tbsp. butter
- 2 tsp. powdered sweetener swerve or monk fruit
- 1 tsp. lime extract
- 1/2 tsp. lime zest

Directions:
Preheat the mini waffle iron.

In a blender, add all the waffle ingredients and blend on high until the mixture is smooth and creamy.

Cook each waffle for about 3–4 min. until it's golden brown. While the waffles are cooking, make the frosting.

In a small bowl, combine all the ingredients for the frosting and mix it until it's smooth.

Allow the waffles to completely cool before frosting them.

Nutrition:
Calories: 201
Fat: 7 g.

Carbohydrate: 5 g.
Protein: 8 g.

309. WAFFLE CREPES
Preparation time: 20 min.
Cooking time: 11 min.
Servings: 3
Ingredients:
- 1 egg
- 1 tbsp. almond flour
- 1/4 tsp. vanilla extract
- 1/2 tbsp. Swerve Confectioners
- 1 tbsp. cream cheese softened
- 1 tsp. heavy cream
- Pinch of cinnamon

Directions:
Mix all the ingredients in a small blender. Let the batter rest for 5 min.

Pour 1 1/2 tbsp. of the batter in the preheated dash griddle. Cook for 30 sec.

Flip with tongs and cook a few more seconds.

Place 1 slice of the cheese, 1 slice of ham, and 1 slice of turkey on each crepe. If desired, microwave for a few seconds to slightly melt the cheese.

Roll the crepes with the filling on the inside.

Serve the filled crepes sprinkled with Swerve Confectioners and drizzled with low-carb raspberry jam.

Nutrition:
Calories: 63
Fat: 6 g.
Carbohydrate: 5 g.
Protein: 5 g.

310. RICE KRISPIE TREAT WAFFLE (COPYCAT RECIPE)

Preparation time: 7 min.
Cooking time: 9 min.
Servings: 2
Ingredients:
For the waffle:

- 1 large egg room temp
- 2 oz. cream cheese softened
- 1/4 tsp. pure vanilla extract
- 2 tbsp. lakanto confectioners sweetener
- 1 oz. pork rinds crushed
- 1 tsp. baking powder

For the marshmallow frosting:

- 1/4 c. heavy whipping cream
- 1/4 tsp. pure vanilla extract
- 1 tbsp. lakanto confectioners sweetener
- 1/2 tsp. xanthan gum

Directions:
Plug in the mini waffle maker to preheat.
In a medium mixing bowl, add the egg, cream cheese, and vanilla. Whisk until blended well.
Add sweetener, crushed pork rinds, and baking powder. Mix until well incorporated.
Sprinkle extra crushed pork rinds onto the waffle maker (optional).
Then add about 1/4 scoop of the batter, sprinkle a bit more pork rinds.
Cook 3–4 min., then remove and cool on a wire rack.
Repeat for the remaining batter.

Nutrition:
Calories: 321
Fat: 18 g.
Carbohydrate: 15 g.
Protein: 14 g.

311. COFFEE FLAVORED WAFFLE

Preparation time: 5 min.
Cooking time: 8 min.
Servings: 4
Ingredients:

- 4 eggs
- 4 oz. cream cheese
- 1/2 tsp. vanilla extract
- 6 tbsp. strong boiled espresso
- 1/4 c. stevia
- 1/2 c. almond flour
- 1 tsp. baking powder
- Pinch of salt
- 2 tbsp. butter to brush the waffle maker

Directions:
Preheat the waffle maker.
Add the eggs and cream cheese to a bowl and stir in the vanilla extract, espresso, stevia, almond flour, baking powder, and a pinch of salt.
Stir just until everything is combined and fully incorporated.
Brush the heated waffle maker with butter and add a few tablespoons of the batter.
Close the lid and cook for about 7–8 min. depending on your waffle maker.
Serve and enjoy.

Nutrition:
Calories: 303
Fat: 26 g.
Carbohydrate: 3 g.
Protein: 10 g.

312. KETO BOSTON CREAM PIE WAFFLE CAKE

Preparation time: 7 min.
Cooking time: 5 min.
Servings: 4
Ingredients:
For the cake:

- 2 eggs

- 1/4 c. almond flour
- 1 tsp. coconut flour
- 2 tbsp. melted butter
- 2 tbsp. cream cheese room temp
- 20 drops Boston Cream extract
- 1/2 tsp. vanilla extract
- 1/2 tsp. baking powder
- 1/4 tsp. Xanthan powder
- 2 tbsp. swerve confectioners sweetener

For the custard:
- 1/2 c. heavy whipping cream
- 1/2 tsp. vanilla extract
- 1 /2 tbsp. swerve confectioners sweetener
- 2 egg yolks
- 1/8 tsp. xanthan gum

For the ganache:
- 2 tbsp. heavy whipping cream
- 2 tbsp. Unsweetened baking chocolate bar chopped
- 1 tbsp. Swerve Confectioners Sweetener

Directions:
Preheat the mini waffle iron to make the cake waffles first.

In a blender, combine all the cake ingredients and blend it on high until it's smooth and creamy. This should only take a couple of minutes.

On the stovetop, heat the heavy whipping cream to a boil. While it's heating, whisk the egg yolks and Swerve together in a separate small bowl.

Once the cream is boiling, pour half of it into the egg yolks. Make sure you are whisking it together while you pour in the mixture slowly.

Pour the egg and cream mixture back into the stovetop pan into the rest of the cream and stir continuously for another 2–3 min.

Take the custard off the heat and whisk in your vanilla and xanthan gum. Then set it aside to cool and thicken.

Put the ingredients for the ganache into a small bowl. Microwave for 20 sec., stir. Repeat if needed. Be careful not to overheat the ganache and burn it.

Serve your Boston Cream Pie Waffle Cake and Enjoy!

Nutrition:
Calories: 139
Fat: 14 g.
Carbohydrate: 8 g.
Protein: 13 g.

313. COCONUT CREAM CAKE WAFFLE
Preparation time: 10 min.
Cooking time: 7 min.
Servings: 6
Ingredients:
For the waffles:
- 2 eggs
- 1-oz. cream cheese softened to room temperature
- 2 tbsp. finely shredded unsweetened coconut
- 2 tbsp. powdered sweetener blends such as Swerve or Lakanto
- 1 tbsp. melted butter or coconut oil
- 1/2 tsp. coconut extract
- 1/2 tsp. vanilla extract

For the filling:
- 1/3 c. coconut milk
- 1/3 c. unsweetened almond or cashew milk
- 2 eggs yolks
- 2 tbsp. powdered sweetener blends such as Swerve or Lakanto
- 1/4 tsp. xanthan gum
- 2 tsp. butter
- Pinch of salt
- 1/4 c. finely shredded unsweetened coconut

Optional toppings:
- Sugar-free whipped cream
- 1 tbsp. finely shredded unsweetened coconut toasted until lightly brown

Directions:

For the waffles:

Heat the mini waffle iron until thoroughly hot.

Beat all the waffle ingredients together into a small bowl.

Add a heaping 2 tbsp. batter to the waffle iron and cook until golden brown and the waffle iron stops steaming, about 5 min.

Repeat 3 times to make 4 waffles. You only need 3 for the recipe.

For the filling:

Heat the coconut and almond milk in a small saucepan over medium-low heat. It should be steaming hot, but not simmering or boiling.

In a separate bowl, beat the egg yolks together lightly. While whisking the milk constantly, slowly drizzle the egg yolks into the milk.

Heat, constantly stirring until the mixture thickens slightly. Do not boil. Whisk in the sweetener. While constantly whisking, slowly sprinkle in the xanthan gum. Continue to cook for 1 min. Remove from the heat and add the remaining ingredients.

Pour coconut cream filling into a container, cover the surface with plastic wrap and refrigerate until cool. The plastic wrap prevents skin from forming on the filling. The mixture will thicken as it cools.

For the cake assembly:

Spread 1/3 of the filling over each of the 3 waffles, stack them together to make a cake.

Top with whipped cream and garnish with toasted coconut.

Nutrition:

Calories: 153

Fat: 15 g.

Carbohydrate: 7 g.

Protein: 15 g.

314. HOT CHOCOLATE BREAKFAST WAFFLE

Preparation time: 5 min.
Cooking time: 13 min.
Servings: 2
Ingredients:
- 1 egg, beaten
- 2 tbsp. almond flour
- 1 tbsp. unsweetened cocoa powder
- 2 tbsp. cream cheese, softened
- 1/4 c. finely grated Monterey Jack cheese
- 2 tbsp. sugar-free maple syrup
- 1 tsp. vanilla extract

Directions:

Preheat the waffle iron.

In a medium bowl, mix all the ingredients.

Open the iron, lightly grease it with cooking spray, and pour in half of the mixture.

Close the iron and cook until crispy, 7 min.

Remove the waffle onto a plate and set it aside.

Pour the remaining batter into the iron and make the second waffle.

Allow cooling and serve afterward.

Nutrition:

Calories: 174

Fat: 16 g.

Carbohydrate: 3 g.

Protein: 12 g.

315. PUMPKIN-CINNAMON CHURRO STICKS

Preparation time: 7 min.
Cooking time: 7 min.
Servings: 2
Ingredients:
- 3 tbsp. coconut flour
- 1/4 c. pumpkin puree
- 1 egg, beaten
- 1/2 c. finely grated mozzarella cheese
- 2 tbsp. sugar-free maple syrup + more for serving

- 1 tsp. baking powder
- 1 tsp. vanilla extract
- 1/2 tsp. pumpkin spice seasoning
- 1/8 tsp. salt
- 1 tbsp. cinnamon powder

Directions:

Preheat the waffle iron.

Mix all the ingredients into a medium bowl until well combined.

Open the iron and add half of the mixture. Close and cook until golden brown and crispy for 7 min.

Remove the waffle onto a plate and make 1 more with the remaining batter.

Cut each waffle into sticks, drizzle the top with more maple syrup and serve after.

Nutrition:

Calories: 213
Fat: 10 g.
Carbohydrate: 2 g.
Protein: 25 g.

316. PUMPKIN WAFFLE WITH MAPLE SYRUP

Preparation time: 5 min.
Cooking time: 15 min.
Servings: 2
Ingredients:

- 2 eggs, beaten
- 1/2 c. mozzarella cheese, shredded
- 1 tsp. coconut flour
- 3/4 tsp. baking powder
- 3/4 tsp. pumpkin pie spice
- 2 tsp. pureed pumpkin
- 4 tsp. heavy whipping cream
- 1/2 tsp. vanilla
- Pinch salt
- 2 tsp. maple syrup (sugar-free)

Directions:

Turn your waffle maker on.

Mix all the ingredients except maple syrup in a large bowl.

Pour half of the batter into the waffle maker.

Close and cook for 4–5 min.

Transfer to a plate to cool for 2 min.

Repeat the steps with the remaining mixture.

Drizzle the maple syrup on top of the waffles before serving.

Nutrition:

Calories: 222
Fat: 16 g.
Carbohydrate: 8 g.
Protein: 18 g.

317. ALMOND JOY CAKE WAFFLE

Preparation time: 7 min.
Cooking time: 4 min.
Servings: 6
Ingredients:
For the waffles:

- 1 egg
- 1-oz. cream cheese
- 1 tbsp. almond flour
- 1 tbsp. unsweetened cocoa powder
- 1 tbsp. erythritol sweeteners blends such as Swerve, Pyure, or Lakanto
- 1/2 tsp. vanilla extract
- 1/4 tsp. instant coffee powder

For the filling:

- 1 1/2 tsp. coconut oil melted
- 1 tbsp. heavy cream
- 1/4 c. unsweetened finely shredded coconut
- 2 oz. cream cheese
- 1 tbsp. confectioner's sweetener such as Swerve
- 1/4 tsp. vanilla extract
- 14 whole almonds

Directions:
For the waffles:
Reheat the mini Dash waffle iron until thoroughly hot.

In a medium bowl, whisk all the waffle ingredients together until well combined. Pour half of the batter into the waffle iron.

Close and cook 3–5 min., until done. Remove to a wire rack. Repeat for the second waffle.

For the filling:
Soften cream to room temperature or warm in the microwave for 10 sec.

Add all the ingredients to a bowl and mix until smooth and well-combined.

For the assembly:
Spread half the filling on one waffle and place 7 almonds evenly on top of the filling.

Repeat with the second waffle and stack together.

Nutrition:
Calories: 139

Fat: 10 g.

Carbohydrate: 3 g.

Protein: 14 g.

318. CINNAMON ROLL WAFFLES

Preparation time: 15 min.

Cooking time: 20 min.

Servings: 3

Ingredients:

For the batter:
- 1/2 c. shredded mozzarella cheese
- 2 tbsp.golden monk fruit sweetener
- 2 tbsp.SunButter
- 1 egg
- 1 tbsp.coconut flour
- 2 tsp. cinnamon
- 1/4 tsp. vanilla extract
- 1/8 tsp. baking powder

For the frosting:
- 1/4 c. powdered monk fruit sweetener
- 1 tbsp.cream cheese
- 3/4 tbsp. butter, melted
- 1/4 tsp. vanilla extract
- 1 tbsp.unsweetened coconut milk

For the coating:
- 1 tsp. cinnamon
- 1 tsp. golden monk fruit sweetener

Directions:
Turn on the waffle maker to heat and oil it with cooking spray.

Combine all the batter components in a bowl, then set aside and leave for 3–5 min. In another bowl, whisk all the frosting components until well-combined.

Divide the batter into 3 portions and spoon 1 part into the waffle maker.

Cook for 2–4 min., until golden brown.

Open and let the waffle cool for 30 sec. in the waffle maker before you transfer it to a plate.

Repeat with the remaining batter.

While the waffles are warm, sprinkle with cinnamon and the sweetener coating.

When cooled a little, drizzle with the icing.

Nutrition:
Calories: 195

Fat: 15 g.

Carbohydrate: 4 g.

Protein: 10 g

319. RED VELVET WAFFLE

Preparation time: 5 min.

Cooking time: 15 min.

Servings: 3

Ingredients:
- 1 egg
- 1/4 c. mozzarella cheese, shredded
- 1 oz. cream cheese
- 4 tbsp. almond flour
- 1 tsp. baking powder
- 2 tsp. sweetener

- 1 tsp. red velvet extract
- 2 tbsp. cocoa powder

Directions:

Combine all the ingredients into a bowl.

Plug in your waffle maker.

Pour 1/3 of the batter into the waffle maker.

Seal and cook for 4–5 min.

Open and transfer to a plate.

Repeat the steps with the remaining batter.

Nutrition:

Calories: 125

Fat: 10 g.

Carbohydrate: 3 g.

Protein: 10 g.

320. SWEET RASPBERRY WAFFLE

Preparation time: 5 min.

Cooking time: 5 min.

Servings: 2

Ingredients:

- 1 tsp. baking powder
- 2 eggs
- 1 c. mozzarella cheese
- 2 tbsp. almond flour
- 4 raspberries, chopped
- 1 tsp. cinnamon
- 10 drops Stevia, liquid

Directions:

Reheat the mini waffle maker until hot

Whisk the eggs in a bowl, add the cheese, then mix well

Stir in the remaining ingredients (except toppings, if any)

Grease the preheated waffle maker with non-stick cooking spray

Scoop 1/2 of the batter onto the waffle maker, spread across evenly

Cook until a bit browned and crispy, about 4 min.

Cook 3–4 min., until done as desired (or crispy)

Gently remove from the waffle maker and let it cool

Repeat with the remaining batter

Top with keto syrup

Serve and enjoy!

Nutrition:

Calories: 116

Net carbs: 1 g.

Fat: 8 g.

Protein: 8 g.

321. OREO WAFFLE

Preparation time: 10 min.

Cooking time: 20 min.

Servings: 2 mini waffles

Ingredients:

- 2 tsp. coconut flour
- 3 tbsp. cocoa, unsweetened
- 1 tsp. baking powder
- 4 tbsp. swerve sweetener
- 1 tsp. vanilla extract, unsweetened
- 2 tbsp. heavy cream
- 2 eggs, at room temperature
- 2 tbsp. whipped cream

Directions:

Take a non-stick waffle iron, plug it in, select the medium or medium-high heat setting and let it preheat until ready to use; it could also be indicated with an indicator light changing its color.

Meanwhile, prepare the batter, and for this, take a large bowl, add flour in it along with the other ingredients and mix with an electric mixer until smooth.

Use a ladle to pour 1/4 of the prepared batter into the heated waffle iron in a spiral direction, starting from the edges, then shut the lid and cook for 5 min. or more until solid and nicely browned; the cooked waffle will look like a cake. When done, transfer the waffle to a plate with a silicone spatula and repeat with the remaining batter.

When done, prepare the Oreo sandwiches, and for this, spread 1 tbsp. whipped cream on one side of two waffles and then cover with the remaining waffles.

Serve immediately.

Nutrition:
Cal: 400
Fat: 38.8 g.
Protein: 9.6 g.
Carb: 7.5 g.
Fiber: 2.6 g.
Net Carb: 4.9 g.

322. BROWNIE BATTER WAFFLE

Preparation time: 10 min.
Cooking time: 25 min.
Servings: 16 mini waffles
Ingredients:
- 1/2 c./50 g. almond flour
- 1/2 c./75 g. chopped chocolate, unsweetened
- 1 tsp. baking powder
- 1/4 tsp. salt
- 1/4 c./40 g. cocoa powder, unsweetened
- 1/4 tsp. liquid stevia
- 1/2 c./100 g. Swerve Sweetener
- 1/2 tsp. vanilla extract, unsweetened
- 12 tbsp. coconut butter
- 5 eggs, at room temperature

Directions:
Take a non-stick waffle iron, plug it in, select the medium or medium-high heat setting and let it preheat until ready to use; it could also be indicated with an indicator light changing its color.

Meanwhile, prepare the batter and for this, take a saucepan, place it over medium heat, add cocoa powder, chocolate, and butter and cook for 3–4 min. until the butter has melted, whisking frequently.

Then add sweetener, stevia, and vanilla into the pan, stir until combined, remove the pan from the heat and let it stand for 5 min.

Take a medium bowl, add flour in it and then stir in baking powder and salt until mixed.

After 5 min., beat the egg into the chocolate-butter mixture and stir the flour until incorporated.

Use a ladle to pour 1/4 c. of the prepared batter into the heated waffle iron in a spiral direction, starting from the edges, then shut the lid and cook for 5 min. or more until solid and nicely browned; the cooked waffle will look like a cake. When done, transfer the waffle to a plate with a silicone spatula and repeat with the remaining batter.

Let the waffles stand for some time until crispy and serve straight away.

Nutrition:
Cal: 170
Fat: 16 g.
Protein: 4.2 g.
Carb: 4 g.
Fiber: 2 g.
Net Carb: 2 g.

323. BLUEBERRY WAFFLE

Preparation time: 10 min.
Cooking time: 25 min.
Servings: 5 mini waffles
Ingredients:
- 3 tbsp. frozen blueberries
- 2 tbsp. almond flour
- 2 tsp. Swerve sweetener
- 1 tsp. baking powder
- 1 tsp. cinnamon
- 2 eggs, at room temperature
- 1 c./135 g. shredded mozzarella cheese

Directions:
Take a non-stick mini waffle iron, plug it in, select the medium or medium-high heat setting and let it preheat until ready to use; it could also

be indicated with an indicator light changing its color.

Meanwhile, prepare the batter and for this, take a large bowl, add flour in it, then add the remaining ingredients and stir well until smooth and incorporated.

Use a ladle to pour 1/5 of the prepared batter into the heated waffle iron in a spiral direction, starting from the edges, then shut the lid and cook for 4 min. or more until solid and nicely browned; the cooked waffle will look like a cake.

When done, transfer the waffle to a plate with a silicone spatula and repeat with the remaining batter.

Let the waffles stand for some time until crispy, then sprinkle swerve confectioner over them and serve straight away.

Nutrition:
Cal: 119
Fat: 8.2 g.
Protein: 8.5 g.
Carb: 3.6 g.
Fiber: 1 g.
Net Carb 2.6 g.

324. CREAM CHEESE WAFFLE

Preparation time: 10 min.
Cooking time: 20 min.
Servings: 4 mini waffles
Ingredients:

- 4 tsp. coconut flour
- 8 tsp. swerve sweetener
- 1/2 tsp. baking powder
- 1 tsp. vanilla extract, unsweetened
- 4 tbsp. cream cheese, softened
- 2 eggs, at room temperature

Directions:
Take a non-stick waffle iron, plug it in, select the medium or medium-high heat setting and let it preheat until ready to use; it could also be indicated with an indicator light changing its color.

Meanwhile, prepare the batter and for this, take a large bowl, add flour in it, stir in baking powder, and sweetener until mixed.

Then add vanilla, egg, and cream cheese and mix with an electric mixer until smooth.

Use a ladle to pour one-fourth of the prepared batter into the heated waffle iron in a spiral direction, starting from the edges, then shut the lid and cook for 5 min. or more until solid and nicely browned; the cooked waffle will look like a cake.

When done, transfer the waffles to a plate with a silicone spatula and repeat with the remaining batter.

Let waffles stand for some time until crispy, and serve with your favorite toppings.

Nutrition:
Calories 175
Fat 14.3 g.
Protein 8.2 g.
Carb 1.5 g.
Fiber 0 g.
Net Carb 1.5 g.

325. KETO RED VELVET WAFFLE CAKE

Preparation time: 10 min.
Cooking time: 5 min.
Servings: 2
Ingredients:

- 2 tbsp. dutch-processed cocoa
- 2 tbsp. monk fruit confectioner's
- 1 egg
- 2 drops of optional super drop food coloring
- 1/4 tsp. baking powder
- 1 tbsp. heavy whipped cream

Frosted ingredients:

- 2 tbsp. monk fruit confectioners

- 2 tbsp. cream cheese softens, room temperature
- 1/4 tsp. transparent vanilla

Directions:
Put the eggs into a small bowl.
Add the remaining ingredients and mix well until smooth and creamy.
Put half of the butter in a mini waffle pan and cook for 2 1/2–3 min. until completely cooked.
Put the sweetener, cream cheese, and vanilla in separate small pots. Mix the frosting until everything mixes well.
When the waffle cake has completely cooled to room temperature, spread the frosting.

Nutrition:
Calories 75
Total Fat: 5.8 g.
Cholesterol 101.5 mg.
Sodium 39.8 mg.
Total Carbohydrate 4.1 g.
Dietary Fiber 2 g.
Sugars 0.4 g.
Protein: 4.4 g.
Vitamin A 70.8µg
Vitamin C 0 mg.

326. KETO CHOCOLATE FUDGE WAFFLE

Preparation time: 10 min.
Cooking time: 14 min.
Servings: 2
Ingredients:
- 1 egg, beaten
- 1/4 c. finely grated gruyere cheese
- 2 tbsp. unsweetened cocoa powder
- 1/4 tsp. baking powder
- 1/4 tsp. vanilla extract
- 2 tbsp. erythritol
- 1 tsp. almond flour
- 1 tsp. heavy whipping cream
- A pinch of salt

Directions:
Preheat the waffle iron.
Add all the ingredients to a medium bowl and mix well.
Open the iron and add half of the mixture. Close and cook until golden brown and crispy, 7 min.
Remove the waffle onto a plate and make another with the remaining batter.
Cut each waffle into wedges and serve after.

Nutrition:
Calories 173
Fats 13.08 g.
Carbs 3.98 g.
Net carbs 2.28 g.
Protein 12.27 g.

327. NUTMEG RAISINS CAKE WAFFLE

Preparation time: 10 min.
Cooking time: 10 min.
Servings: 4
Ingredients:
- 1/2 c. coconut flour
- 1/2 c. coconut cream
- 3 tbsp. cream cheese, soft
- 1 tsp. nutmeg, ground
- 1/4 c. raisins
- 4 eggs, whisked
- 1 tsp. baking soda
- 2 tbsp. stevia

Directions:
In a bowl, mix the cream cheese with the flour and the other ingredients except for the coconut cream, raisins, and stevia and whisk well.
Heat up the waffle iron, pour 1/4 of the batter, cook for 10 min., and transfer to a plate.
Repeat with the rest of the batter and cool the waffles down.

In a bowl, mix the rest of the ingredients and stir really well.

Layer the waffles and the raisins mix and serve the cake cold.

Nutrition:

Calories 324

Fat 12 g.

Fiber 3 g.

Carbs 4 g.

Protein 11 g.

328. CHOCOLATE CHERRY CAKE WAFFLES

Preparation time: 10 min.

Cooking time: 10 min.

Servings: 4

Ingredients:

- 2 tbsp. dark chocolate chips, unsweetened and melted
- 2 tbsp. ghee, melted
- 1/2 c. cherries, pitted and chopped
- 2 tbsp. stevia
- 1 egg, whisked
- 1 tbsp. cream cheese, soft
- 1/2 tsp. baking soda
- 1/2 c. almond flour
- 1/4 c. almond milk

Directions:

In a bowl, mix the flour with the egg, milk, and the other ingredients, except the cherries, ghee, and chocolate, and whisk well.

Heat up the waffle iron, divide the batter into 4 servings and cook the waffles.

In a bowl, mix the rest of the ingredients and whisk.

Layer the waffles and the cherry mix and serve.

Nutrition:

Calories 151

Fat 13 g.

Fiber 2 g.

Carbs 5 g.

Protein 8 g.

329. WAFFLE STRAWBERRY SANDWICH

Preparation time: 5 min.

Cooking time: 0 min.

Servings: 2

Ingredients:

- 1/4 c. heavy cream
- 4 oz. strawberry slice

For the waffle:

- 1 egg
- 1/2 c. mozzarella cheese

Directions:

Make 2 waffles with the waffle ingredients Meanwhile, mix together the cream and strawberries.

Spread this mixture over the waffle slice.

Drizzle the chocolate sauce over a sandwich.

Serve and enjoy!

Nutrition:

Amount per serving 80 g.

Total calories 253

Fats 22.15 g.

Protein 11.34 g.

Net carbs 0.42 g.

Fiber 0.9 g.

Starch 0 g.

330. CRUNCHY COCONUT WAFFLES CAKE

Preparation time: 5 min.

Cooking time: 15 min.

Servings: 4

Ingredients:

- 4 large eggs
- 1 c. shredded cheese
- 2 tbsps. coconut cream
- 2 tbsps. coconut flour.
- 1 tsp. stevia

For the topping:

- 1 c. heavy cream
- 8 oz. raspberries
- 4 oz. blueberries
- 2 oz. cherries

Directions:

Make 4 thin round waffles with the waffle ingredients. Once the waffles are cooked, set in layers on a plate.

Spread heavy cream in each layer.

Top with raspberries then blueberries and cherries.

Serve and enjoy!

Nutrition:

Amount per serving 216 g.
Total calories 318
Fats 26.05 g.
Protein 15.72 g.
Net carbs 0.26 g.
Fiber 1.1 g.
Starch 0 g.

331.   DOUBLE   DECKER WAFFLE

Preparation time: 5 min.
Cooking time: 10 min.
Servings: 2
Ingredients:

- 1 large egg
- 1 c. shredded cheese

For the topping:

- 1 keto chocolate ball
- 2 oz. cranberries
- 2 oz. blueberries

Directions:

Make 2 mini dash waffles.

Put the cranberries and blueberries in the freezer for about 2 hours.

For serving, arrange the keto chocolate ball between 2 waffles.

Top with frozen berries.

Serve and enjoy!

Nutrition:

Amount per serving 148 g.
Total calories 333
Fats 24.83 g.
Protein 19.33 g.
Net carbs 2.37 g.
Fiber 2 g.
Starch 0.01 g.

332.   YOGURT WAFFLE

Preparation time: 5 min.
Cooking time: 10 min.
Servings: 4
Ingredients:

- 1/2 c. mozzarella cheese, shredded
- 1/2 c. cheddar cheese, shredded
- 1 egg
- 2 tbsps. ground almonds
- 1 tsp. psyllium husk
- 1/4 tsp. baking powder
- 1 tbsp. Greek yogurt

For the topping:

- 1 scoop heavy cream, frozen
- 1 scoop raspberry puree, frozen
- 2 raspberries

Directions:

Mix together all of the waffle ingredients and heat up your waffle maker.

Let the batter stand for 5 min.

Spray the waffle maker with cooking spray.

Spread some cheese on the waffle maker and pour the waffle mixture into a heart-shaped Belgian waffle maker.

Close the lid and cook for about 4–5 min.

For serving, scoop the frozen cream and puree in the middle of the waffle.

Top with a raspberry.

Serve and enjoy!

Nutrition:

Amount per serving 45 g.
Total calories 133
Fats 9.75 g.

Protein 10.02 g.
Net carbs 1.59 g.
Fiber 0.1 g.
Starch 0 g.

333.   KETO WAFFLE WITH ICECREAM

Preparation time: 5 min.
Cooking time: 5 min.
Servings: 2
Ingredients:

- 1 egg
- 1/2 c. cheddar cheese, shredded
- 1 tbsp. almond flour
- 1/2 tsp. baking powder

For serving:

- 1/2 c. heavy cream
- 1 tbsp. keto chocolate chips
- 2 oz. raspberries
- 2 oz. blueberries

Directions:
Preheat your mini waffle maker according to the manufacturer's instructions.
Mix together the waffle ingredients into a small bowl and make 2 mini waffles.
For an ice cream ball, mix cream and chocolate chips in a bowl and pour this mixture into 2 silicone molds.
Freeze the ice cream balls in a freezer for about 2–4 hours.
For serving, set the ice cream ball on the waffle.
Top with berries and enjoy!
Nutrition:
Amount per serving 87 g.
Total calories 273
Fats 24.61 g.
Protein 11.42 g.
Net carbs 1 g.
Fiber 0.1 g.
Starch 0 g.

334.   WAFFLES ICECREAM FOR THE TOPPING

Preparation time: 5 min.
Cooking time: 0 min.
Servings: 2
Ingredients:

- 1/4 c. coconut cream, frozen
- 1 c. coconut flour
- 1/4 c. strawberries chunks
- 1 tsp. vanilla extract
- 1 oz. chocolate flakes
- 4 keto the waffles

Directions:
Mix together all ingredients in a mixing bowl.
Spread the mixture between 2 waffles and freeze in the freezer for 2 hours.
Servings chill and enjoy!
Nutrition:
Amount per serving 125 g.
Total calories 263
Fats 20.98 g.
Protein 16.26 g.
Net carbs 0.59 g.
Fiber 0.1 g.
Starch 0.1 g.

335.   WAFFLES WITH STRAWBERRY FROSTY

Preparation time: 5 min.
Cooking time: 0 min.
Servings: 2
Ingredients:

- 1 c. frozen strawberries
- 1/2 c. heavy cream
- 1 tsp. stevia
- 1 scoop protein powder
- 3 keto the waffles

Directions:
Mix together all ingredients in a mixing bowl.

192

Pour the mixture into silicone molds and freeze in a freezer for about 4 hours to set. Once the frosty is set, top on keto the waffles and enjoy!

Nutrition:
Amount per serving 141 g.
Total calories 142
Fats 11.22 g.
Protein 1.09 g.
Net carbs 0.95 g.
Fiber 0.4 g.
Starch 0 g.

336.   CHOCOLATE BROWNIE WAFFLES

Preparation time: 5 min.
Cooking time: 5 min.
Servings: 2
Ingredients:

*   2 tbsp. cocoa powder
*   1 egg
*   1/4 tsp. baking powder
*   1 tbsp. heavy whipping cream
*   1/2 c. mozzarella cheese

Directions:
Beat the egg with a fork in a small mixing bowl.
Add the remaining ingredients to a beaten egg and beat well with a beater until the mixture is smooth and fluffy.
Pour the batter into a greased preheated waffle maker.
Close the lid.
Cook the waffles for about 4 min. until they are thoroughly cooked.
Servings with berries and enjoy!

Nutrition:
Amount per serving 69 g.
Total calories 162
Fats 11.22 g.
Protein 12.97 g.
Net carbs 2.45 g.

Fiber 1.6 g.
Starch 0 g.

337.   CREAM   PUFF WAFFLES

Preparation time: 5 min.
Cooking time: 12 min.
Servings: 4
Ingredients:

*   2 eggs
*   2 oz. cream cheese, softened
*   1 tbsp. coconut flour
*   1 tbsp. heavy cream
*   1 tsp. vanilla extract
*   1/2 tsp. baking powder
*   1/4 tsp. stevia powder
*   1/2 tsp. ground cinnamon

For the custard filling:

*   4 egg yolks
*   1 tbsp. stevia powder
*   1/4 tsp. xanthan gum
*   1 c. heavy cream
*   1 tbsp. vanilla extract

For dusting:
*   1/2 tsp. confectioner's sweetener

Directions:
Preheat the waffle maker.
Blend all the waffle ingredients together.
Into the preheated waffle maker, pour about 1/4 of the batter.
Close the lid. Cook for 5–6 min.
Remove the cooked waffle using a pair of tongs.
Repeat step 3 to cook the remaining batter.
Prepare the custard filling by whisking stevia and egg yolks. Add in the xanthan gum and combine well.
Place a saucepan over medium heat. Add in the heavy cream and bring to a simmer.
Add the heavy cream to the egg yolk mixture and whisk quickly.

Transfer the mixture onto the saucepan and continue stirring with a spatula or whisk. Continue whisking until the mixture thickens.

Turn off the heat. Continue to stir for 20 or 30 sec.

Mix in the vanilla.

Using a fine-mesh sieve, strain the custard cream. Place a cling wrap over it and refrigerate for an hour.

Take out the cold custard from the fridge. Remove the wrap and transfer to a bowl. Cut it using a whisk and place it in a piping bag.

Using a knife, cut small pockets in each waffle.

Begin piping the custard cream into the waffle pockets.

Dust the waffles with the powdered sweetener.

Nutrition:
Calories: 390
Carbohydrates: 3.2 g.
Fat: 37.7 g.
Protein: 9.1 g.

338. CHOCOLATE CHIP CANNOLI WAFFLES

Preparation time: 5 min.
Cooking time: 12 min.
Servings: 4
Ingredients: for the chocolate chip waffle:

- 1 tbsp. butter, melted
- 1 tbsp. monk fruit
- 1 egg yolk
- 1/8 tsp. vanilla extract
- 3 tbsp. almond flour
- 1/8 tsp. baking powder
- 1 tbsp. chocolate chips, sugar-free

For the cannoli topping:

- 2 oz. cream cheese
- 2 tbsp. low-carb confectioners sweetener
- 6 tbsp. ricotta cheese, full fat
- 1/4 tsp. vanilla extract
- 5 drops lemon extract

Directions:
Preheat the mini waffle maker.

Mix all the ingredients for the chocolate chip waffle in a mixing bowl. Combine well to make a batter.

Place half the batter on the waffle maker. Allow cooking for 3–4 min.

While waiting for the waffles to cook, start making your cannoli topping by combining all ingredients until the consistency is creamy and smooth.

Place the cannoli topping on the cooked waffles before serving.

Nutrition:
Calories: 187
Carbohydrates: 7 g.
Fat: 13 g.
Protein: 7 g.

339. SUPER EASY CHOCOLATE WAFFLES

Preparation time: 5 min.
Cooking time: 5 min.
Servings: 2
Ingredients:

- 1/4 c. unsweetened chocolate chips
- 1 egg
- 2 tbsps. almond flour
- 1/2 c. mozzarella cheese
- 1 tbsp. Greek yogurts
- 1/2 tsp. baking powder
- 1 tsp. stevia

Directions:
Switch on your square waffle maker.

Spray the waffle maker with cooking spray.

Mix together all the recipe ingredients in a mixing bowl.

Spoon the batter in a greased waffle maker and make two waffles.

Once the waffle is cooked, remove it from the maker.

Serve with coconut cream, shredded chocolate, and nuts on top.

Enjoy!

Nutrition:

Amount per serving 78 g.

Total calories 170

Fats 11.08 g.

Protein 14.25 g.

Net carbs 1.39 g.

Fiber 0.2 g.

Starch 0.01 g.

340. DOUBLE CHOCOLATE WAFFLES

Preparation time: 5 min.

Cooking time: 5 min.

Servings: 2

Ingredients:

- 1/4 c. unsweetened chocolate chips
- 2 tbsps. cocoa powder
- 1 c. egg whites
- 1 tsp. coffee powder
- 2 tbsps. almond flour
- 1/2 c. mozzarella cheese
- 1 tbsp. coconut milk
- 1 tsp. baking powder
- 1 tsp. stevia

Directions:

Switch on your Belgian waffle maker.

Spray the waffle maker with Cooking spray.

Beat the egg whites with an electric beater until fluffy and white.

Add the rest of the ingredients to the egg whites and mix them again.

Pour the batter into a greased waffle maker and make two fluffy waffles.

Once the waffles are cooked, remove them from the maker.

Servings with coconut cream and berries

Enjoy!

Nutrition:

Amount per serving 167 g.

Total calories 188

Fats 8.28 g.

Protein 22.84 g.

Net carbs 2.59 g.

Fiber 0.7 g.

Starch 0.01 g.

341. OREO COOKIES WAFFLES

Preparation time: 5 min.

Cooking time: 5 min.

Servings: 3

Ingredients:

- 1 egg
- 2 tbsps. almond flour
- 1 tbsp. peanut butter
- 1/2 tsp. baking powder
- 1 tsp. stevia
- 2 tbsps. cream cheese
- 2 tbsps. black cocoa powder
- 1 tbsp. mayonnaise
- 2 tbsps. chocolate chips

Directions:

In a small bowl, beat an egg with an electric beater.

Add the remaining ingredients and mix well until the batter is smooth and fluffy.

Divide the batter into 3 portions.

Pour the batter into a mini round greased waffle maker.

Cook the oreo waffle cookies for about 2–3 min. until cooked.

Drizzle coconut flour on top.

Serve and enjoy!

Nutrition:

Amount per serving 46 g.

Total calories 134
Fats 10.66 g.
Protein 7.18 g.
Net carbs 0.88 g.
Fiber 0.3 g.
Starch 0.01 g.

342. CHOCO AND STRAWBERRIES WAFFLES

Preparation time: 5 min.
Cooking time: 5 min.
Servings: 2
Ingredients:

- 1 tbsp. almond flour
- 1/2 c. strawberry puree
- 1/2 c. cheddar cheese
- 1 tbsp. cocoa powder
- 1/2 tsp. baking powder
- 1 large egg.
- 2 tbsps. coconut oil
- 1/2 tsp. vanilla extract optional

Directions:
Preheat the waffle iron while you are mixing the ingredients.
Melt oil in a microwave.
In a small mixing bowl, mix together flour, baking powder, cocoa powder, and vanilla until well combined.
Add the egg, melted oil, 1/2 c. cheese and strawberry puree to the flour mixture.
Pour 1/8 c. cheese in a waffle maker and then pour the mixture in the center of the greased waffle.
Again, sprinkle cheese on the batter.
Close the waffle maker.
Cook the waffles for about 4–5 min. until cooked and crispy.
Once the waffles are cooked, remove and enjoy!
Nutrition:
Amount per serving 113 g.
Total calories 312

Fats 27.91 g.
Protein 11.93 g.
Net carbs 2.06 g.
Fiber 1.6 g.
Starch 0.02 g.

343. CHOCO AND SPINACH WAFFLES

Preparation time: 5 min.
Cooking time: 5 min.
Servings: 2
Ingredients:

- 1 tbsp. almond flour
- 1/2 c. chopped spinach
- 1/2 c. cheddar cheese
- 1 tbsp. cocoa powder
- 1/2 tsp. baking powder
- 1 large egg.
- 2 tbsps. almond butter
- 1/2 tsp. salt
- 1/2 tsp. pepper

Directions:
Preheat the waffle iron while you are mixing the ingredients.
Blend all ingredients in a blender until mixed.
Pour 1/8 c. cheese in a waffle maker and then pour the mixture in the center of a greased waffle.
Again, sprinkle cheese on the batter.
Close the waffle maker.
Cook the waffles for about 4–5 min. until cooked and crispy.
Once the waffles are cooked, remove and enjoy.
Nutrition:
Amount per serving 83 g.
Total calories 187
Fats 14.25 g.
Protein 12.13 g.
Starch 0 g
Net carbs 2.19 g.

Fiber 1.2 g.

344. WAFFLES AND ICECREAM PLATTER

Preparation time: 5 min.
Cooking time: 5 min.
Servings: 2
Ingredients:

- 2 keto brownie waffles
- 2 scoop of vanilla keto ice cream
- 8 oz. strawberries, sliced
- Keto chocolate sauce
- **Directions:**

Arrange the waffles, ice cream, strawberries slice in a serving plate.
Drizzle chocolate sauce on top.
Serve and enjoy!

Nutrition:
Amount per serving 83 g.
Total calories 187
Fats 14.25 g.
Protein 12.13 g.
Net carbs 2.19 g.
Fiber 1.2 g.
Starch 0 g.

345. WAFFLES ICECREAM TOPPING

Preparation time: 5 min
Cooking time: 0 minute
Servings: 2
Ingredients

- 1/4 cup coconut cream, frozen
- 1 cup coconut flour
- ¼ cup strawberries chunks
- 1 tsp. Vanilla extract
- 1 oz. Chocolate flakes
- 4 keto chaffles

Directions
Mix together all Ingredients in a mixing bowl.
Spread mixture between 2 chaffles and freeze in the freezer for 2 hours.
Servings chill and enjoy!

Nutrition:
Amount per serving 125 g
Total calories263 kcal
Fats20.98 g
Protein16.26 g
Net carbs0.59 g
Fiber0.1 g
Starch0.1 g

CHAPTER 10. WAFFLE CAKE RECIPES

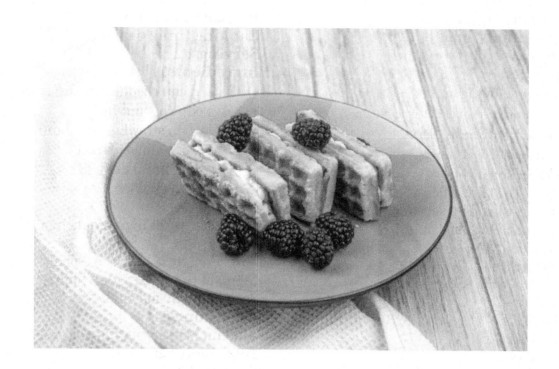

346. KETO WAFFLE BIRTHDAY CAKE

Preparation time: 10 min.
Cooking time: 10 min.
Servings: 4
Ingredients:
For the icing:
- Buttercream Icing

For the waffle:
- tbsp. room temperature cream cheese
- tbsp. almond flour
- tbsp. coconut flour
- 1 tsp. baking powder
- eggs
- tbsp. birthday cake syrup

Directions:

Mix all of the waffle ingredients in a medium-sized mixing bowl and stir until a pancake-like appearance is achieved.

Place 2–3 tbsp. of the batter in your waffle maker. Remove after 2 min. of cooking.

You can now put the cake together after you've made four cake waffles. You'll start with your base cake, then add a layer of buttercream icing, and so on, just like every other cake.

It's really easy to include a surprise inside. Fill the middle with bright shredded coconut or sugar-free sprinkles after piping the icing around the outside.

When you've finished all of the layers, cover with more icing and sprinkles.

Enjoy!

Nutrition:

Calories 384
Fat 35 g.
Total Carbs 23 g.
Fiber 3 g.
Sugar Alcohol 16 g
Protein 11 g.
Net Carbs 4 g.

347. KETO PUMPKIN WAFFLE CAKE

Preparation time: 10 min.
Cooking time: 12 min.
Servings: 4
Ingredients:
For the cake:
- 2 large eggs
- 1/4 c. pumpkin puree
- 2 tbsp. brown sugar substitute
- 2 tsp. pumpkin pie spice
- 2 tsp. coconut flour
- 1/2 tsp. vanilla
- 1 c. finely shredded mozzarella cheese

For the frosting:
- 4 oz. room temperature cream cheese
- 1/4 c. room temperature butter
- 1/2 c. powdered sweetener
- 1 tsp. vanilla
- 1/4 c. chopped pecans

Directions:

Turn on the waffle cooker. Using a non-stick spray, coat the surface.

In a shallow mixing cup, whisk together the eggs, pumpkin puree, sweetener, pumpkin pie spice, coconut flour, and vanilla.

Add the cheese and mix well.

1/4 of the batter can be spooned onto the heated waffle iron and smoothed down to the edges.

Cook for 3 min. after closing the iron.

Remove the waffle from the pan and set it aside. Continue for the last batter.

Allow the waffles to cool completely before frosting them.

To make the frosting, use an electric mixer to whip together the cream cheese and butter until smooth and fluffy. Blend in the powdered sweetener and vanilla extract until smooth.

Place the frosting on top of one waffle and top with another waffle. Repeat the layers, finishing with a frosting coat.

To finish, scatter chopped pecans on top.

Nutrition:
Calories 455
Fat 34.98 g.
Total Carbs 27.29 g.
Fiber 1.6 g.
Sugar 21.31 g.
Protein 9.6 g.
Net Carbs 4 g.

348.   CHOCOLATE WAFFLE CAKE

Preparation time: 2 min.
Cooking time: 8 min.
Servings: 2
Ingredients:
For the waffle cake:
- 2 tbsp. cocoa powder
- 2 tbsp. swerve granulated sweetener
- 1 egg
- 1 tbsp. heavy whipping cream
- 1 tbsp. almond flour
- 1/4 tsp. baking powder
- 1/2 tsp. extract of vanilla

For the frosting:
- 2 tbsp. cream cheese
- 2 tsp. swerve confectioners
- 1/8 tsp. extract of vanilla
- 1 tsp. heavy cream

Directions:
Whisk together chocolate powder, swerve, almond flour, and baking powder in a shallow bowl.

Mix in the vanilla extract and heavy whipping cream until well mix.

Mix up the egg thoroughly. Scrape the sides of the bowl to ensure that all of the ingredients are thoroughly mixed.

Allow 3–4 min. for the mini waffle maker to heat up.

Cook for 4 min. with half of the waffle mixture in the waffle maker. Cook the second waffle after that. Create the frosting while the second chocolate keto waffle is baking.

For the frosting:
tsp. cream cheese in a shallow microwave-safe bowl. To melt the cream cheese, place it in the microwave for 8 sec.

Using a handheld hand mixer to thoroughly mix the hard whipping cream and vanilla extract.

Then, using the hand mixer, incorporate the confectioners' swerve and fluffy the frosting.

For the waffle cake:
On a pan, place one chocolate waffle and a layer of frosting on top. You may use a knife to scatter it or a pastry bag to pipe the frosting.

Place the second chocolate waffle on top of the frosting layer before spreading or piping the remaining frosting on top.

Nutrition:
Calories: 151
Carbohydrates: 5 g.
Protein: 6 g.
Fat: 13 g.
Cholesterol: 111 mg.
Sodium: 83 mg.
Potassium: 190 mg.

349.   KETO STRAWBERRY SHORTCAKE WAFFLE

Preparation time: 5 min.
Cooking time: 2 min.
Servings: 2
Ingredients:
- 2 tbsp. room temperature cream cheese
- 2 room temperature eggs
- 1tsp butter extract of vanilla
- 1 tbsp. almond flour
- 2 tbsp. coconut flour
- 1 tbsp. monk fruit sweetener

- 1/2 tsp. baking powder
- 1/4 tsp. salt

For the whipped cream:
- 1/2 c. heavy whipping cream
- 2 tsp. monk fruit sweetener
- 1 tsp. extract of vanilla

For the topping:
- 5 sliced strawberries
- 1 tbsp. sugar-free strawberry syrup

Directions:

Mix all the waffle ingredients in a medium mixing bowl and stir until a pancake-like batter forms.

Fill your mini waffle maker with 3 tsp. or 1 big ice cream scoop of the batter. Remove after 2 min. of cooking.

Mix the ingredients for the whipped cream in a bowl. Mix with medium to high speed with a handheld mixer until rigid peaks form. It takes about 2–3 min. to complete this task.

After you've made two shortcake waffles and the whipped cream, it's time to put it all together. Start with a waffle foundation, then top with whipped cream and sliced strawberries. Finish with whipped cream and a few strawberry slices for the second layer.

If desired, drizzle with sugar-free strawberry syrup and serve.

Nutrition:

Calories: 393
Carbohydrates: 25.67 g.
Protein: 11.16 g.
Fat: 27.46 g.
Cholesterol: 678 mg.
Sodium: 510 mg.
Potassium: 176 mg.
Fiber: 1 g.

350. KETO CHOCOLATE WAFFLE

Preparation time: 5 min.
Cooking time: 4 min.
Servings: 2
Ingredients:
- 1 large egg
- 1 tbsp. melted butter
- 1/2 tsp. vanilla extract
- 2 tbsp. almond flour
- 2 tbsp. unsweetened cocoa powder
- 1/4 tsp. baking powder
- 1 tbsp. erythritol
- 1/4 c. Shredded mozzarella or 1/3 c. for extra-crispiness (optional)
- 1 tsp. sugar-free chocolate chip (serving suggestion per chaffle)

Directions:

Heat a mini waffle iron for about 5 min., and grease it with coconut oil with a pastry brush.

Mix the egg, melting butter, and vanilla extract in a medium mixing bowl.

Mix almond flour, cocoa powder, baking powder, and erythritol in a large mixing bowl.

You have two alternatives now that the batter is smooth.

Stir in the melted mozzarella for a crispy waffle or fry the waffle without cheese for a light chocolate waffle. For a mild crispy texture, I use 1/4 c. shredded mozzarella; for a super crispy waffle, I use 1/3 c.

Pour enough batter to completely coat the iron's top, leaving some space along the edges to keep the batter from spilling during baking. I used about 2 1/2 tbsp. of the batter for one mini iron the waffle maker.

To stop dry waffles, cook for no more than 3–4 min. When you open the iron, the waffle will not be crispy, but it will be set, not runny, and it will not stick to the iron.

To clear the border from the waffle iron, use the tip of a knife or fork to loosen it. Yes, the waffle is really fluffy, but that's fine! When they cool off, they crisp up!

Crisp the waffle by placing it on a cooling rack for 5 min. In the meantime, bake the remaining batter to make two more mini waffles.

Nutrition:
Calories: 210
Carbohydrates: 16.49 g.
Protein: 11.16 g.
Fat: 14.61 g.
Cholesterol: 133 mg.
Sodium: 243 mg.
Potassium: 282 mg.
Fiber: 2.3 g.

351. KETO ITALIAN CREAM CAKE

Preparation time: 10 min.
Cooking time: 30 min.
Servings: 2
Ingredients:
For the cake:
- 2 1/2 c. almond flour
- 6 large eggs
- 2 sticks of butter
- 1 c. 0% Greek yogurt
- 1/2 c. almond milk
- 1/4 c. swerve
- 2 tsp. vanilla
- 1 tsp. baking soda
- 3/4 tsp. baking powder
- 1 tsp. cinnamon
- 1/2 tsp. nutmeg
- 1/2 tsp. salt
- 1 c. chopped walnuts
- 1 c. shredded unsweetened coconut

For the icing:
- 16 oz. cream cheese
- 1 stick unsalted butter
- 4 tsp. THM Sweet Blend
- 2 tsp. vanilla
- 1/2 tsp. salt
- 1 tsp. cinnamon
- 1/2 tsp. nutmeg
- 1 c. almonds
- 1 c. shredded coconut

Directions:
For the cake:
Both of the dry ingredients (except the sweetener) should be thoroughly mixed.

Blend butter and sweetener thoroughly in a blender.

After that, add the yogurt, eggs, and almond milk.

Mix the dry ingredients into the wet ingredients slowly.

Two 9-in. circular cake pans should be well greased.

Pour the flour into both pans equally.

Heat the oven at 350 °F and then bake for 30–35 min. The knife would be spotless.

Allow for full cooling before transferring to a cake tray.

For the icing:
Mix the cream cheese and butter in a mixing bowl.

Mix the sweetener, vanilla, salt, almonds, and coconut in a mixing bowl.

Mix well.

Later, there would be an ice bottom.

Place the top layer on top.

Ice the cake's top and bottom.

Have fun!

Nutrition:
Calories: 1561
Carbohydrates: 41.76 g.
Protein: 37.48 g.
Fat: 142.54 g.
Cholesterol: 133 mg.
Sodium: 3104 mg.
Potassium: 1573 mg.

Fiber: 12.2 g.

352. KETO NUT FREE ITALIAN LEMON CREAM CAKE

Preparation time: 30 min.
Cooking time: 30 min.
Servings: 2
Ingredients:
For the cake:
- 1 c. coconut flour
- 1/2 c. swerve confectioners
- 1 tsp. baking soda
- 1 tsp. baking powder
- 1/4 tsp. salt
- 1 tsp. glucomannan or xanthan gum
- 1/2 c. sour cream
- 1/2 c. butter softened
- 1/2 c. heavy cream
- 1 tsp. lemon extract
- 1/2 tsp. lemon liquid stevia
- 6 large eggs

For the filling:
- 8 oz. softened mascarpone cheese or cream cheese
- 1/2 c. Swerve confectioners
- 1/2 tsp. lemon zest
- 1 tbsp. lemon juice
- 1 c. heavy cream

For the topping:
- 1/2 c. coconut flour
- 1 tsp. lemon juice
- 1/3 c. Swerve confectioners
- 1/4 tsp. vanilla liquid stevia
- 1 stick cold butter, cut into pieces or 1/2 c. of

Directions:
For the cake:
Heat oven to 350 °F. Put aside two 9-in. spring-shaped pans that have been greased.

Mix coconut flour, Swerve, baking soda, baking powder, salt, and glucomannan or xanthan gum in a large mixing bowl. Remove from the equation.

Mix the sour cream, melted butter, heavy cream, lemon extract, and stevia in a stand mixer or an electric hand mixer and blend until smooth. Add one egg at a time before it is well mixed. Blend in half of the dry ingredients until thoroughly mixed. Mix in the remaining dry ingredients until well mixed.

Fill every cake pan uniformly with cake batter. Cook for 25–30 min., or until a toothpick inserted in the middle comes out clean. Allow 5 min. to cool before loosening the sides of the cake with a butter knife. Allow the spring shape pan to cool fully before removing the sides.

For the filling:
Blend all of the ingredients, except the heavy cream, until smooth in a clean bowl or stand mixer with the paddle attachment. Taste and, if necessary, change the sweetener. Pour in the heavy cream and whisk on medium-high until smooth and thickened, using the whisk attachment. Refrigerate until the cake has finished cooking and has cooled.

For the topping:
In a food processor, mix the dry ingredients and process until smooth. Pour in the cool butter. Pulse till you have crumbs.

For the assemble:
Place one layer of cake on a serving tray. 3/4 of the filling can be spread on the cake, with 1/4 reserved for the top layer. Cover the filling with the second cake layer. Cover the top of the remaining filling. Sprinkle the crumb topping over the top and sides of the cake with your

fingertips, gently pressing it into the cake. Keep chilled until ready to serve.

Nutrition:
Calories: 2779
Carbohydrates: 97.56 g.
Protein: 25.75 g.
Fat: 258.59 g.
Cholesterol: 1171 mg.
Sodium: 2,936 mg.
Potassium: 1,212 mg.
Fiber: 2.1 g.

353. CHOCOLATE CUP OF WAFFLE CAKE

Preparation time: 3 min.
Cooking time: 3 min.
Servings: 2
Ingredients:

- 1 beaten large egg
- 2 tbsp. dark cocoa powder
- 2 tbsp. granulated sweetener
- 1/4 tsp. baking powder
- 1/2 tsp. extract of vanilla
- 1 tbsp. heaving whipping cream

Directions:
Mix all of the ingredients in a bowl.
Pour half of the batter into a mini waffle maker and cook for 3 min., or until the waffle maker is no longer steaming.
Allow for cooling on a cooling rack for 5–10 min.
For a second waffle, repeat steps 2 and 3.
Create a frosting of 2 tbsp. cream cheese, 2 tbsp. Swerve confectioners, and 1/4 tsp. vanilla extract and spread it between two of these waffles for a delicious dessert sandwich. There will be enough frosting to make two "sandwiches."

Nutrition:
Calories: 31
Carbohydrates: 0.74 g.
Protein: 1.35 g.
Fat: 2.26 g.
Cholesterol: 92 mg.

Sodium: 5 mg.
Potassium: 76 mg.
Fiber: 0 g.

354. GERMAN CHOCOLATE WAFFLE CAKE

Preparation time: 20 min.
Cooking time: 30 min.
Servings: 2
Ingredients:

- 2 eggs
- 1 tbsp. melted butter
- 1 tbsp. cream cheese softened to room temperature
- 2 tbsp. unsweetened cocoa powder or unsweetened raw cacao powder
- 2 tbsp. almond flour
- 2 tsp. coconut flour
- 2 tbsp. Pyure granulated sweetener blend
- 1/2 tsp. baking powder
- 1/2 tsp. instant coffee granules dissolved in 1 tbsp. hot water
- 1/2 tsp. extract of vanilla
- 2 pinches salt

For the filling:

- 1 egg yolk
- 1/4 c. heavy cream
- 2 tbsp. Pyure granulated sweetener blend
- 1 tbsp. butter
- 1/2 tsp. caramel extract
- 1/4 c. chopped pecans
- 1/4 c. unsweetened flaked coconut
- 1 tsp. coconut flour

Directions:
For the waffle:
Heat the mini waffle iron.

In a bowl, whisk together all of the ingredients until well mixed.

Fill a waffle iron halfway with batter, close it, and cook for 3–5 min., or until baked.

Place on a wire rack to cool.

Repeat 3 times more.

For the filling:

Mix the egg yolk, heavy cream, butter, caramel extract, and sweetener in a shallow saucepan over medium heat.

Simmer for 5 min., stirring continuously.

Take out from the heat and whisk in the coconut flour, pecans, and flaked coconut.

Nutrition:

Calories: 3159

Carbohydrates: 367.13 g.

Protein: 39.12 g.

Fat: 184.9 g.

Cholesterol: 900 mg.

Sodium: 2463 mg.

Potassium: 2439 mg.

Fiber: 21.1 g.

355. KETO STRAWBERRY CAKE WAFFLE

Preparation time: 10 min.

Cooking time: 35 min.

Servings: 2

Ingredients:

- 1 egg
- 1-oz. cream cheese
- 1/2 tsp. vanilla
- 1 tbsp. almond flour
- 1 tbsp. monk fruit confectioners blend
- 10 drops OOOFlavors Strawberry Souffle
- 10 drops OOOFlavors Cake Batter
- 2 drops red food coloring
- Top with sliced strawberries

For the frosting:

- 1 tbsp. cream room temp cheese
- 1 tbsp. room temp butter
- 1 tbsp. monk fruit confectioners blend
- 9 drops OOOFlavors Strawberry Souffle

Directions:

Add the egg to a bowl and then whisk it with a hand whisk until moist.

Mix with the remaining ingredients until all is well mixed.

Heat the waffle maker for mini waffles.

Pour half of the batter into a mini waffle maker (or all of the batter into a big waffle maker) and cook for 3 min., or until finished.

Cook the other strawberry cake waffle in the same manner.

Allow the waffle cakes to cool completely before frosting.

To make a larger cake, double the recipe.

When the waffles are cooling, make the strawberry frosting.

Mix all of the ingredients in a deep mixing bowl and mix with a small hand mixer. If you like more frosting, you can double or triple the recipe.

After the cake has cooled, frost it and line it with strawberries!

Enjoy!

Nutrition:

Calories: 5036

Carbohydrates: 1047.75 g.

Protein: 98.82 g.

Fat: 37.84 g.

Cholesterol: 344 mg.

Sodium: 5990 mg.

Potassium: 2163 mg.

Fiber: 21.2 g.

356. LOW-CARB CAKE BATTER WAFFLES

Preparation time: 5 min.

Cooking time: 5 min.

Servings: 3

Ingredients:

- 3 tbsp. egg whites

- 1/2-oz. mozzarella cheese
- 1/2 tsp. baking powder
- 1/2 tsp. cake batter flavoring
- 1 tsp. sprinkles
- 2 tbsp. whipped topping optional

Directions:

Except for the sprinkles, mix all the ingredients in a mixing bowl. Spray a mini waffle maker or a regular waffle maker with cooking spray.

Fill the waffle maker halfway with batter and top with sprinkles. Cook for 4–5 min.

Nutrition:

Calories: 74
Carbohydrates: 4 g.
Protein: 8 g.
Fat: 2 g.

357. STRAWBERRY CHEESECAKE SWEETHEART WAFFLE

Preparation time: 15 min.
Cooking time: 10 min.
Servings: 2
Ingredients:

- 3 tbsp. egg white
- 1 tbsp. + 1 tsp. coconut flour
- 1 tsp. oat fiber
- 2 drops graham cracker crust flavoring
- 1 tbsp. cream cheese
- 1 pinch baking powder
- 1–2 pinch of pink Himalayan salt

For the cheesecake mixture:

- 1/4 c. heavy whipping cream
- 2 drops strawberry extract
- 15–20 drops cheese-cake flavor drops
- 1 tsp. classic monk fruit
- 1 tbsp. lily's choco chips
- 2–3 tbsp. cream cheese
- 1 tsp. coconut oil
- 1 chopped strawberry

Directions:

Add the choco chips in a shallow microwaveable bowl; microwave in 10–15 sec. intervals, stirring frequently, until fully melted

To set the strawberry, dip it in the chocolate and put it on parchment paper.

Assemble the waffles

Place your chocolate-dipped strawberry on top or on the side and decorate with whipped topping if desired.

Enjoy!

Nutrition:

Calories: 1,106
Carbohydrates: 120.85 g.
Protein: 17.46 g.
Fat: 61.68 g.

358. 10 MINUTE KETO RED VELVET WAFFLE CAKE

Preparation time: 15 min.
Cooking time: 15 min.
Servings: 2
Ingredients:

- 2 eggs
- 2 oz. cream cheese
- 1/4 c. coconut flour
- 2 tbsp. buttermilk
- 1 1/2 tbsp. monk fruit
- 1 tsp. baking powder
- 1/2 tsp. cocoa powder
- Red food coloring

For the frosting:

- 4 oz. cream cheese
- 6 tbsp. softened unsalted butter
- 2 tsp. vanilla
- 1/2 c. Sugar-free White Chocolate Chips, melted
- 1 c. powdered sugar substitute

Directions:

In a shallow mixing bowl, mix all of the ingredients for the red velvet waffle. Stir all together with an electric mixer.

Pour 1/4 of the batter into a preheated waffle maker. Cook for 3–5 min. or until the sauce has thickened.

Remove the batter and do the same for the remaining batter.

For the frosting:

To make the frosting, whisk together cream cheese, butter, and vanilla extract in a medium mixing bowl until smooth.

Slowly beat in the white chocolate and powdered sugar replacement until smooth.

Assemble your cake:

Start assembling your cake until your red velvet waffles have cooled.

Place one waffle on the baking sheet, sprinkle cream cheese frosting on top, and top with a second waffle.

Continue laying out the cake tiers until you've used up enough of your waffles.

Serve with a cream cheese frosting on the outside.

Nutrition:

Calories: 617
Carbohydrates: 7.8 g.
Protein: 17.2 g.
Fat: 57.37 g.

359.   CAKE WAFFLE

Preparation time: 10 min.
Cooking time: 8 min.
Servings: 4
Ingredients:

- 1/4 c. almond flour
- 2 eggs, whisked
- 2 tbsp. cream cheese, soft
- 2 tbsp. ghee, melted
- 1/2 tsp. vanilla extract
- 1/2 tsp. baking powder

- 2 tbsp. stevia
- 1/2 c. whipping cream
- 2 tbsp. swerve
- 1/2 tsp. almond extract

Directions:

In a bowl, mix the flour with the eggs and the other ingredients except for the whipping cream, swerve, and almond extract and whisk well.

Heat up the waffle iron, divide the batter into 4 parts, cook the waffles one at a time and cool them down.

In a bowl, mix the remaining ingredients and whisk well.

Layer the waffles and the frosting mix and serve the cake cold.

Nutrition:

Calories 140
Fat 10.2 g.
Fiber 1 g.
Carbs 4.7 g.
Protein 4.7 g.

360.   CREAMY   VANILLA CAKE WAFFLE

Preparation time: 10 min.
Cooking time: 10 min.
Servings: 2
Ingredients:

- 1-oz. cream cheese, soft
- 1 egg, whisked
- 2 tbsp. coconut flour
- 4 tbsp. heavy cream
- 2 tsp. stevia
- 1/2 tsp. vanilla extract
- 1/2 tsp. cake batter extract
- 1/2 tsp. baking soda
- 1/2 c. ghee, melted
- 1/2 c. swerve

Directions:

In a bowl, mix the cream cheese with the egg, 1 tbsp. heavy cream, flour, stevia, vanilla, cake batter extract, and baking soda and whisk well.

Heat up the waffle iron, pour half of the batter, cook for 10 min. and transfer to a plate.

Repeat with the rest of the batter and cool the waffles down.

In a bowl, mix the ghee with the remaining heavy cream and the other ingredients and whisk.

Layer the waffles and the frosting mix and serve the cake.

Nutrition:

Calories 252
Fat 9.3 g.
Fiber 2.3 g.
Carbs 12 g.
Protein 3.4 g.

361. COCONUT CAKE WAFFLE

Preparation time: 10 min.
Cooking time: 10 min.
Servings: 4
Ingredients:

- 3 tbsp. heavy cream
- 1/2 c. coconut cream
- 3 tbsp. cream cheese, soft
- 4 tbsp. coconut flour
- 1 tbsp. almond flour
- 4 eggs, whisked
- 1 tsp. baking powder
- 2 tbsp. swerve

Directions:

In a bowl, mix the cream cheese with the flour and the other ingredients except for the coconut and heavy cream and whisk.

Heat up the waffle iron, pour 1/4 of the batter, cook for 10 min. and transfer to a plate.

Repeat with the rest of the batter and cool the waffles down.

In a bowl, mix the cream with the coconut cream and whisk.

Layer the waffles and the coconut cream mixture and serve the cake cold.

Nutrition:

Calories 384
Fat 32 g.
Fiber 3 g.
Carbs 23 g.
Protein 11 g.

362. CHOCOLATE CAKE WAFFLES

Preparation time: 10 min.
Cooking time: 10 min.
Servings: 4
Ingredients:

- 2 tbsp. cocoa powder
- 2 tbsp. stevia
- 1 egg, whisked
- 1 tbsp. heavy cream
- 1/2 tsp. baking soda
- 1 tbsp. almond flour
- 1/2 c. cream cheese, soft
- 1 tbsp. swerve

Directions:

In a bowl, mix the cocoa with the stevia and the other ingredients except for the cream cheese and swerve and whisk.

Heat up the waffle iron, divide the batter into 4 parts, and cook the waffles.

In a bowl, mix the cream cheese with the swerve and whisk.

Layer the waffles and the cream cheese mix and serve the cake cold.

Nutrition:

Calories 151
Fat 13 g.
Fiber 2 g.
Carbs 5 g.
Protein 6 g.

363. BUTTERY CAKE WAFFLES

Preparation time: 10 min.
Cooking time: 10 min.
Servings: 4
Ingredients:

- 1 c. almond flour
- 1 c. almond milk
- 2 tsp. baking powder
- 2 eggs, whisked
- 1/2 c. Greek yogurt
- 1/2 tsp. almond extract
- 1/2 tsp. vanilla extract
- 4 oz. cream cheese, soft
- 1/4 c. butter, melted
- 3 tbsp. swerve

Directions:

In a bowl, mix the flour with the milk and the other ingredients except for the cream cheese, butter, and swerve and whisk.

Heat up the waffle iron, pour 1/4 of the batter, cook for 7 min., and transfer to a platter.

Repeat with the rest of the waffle batter and cool them down.

In a bowl, mix the rest of the ingredients and whisk.

Layer the waffles and the buttery mix and serve the cake cold.

Nutrition:

Calories 520
Fat 22 g.
Fiber 1 g.
Carbs 32 g.
Protein 10 g.

364. KETO CHOCOLATE WAFFLE CAKE

Preparation time: 5 min.
Cooking time: 5 min.
Servings: 3
Ingredients:

- 2 tbsp. cocoa
- 2 tbsp. monk fruit confectioner's
- 1 egg
- 1/4 tsp. baking powder
- 1 tbsp. heavy whipped cream

For the frosting:

- 2 tbsp. monk fruit confectioners
- 2 tbsp. cream cheese softens, room temperature
- 1/4 tsp. transparent vanilla

Directions:

Whip the egg into a small bowl.

Add the rest of the ingredients and mix well until smooth and creamy.

Pour half of the batter into a mini waffle maker and cook until fully cooked for 2 1/2–3 min.

Add the sweetener, cream cheese, and vanilla in a separate small bowl. Mix the frosting until all is well embedded.

Spread the frosting on the cake after it has cooled down to room temperature.

Nutrition:

Calories 120
Total Fat 10.5 g.
Cholesterol 87.2 mg.
Sodium 87.3 mg.
Total carbohydrate 9.2 g.
Dietary Fiber 1.4 g.
Sugars 1.1 g.
Protein 4.1 g.

365. KETO VANILLA TWINKIE COPYCAT WAFFLE

Preparation time: 5 min.
Cooking time: 4 min.
Servings: 4
Ingredients:

- 2 tbsp. butter (cooled)
- 2 oz. cream cheese softened
- 2 large eggs at room temperature
- 1 tsp. vanilla essence
- Optional 1/2 tsp. vanilla cupcake extract
- 1/4 c. lakanto confectionery
- Pinch of salt
- 1/4 c. almond flour
- 2 tbsp. coconut powder
- 1 tsp. baking powder

Directions:

Preheat the corndog maker.

Melt the butter and let cool for 1 min.

Whisk the butter until the eggs are creamy.

Add vanilla, extract, sweetener, and salt and mix well.

Add almond flour, coconut flour, baking powder.

Mix until well incorporated.

Add 2 tbsp. batter to each well and spread evenly.

Close and lock the lid and cook for 4 min.

Remove and cool the rack.

Nutrition:

Calories 152
Total Fat: 9 g.
Cholesterol 100.7 mg.
Sodium 727.7 mg.
Total carbohydrate 6.5 g.
Dietary Fiber 1.6 g.
Sugars 2.4 g.
Protein: 6.1 g.

366. EASY SOFT CINNAMON ROLLS WAFFLE CAKE

Preparation time: 5 min.
Cooking time: 12 min.
Servings: 3
Ingredients:

- 1 egg
- 1/2 c. mozzarella cheese
- 1/2 tsp. vanilla
- 1/2 tsp. cinnamon
- 1 tbsp. monk fruit confectioners blend

Directions:

Put the egg into a small bowl.

Add the remaining ingredients.

Spray to the waffle maker with a non-stick cooking spray.

Make two waffles.

Separate the mixture.

Cook half of the mixture for about 4 min. or until golden.

Notes added glaze: 1 tbsp. cream cheese melted in a microwave for 15 sec., and 1 tbsp. of monk fruit confectioners mix. Mix it and spread it over the moist fabric.

Additional frosting: 1 tbsp. cream cheese (high temp), 1 tbsp. room temp butter (low-temp), and 1 tbsp. monk fruit confectioners' mix. Mix all the ingredients together and spread to the top of the cloth.

Top with optional frosting, glaze, nuts, sugar-free syrup, whipped cream, or simply dust with monk fruit sweets.

Nutrition:

Calories 106
Total Fat: 6.6 g.
Cholesterol 107 mg.
Sodium 182.3 mg.
Total carbohydrate 4.6 g.
Dietary Fiber 0.3 g.
Sugars 2.7 g.

Protein: 8.2 g.

367. KETO PEANUT BUTTER WAFFLE CAKE

Preparation time: 5 min.
Cooking time: 5 min.
Servings: 2
Ingredients:
For the waffle:

- 2 tbsp. sugar-free peanut butter powder
- 2 tbsp. monk fruit confectioner's
- 1 egg
- 1/4 tsp. baking powder
- 1 tbsp. heavy whipped cream
- 1/4 tsp. peanut butter extract

For the frosting:

- 2 tbsp. monk fruit confectioners
- 1 tbsp. sugar-free natural peanut butter or peanut butter powder
- 2 tbsp. cream cheese softens, room temperature
- 1/4 tsp. vanilla

Directions:

Put the egg into a small bowl.

Add the remaining ingredients and mix well until the dough is smooth and creamy.

If you don't have peanut butter extract, you can skip it. It adds absolutely wonderful, more powerful peanut butter flavor and is worth investing in this extract.

Pour half of the butter into a mini waffle maker and cook for 2–3 min. until it is completely cooked.

In another small bowl, add sweetener, cream cheese, sugar-free natural peanut butter, and vanilla. Mix the frosting until everything is well incorporated.

When the waffle cake has completely cooled to room temperature, spread the frosting.

Or you can even pipe the frost!

Or you can heat the frosting and add 1/2 tsp. water to make the peanut butter are pill and drizzle over the waffle! I like it anyway!

Nutrition:

Calories 92
Total Fat: 7 g.
Cholesterol 97.1 mg.
Sodium 64.3 mg.
Total carbohydrate 3.6 g.
Dietary Fiber 0.6 g.
Sugars 1.8 g.
Protein: 5.5 g.

368. KETO ITALIAN CREAM WAFFLE CAKE

Preparation time: 5 min.
Cooking time: 3 min.
Servings: 1
Ingredients:
For a sweet waffle:

- 4 oz. cream cheese softens, room temperature
- 4 eggs
- 1 tbsp. butter
- 1 tsp. vanilla essence
- 1/2 tsp. cinnamon
- 1 tbsp. monk fruit sweetener or favorite keto-approved sweetener
- 4 tbsp. coconut powder
- 1 tbsp. almond flour
- 1 1/2 c. baking powder
- 1 tbsp. coconut
- 1 walnut chopped

For the frosting:

- 2 oz. cream cheese softens, room temperature
- 2 c. butter room temp
- 2 tbsp. monk fruit sweetener or favorite keto-approved sweetener
- 1/2 tsp. vanilla

Directions:

In a medium blender, add cream cheese, eggs, melted butter, vanilla, cinnamon, sweeteners, coconut flour, almond flour, and baking powder. Optional: add shredded coconut and walnut to the mixture or save them for matting. Both methods are great!

Mix the ingredients high until smooth and creamy.

Reheat the mini waffle maker.

Add the ingredients to the preheated waffle maker.

Cook for about 2–3 min. until the waffle is done. Remove the waffle and let cool.

In a separate bowl, add all the ingredients together and start the frosting. Stir until smooth and creamy.

When the waffle has cooled completely, frost the cake.

Note: Create 8 mini waffles or 3–4 large waffles.

Nutrition:

Calories 127
Total Fat: 9.7 g.
Cholesterol 102.9 mg.
Sodium 107.3 mg.
Total carbohydrate 5.5 g.
Dietary Fiber 1.3 g.
Sugars 1.5 g.
Protein: 5.3 g.

369.   SLOPPY JOE WAFFLE

Preparation time: 10 min.
Cooking time: 5 min.
Servings: 4
Ingredients:
For the Sloppy Joe:

- 1 lb. ground beef
- 1 tsp. onion powder
- 1 tsp. garlic
- 3 tbsp. tomato paste
- 1/2 tsp. salt
- 1/4 tsp. pepper
- 1 tbsp. chili powder
- 1 tsp. cocoa powder (this is optional but highly recommended! It enhances the flavor!)
- 1/2 c. bone soup beef flavor
- 1 tsp. coconut amino or soy sauce as you like
- 1 tsp. mustard powder
- 1 tsp. brown or golden sugar
- 1/2 tsp. paprika

For the waffle:

- 1 egg
- 1/2 c. cheddar cheese
- 5-slice jalapeno, very small diced (pickled or fresh)
- 1 tsp. Frank Red-Hot sauce
- 1/4 tsp. corn extract is optional, but tastes like real cornbread!
- A pinch of salt

Directions:

First, cook the minced meat with salt and pepper.

Add all the remaining ingredients.

Cook the mixture while making the waffle.

Preheating the waffle maker.

Put the eggs into a small bowl.

Add the remaining ingredients.

Spray to the waffle maker with a non-stick cooking spray.

Divide the mixture in half.

Simmer half of the mixture for about 4 min. or until golden.

For a crispy waffle, add 1 tsp. cheese to the waffle maker for 30 sec. before adding the mixture.

Pour the warm Sloppy Joe mix into the hot waffle and finish! Dinner is ready!

Note: You can also add diced jalapenos (fresh or pickled) to this basic waffle recipe to make a jalapeno cornbread waffle recipe!

Nutrition:

Calories 156
Total Fat: 3.9 g.
Cholesterol 67.8 mg.
Sodium 392.6 mg.
Total carbohydrate 3.9 g.
Dietary Fiber 1.2 g.
Sugars 1.6 g.
Protein: 25.8 g
.

370. BACON EGG AND CHEESE WAFFLE

Preparation time: 3 min.
Cooking time: 7 min.
Servings: 2
Ingredients:

- 3/4 c. chopped cheese (i used a blend of sharp cheddar and mozzarella cheese)
- 2 eggs (scrambled)
- 3 slices of thin bacon
- A pinch of salt
- 1/4 tsp. pepper

Directions:

Cut small pieces of bacon. Scramble the egg in a medium-sized bowl and mix salt and pepper in the cheese, then add the pieces of bacon and mix them all together.

Preheat your waffle iron when it is open at the proper cooking temperature and pour the mixture into the center of the iron to ensure that it is distributed evenly.

Close your waffle iron and set the timer for 4 min. and do not open too quickly. No matter how good it begins to smell, let it cook. A good rule to follow is that if the waffle machine stops steaming, the waffle will be done.

When the time is up, gently open the waffle iron and make sure not all of it sticks to the top. If so, use a Teflon or another non-metallic spatula to pry the waffle softly away from the top and then gently pull the waffle from the bottom and onto the plate after you have fully opened the unit.

Nutrition:

Calories 490
Calories: 141
Fat: 15.7 g.
sodium 209 mg.
potassium 128 mg.
carbohydrates 9.9 g.
Fiber 2.9 g.
sugar 0.9 g.
Protein: 11.5 g.

371. CRUNCHY KETO CINNAMON WAFFLE

Preparation time: 5 min.
Cooking time: 10 min.
Servings: 2
Ingredients:

- 1 tbsp. almond flour
- 1 egg
- 1 tsp. vanilla
- A pinch of cinnamon
- 1 tsp. baking powder
- 1 c. mozzarella cheese

Directions:

Mix the egg and vanilla extract in a bowl.

Mix baking powder, almond flour, and cinnamon.

Finally, add the mozzarella and coat with the mixture.

Spray oil on your waffle maker and let it heat up to its maximum setting.

Cook the waffle, test it every 5 min. until it becomes golden and crunchy. A tip: make sure you put half of the batter in it. It can overflow the waffle maker. I suggest you put down a silpat mat to make it easy to clean.

Enjoy with butter and your favorite low-carb syrup.

Nutrition:
Calories 450
Fat: 15.7 g.
Sodium 209 mg.
Potassium 128 mg.
Carbohydrates 9.9 g.
Fiber 2.9 g.
Sugar 0.9 g.
Protein: 11.5 g.

372. CRISPY BURGER BUN WAFFLE

Preparation time: 5 min.
Cooking time: 14 min.
Servings: 1
Ingredients:

- 1 egg
- 1/2 c. mozzarella cheese shredded
- 1/4 tsp. baking powder
- 1/4 tsp. glucomannan powder
- 1/4 tsp. allulose or another sweetener
- 1/4 tsp. caraway seed or other seasonings

Directions:
In a pot, add all the ingredients and blend them together with a fork.

Spoon part of the mixture into the waffle maker, depending on whether you want them soft or crispy, cook for 5–7 min.

Prepare as you usually do your burger. Usually, I cook a bacon strip in a cast iron pan and then fry a burger over medium-low heat with salt and pepper in the bacon fat. I add the cheese a couple of minutes after frying, pour in a 1/4 c. water and place a metal bowl over the burger to steam the cheese. I like my burgers with lettuce, tomato, onion, a bit of ranch dressing, salt, and pepper. But, that's me. You're doing it.

Pop it in the toaster oven when the first waffle comes out to keep it warm while the second waffle is being made, again for 5–7 min.

Nutrition:
Calories 258
Fat: 15.7 g.
Sodium 209 mg.
Potassium 128 mg.
Carbohydrates 9.9 g.
Fiber 2.9 g.
Sugar 0.9 g.
Protein: 11.5 g.

373. VEGAN KETO WAFFLE WAFFLE

Preparation time: 5 min.
Cooking time: 5 min.
Servings: 2
Ingredients:

- 1 tbsp. flaxseed
- 2 glasses of water
- 1/4 c. low-carb vegan cheese
- 2 tbsp. coconut powder
- 1 tbsp. low-carb vegan cream cheese
- A pinch of salt

Directions:
Preheat the waffle maker to medium-high heat.
In a small bowl, mix flaxseed meal and water.
Leave for 5 min. until thick and sticky.
Make the flax eggs.
Whisk all the waffle ingredients together.
Meat the waffle.
Pour the waffle dough into the center of the waffle iron. Close the waffle maker and cook for 3–5 min. or until the waffles are golden and firm. If using a mini waffle maker, pour only half the dough.
Pour the waffle mixture into the waffle maker
Remove the vegan waffle from the waffle maker and serve.
You can eat vegan keto the waffles

Nutrition:
Calories 168
Total Fat: 11.8 g.
Cholesterol 121 mg.

Sodium 221.8 mg.
Total carbohydrate 5.1 g.
Dietary Fiber 1.7 g.
Sugars 1.2 g.
Protein: 10 g.

374. PUMPKIN CAKE WAFFLE WITH CREAM CHEESE FROSTING

Preparation time: 15 min.
Cooking time: 28 min.
Servings: 4
Ingredients:
For the waffles:

- 2 eggs, beaten
- 1/2 tsp. pumpkin pie spice
- 1 c. finely grated mozzarella cheese
- 1 tbsp. pumpkin puree

For the frosting:

- 2 tbsp. cream cheese, softened
- 2 tbsp. swerve confectioner's sugar
- 1/2 tsp. vanilla extract

Directions:
For the waffles:
Preheat the waffle iron.
In a medium bowl, mix the egg, pumpkin pie spice, mozzarella cheese, and pumpkin puree.
Open the iron and add 1/4 of the mixture. Close and cook until crispy, 7 min.
Transfer the waffle to a plate and make 3 more waffles with the remaining batter.

For the frosting:
Add the cream cheese, swerve sugar, and vanilla to a medium bowl and whisk using an electric mixer until smooth and fluffy.
Layer the waffles one on another but with some frosting spread between the layers. Top with a bit of frosting.
Slice and serve.

Nutrition:
Calories 106
Fats 5.17 g.

Carbs: 1.9 g.
Net Carbs: 1.2 g.
Protein: 12.82 g.

375. BIRTHDAY CAKE WAFFLES

Preparation time: 15 min.
Cooking time: 28 min.
Servings: 4
Ingredients:
For the waffles:

- 2 eggs, beaten
- 1 c. finely grated swiss cheese

For the frosting and topping:

- 1/2 c. heavy cream
- 2 tbsp. sugar-free maple syrup
- 1/2 tsp. vanilla extract
- 3 tbsp. funfetti

Directions:
For the waffles:
Preheat the waffle iron.
In a medium bowl, mix the egg and swiss cheese.
Open the iron and add 1/4 of the mixture. Close and cook until crispy, 7 min.
Transfer the waffle to a plate and make 3 more waffles with the remaining batter.

For the frosting and topping:
Add the heavy cream, maple syrup, and vanilla extract to a medium bowl and whisk using an electric mixer until smooth and fluffy.
Layer the waffles one on another but with some frosting spread between the layers.
top with the remaining bit of frosting and garnish with the funfetti.

Nutrition:
Calories 210
Fats 16.82 g.
Carbs: 2.42 g.
Net Carbs: 2.42 g.
Protein: 11.96 g.

376. CHOCOLATE CAKE WAFFLES WITH CREAM CHEESE FROSTING

Preparation time: 10 min.
Cooking time: 28 min.
Servings: 4
Ingredients:
For the waffles:

- 2 eggs, beaten
- 1 c. finely grated gouda cheese
- 2 tsp. unsweetened cocoa powder
- 1/4 tsp. sugar-free maple syrup
- 1 tbsp. cream cheese, softened

For the frosting:

- 3 tbsp. cream cheese, softened
- 1/4 tsp. vanilla extract
- 2 tbsp. sugar-free maple syrup

Directions:
For the waffles:

Preheat the waffle iron.

In a medium bowl, mix all the ingredients for the waffles.

Open the iron and add 1/4 of the mixture. Close and cook until crispy, 7 min.

Transfer the waffle to a plate and make 3 more waffles with the remaining batter.

For the frosting:

In a medium bowl, beat the cream cheese, vanilla extract, and maple syrup with a hand mixer until smooth.

Assemble the waffles with the frosting to make the cake making sure to top the last layer with some frosting.

Slice and serve.

Nutrition:
Calories 78
Fats 6.5 g.
Carbs: 1.24 g.
Net Carbs: 0.94 g.
Protein: 3.99 g.

377. LEMON CAKE WAFFLE WITH LEMON FROSTING

Preparation time: 10 min.
Cooking time: 28 min.
Servings: 4
Ingredients:
For the waffles:

- 2 eggs, beaten
- 1/2 c. finely grated swiss cheese
- 2 oz. cream cheese, softened
- 1/2 tsp. lemon extract
- 20 drops cake batter extract

For the frosting:

- 1/2 c. heavy cream
- 1 tbsp. sugar-free maple syrup
- 1/4 tsp. lemon extract

Directions:
For the waffles:

Preheat the waffle iron.

In a medium bowl, mix all the ingredients for the waffles.

Open the iron and add 1/4 of the mixture. Close and cook until crispy, 7 min.

Transfer the waffle to a plate and make 3 more waffles with the remaining batter.

For the frosting:

In a medium bowl, using a hand mixer, beat the heavy cream, maple syrup, and lemon extract until fluffy.

Assemble the waffles with the frosting to make the cake.

Slice and serve.

Nutrition:
Calories 176
Fats 15.18 g.
Carbs: 2.88 g.
Net Carbs: 2.88 g.
Protein: 7.63 g.

378.   RED VELVET WAFFLE CAKE

Preparation time: 15 min.
Cooking time: 28 min.
Servings: 4
Ingredients:
For the waffles:
- 2 eggs, beaten
- 1/2 c. finely grated parmesan cheese
- 2 oz. cream cheese, softened
- 2 drops red food coloring
- 1 tsp. vanilla extract

For the frosting:
- 3 tbsp. cream cheese, softened
- 1 tbsp. sugar-free maple syrup
- 1/4 tsp. vanilla extract

Directions:
For the waffles:
Preheat the waffle iron.
In a medium bowl, mix all the ingredients for the waffles.
Open the iron and add 1/4 of the mixture. Close and cook until crispy, 7 min.
Transfer the waffle to a plate and make 3 more waffles with the remaining batter.

For the frosting:
In a medium bowl, using a hand mixer, whisk the cream cheese, maple syrup, and vanilla extract until smooth.
Assemble the waffles with the frosting to make the cake.
Slice and serve.

Nutrition:
Calories 147
Fats 9.86 g.
Carbs: 5.22 g.
Net Carbs: 5.22 g.
Protein: 8.57 g.

379.   ALMOND BUTTER WAFFLE CAKE WITH CHOCOLATE BUTTER FROSTING

Preparation time: 20 min.
Cooking time: 28 min.
Servings: 4
Ingredients:
For the waffles:
- 1 egg, beaten
- 1/3 c. finely grated mozzarella cheese
- 1 tbsp. almond flour
- 2 tbsp. almond butter
- 1 tbsp. swerve confectioner's sugar
- 1/2 tsp. vanilla extract

For the frosting:
- 1 1/2 c. butter, room temperature
- 1 c. unsweetened cocoa powder
- 1/2 c. almond milk
- 5 c. swerve confectioner's sugar
- 2 tsp. vanilla extract

Directions:
For the waffles:
Preheat the waffle iron.
In a medium bowl, mix the egg, mozzarella cheese, almond flour, almond butter, swerve confectioner's sugar, and vanilla extract.
Open the iron and add 1/4 of the mixture. Close and cook until crispy, 7 min.
Transfer the waffle to a plate and make 3 more waffles with the remaining batter.

For the frosting:
In a medium bowl, cream the butter and cocoa powder until smooth.
Gradually, whisk in the almond milk and swerve confectioner's sugar until smooth.
Add the vanilla extract and mix well.
Assemble the waffles with the frosting to make the cake.
Slice and serve.

Nutrition:
Calories 838
Fats 85.35 g.
Carbs: 8.73 g.
Net Carbs: 2.03 g.
Protein: 13.59 g.

380. CINNAMON WAFFLES WITH CUSTARD FILLING

Preparation time: 25 min.
Cooking time: 28 min.
Servings: 4
Ingredients:
For the custard filling:

- 4 egg yolks, beaten
- 1 tbsp. erythritol
- 1/4 tsp. xanthan gum
- 1 c. heavy cream
- 1 tbsp. vanilla extract

For the waffles:

- 2 eggs, beaten
- 2 tbsp. cream cheese, softened
- 1 c. finely grated Monterey Jack cheese
- 1 tsp. vanilla extract
- 1 tbsp. heavy cream
- 1 tbsp. coconut flour
- 1/2 tsp. baking powder
- 1/2 tsp. ground cinnamon
- 1/4 tsp. erythritol

Directions:
For the custard filling:
In a medium bowl, beat the egg yolks with the erythritol. Mix in the xanthan gum until smooth. Pour the heavy cream into a medium saucepan and simmer over low heat. Pour the mixture into the egg mixture while whisking vigorously until well mixed.
Transfer the mixture to the saucepan and continue whisking while cooking over low heat until thickened, 20–30 sec. Turn the heat off and stir in the vanilla extract.

Strain the custard through a fine-mesh into a bowl. Cover the bowl with plastic wrap. Refrigerate for 1 hour.
For the waffles:
After 1 hour, preheat the waffle iron.
In a medium bowl, mix all the ingredients for the waffles.
Open the iron and add 1/4 of the mixture. Close and cook until crispy, 7 min.
Transfer the waffle to a plate and make 3 more with the remaining batter.
To serve:
Spread the custard filling between two waffle quarters, sandwich, and enjoy!
Nutrition:
Calories 239
Fats 21.25 g.
Carbs: 3.21 g.
Net Carbs: 3.01 g.
Protein: 6.73 g.

381. TIRAMISU WAFFLES

Preparation time: 20 min.
Cooking time: 28 min.
Servings: 4
Ingredients:
For the waffles:

- 2 eggs, beaten
- 3 tbsp. cream cheese, softened
- 1/2 c. finely grated gouda cheese
- 1 tsp. vanilla extract
- 1/4 tsp. erythritol

For the coffee syrup:

- 2 tbsp. strong coffee, room temperature
- 3 tbsp. sugar-free maple syrup

For the filling:

- 1/4 c. heavy cream
- 2 tsp. vanilla extract
- 1/4 tsp. erythritol
- 4 tbsp. mascarpone cheese, room temperature
- 1 tbsp. cream cheese, softened

218

For dusting:
- 1/2 tsp. unsweetened cocoa powder

Directions:
For the waffles:
Preheat the waffle iron.

In a medium bowl, mix all the ingredients for the waffles.

Open the iron and add 1/4 of the mixture. Close and cook until crispy, 7 min.

Transfer the waffle to a plate and make 3 more with the remaining batter.

For the coffee syrup:
In a small bowl, mix the coffee and maple syrup. Set aside.

For the filling:
Beat the heavy cream, vanilla, and erythritol in a medium bowl using an electric hand mixer until stiff peak forms.

In another bowl, beat the mascarpone cheese and cream cheese until well combined. Add the heavy cream mixture and fold in. Spoon the mixture into a piping bag.

To assemble:
Spoon 1 tbsp. of the coffee syrup on one waffle and pipe some of the cream cheese mixture on top. Cover with another waffle and continue the assembling process.

Generously dust with cocoa powder and refrigerate overnight.

When ready to enjoy, slice, and serve.

Nutrition:
Calories 208
Fats 15.91 g.
Carbs: 4.49 g.
Net Carbs: 4.39 g.
Protein: 10.1 g.

382. COCONUT WAFFLES WITH MINT FROSTING
Preparation time: 15 min.
Cooking time: 28 min.
Servings: 4
Ingredients:
For the waffles:
- 2 eggs, beaten
- 2 tbsp. cream cheese, softened
- 1 c. finely grated Monterey Jack cheese
- 2 tbsp. coconut flour
- 1/4 tsp. baking powder
- 1 tbsp. unsweetened shredded coconut
- 1 tbsp. walnuts, chopped

For the frosting:
- 1/4 c. unsalted butter, room temperature
- 3 tbsp. almond milk
- 1 tsp. mint extract
- 2 drops green food coloring
- 3 c. swerve confectioner's sugar

Directions:
For the waffles:
Preheat the waffle iron.

In a medium bowl, mix all the ingredients for the waffles.

Open the iron and add 1/4 of the mixture. Close and cook until crispy, 7 min.

Transfer the waffle to a plate and make 3 more with the remaining batter.

For the frosting:
In a medium bowl, cream the butter using an electric hand mixer until smooth.

Gradually mix in the almond milk until smooth. Add the mint extract and green food coloring; whisk until well combined.

Finally, mix in the swerve confectioner's sugar a cup at a time until smooth.

Layer the waffles with the frosting.

Slice and serve afterward.

Nutrition:
Calories 141
Fats 13.13 g.
Carbs: 1.31 g.
Net Carbs: 1.03 g.
Protein: 4.31 g.

383. KETO BIRTHDAY CAKE WAFFLE WITH SPRINKLES

Preparation time: 10 min.
Cooking time: 7 min.
Servings: 4
Ingredients:
For the waffle cake:

* 2 eggs
* 1/4 almond flour
* 1 c. coconut powder
* 1 c. melted butter
* 2 tbsp. cream cheese
* 1 tsp. cake butter extract
* 1 tsp. vanilla extract
* 2 tsp. baking powder
* 2 tsp. confectionery sweetener or monk fruit
* 1/4 tsp. xanthan powder whipped cream

For the frosting:

* 1/2 c. heavy whipped cream
* 2 tbsp. sweetener or monk fruit
* 1/2 tsp. vanilla extract

Directions:
Preheat the mini waffle maker.
Add all the ingredients of the waffle cake to a medium-sized blender and blend it to the top until it is smooth and creamy. Allow only a minute to sit with the batter. It may seem a little watery, but it's going to work well.
Add 2–3 tbsp. of the batter to your waffle maker and cook until golden brown for about 2–3 min. Start to frost the whipped vanilla cream in a separate bowl.

Add all the ingredients and mix with a hand mixer until thick and soft peaks are formed by the whipping cream.
Until frosting your cake, allow the keto birthday cake waffles to cool completely. If you frost it too soon, the frosting will be melted.
Enjoy!

Nutrition:
Calories 141
Total Fat: 10.2 g.
Cholesterol 111 mg.
Sodium 55.7 mg.
Total carbohydrate 4.7 g.
Dietary Fiber 0.4 g.
Sugars 0.8 g.
Protein: 4.7 g.

384. CARROT WAFFLE CAKE

Preparation time: 5 min.
Cooking time: 5 min.
Servings: 6
Ingredients:

* 1/2 c. chopped carrot
* 1 egg
* 2 t butter melted
* 2 t heavy whipped cream
* 3/4 c. almond flour
* 1 walnut chopped
* 2 t powder sweetener
* 2 tsp. cinnamon
* 1 tsp. pumpkin spice
* 1 tsp. baking powder

For the frosting:

* 4 oz. cream cheese softened
* 1/4 c. powdered sweetener
* 1 tsp. vanilla essence
* 1–2 t heavy whipped cream according to your preferred consistency

Directions:

Mix the dry ingredients such as almond flour, cinnamon, pumpkin spices, baking powder, powdered sweeteners, and walnut pieces.

Add the grated carrots, eggs, melted butter, and cream.

Add the batter to a preheated mini waffle maker. Cook for 2 1/2–3 min.

Mix the frosted ingredients with a hand mixer with a whisk until well mixed.

Stack waffles and add a frost between each layer!

Nutrition:
Calories 270
Total Fat: 22.07 g.
Cholesterol 111 mg.
Sodium 119 mg.
Total carbohydrate 14.27 g.
Dietary Fiber 2.1 g.
Sugars 9.47 g.
Protein 6.06 g.

385. KETO BIRTHDAY CAKE WAFFLE

Preparation time: 10 min.
Cooking time: 5 min.
Servings: 4
Ingredients:
For the waffle cake:

- 2 eggs
- 1/4 c. almond flour
- 1 tsp. coconut flour
- 2 tbsp. melted butter
- 2 tbsp. cream cheese
- 1 tsp. cake batter extract
- 1/2 tsp. vanilla essence
- 1/2 tsp. baking powder
- 2 tbsp. sweetener or monk fruit
- 1/4 tsp. xanthan powder

For the frosting:

- 1/2 c. fresh cream

- 2 tbsp. 2 tbsp. sweets sweetener or monk fruit
- 1/2 tsp. vanilla essence

Directions:

Reheat the mini waffle maker.

In a medium-sized blender, add all the ingredients of the waffle cake and blend high until smooth and creamy. Let the dough sit for only 1 min. It may look a bit watery, but it works. Add 2–3 tbsp. of dough to the waffle maker and cook for about 2–3 min. until golden.

In another bowl, start making the whipped cream vanilla frosting.

Add all the ingredients and mix with a hand mixer until the whipped cream thickens and soft peaks form.

Let the keto birthday cake waffle cool completely before frosting the cake. If the frosting is too early, the frost will melt.

Enjoy!

Nutrition:
Calories 141
Total Fat: 10.2 g.
Cholesterol 111 mg.
Sodium 55.7 mg.
Total carbohydrate 4.7 g.
Dietary Fiber 0.4 g.
Sugars 0.8 g.
Protein: 4.7 g.

386. BANANA PUDDING WAFFLE CAKE

Preparation time: 5 min.
Cooking time: 5 min.
Servings: 2
Ingredients:

- 1 large egg yolk
- 1/2 c. heavy cream
- 3 tbsp. powder sweetener
- 1/4–1/2 tsp. xanthan gum
- 1/2 tsp. banana extract
- A pinch of salt

For the waffle:
- 1 oz. softened cream cheese
- 1/4 c. mozzarella cheese shredded
- 1 egg
- 1 tsp. banana extract
- 2 tbsp. sweetener
- 1 tsp. baking powder
- 4 tbsp. almond flour

Directions:
Mix heavy cream, powdered sweetener, and egg yolk in a small pot. Whisk constantly until the sweetener has dissolved and the mixture is thick. Cook for 1 min. Add xanthan gum and whisk.

Remove from the heat, add a pinch of salt and banana extract and stir well.

Transfer to a glass dish and cover the pudding with plastic wrap. Refrigerate.

Mix all the banana waffle ingredients together. Cook in a preheated mini waffle maker.

Nutrition:
Calories 337
Total Fat: 23.99 g.
Cholesterol 457 mg.
Sodium 250 mg.
Total carbohydrate 18.63 g.
Dietary Fiber 0.8 g.
Sugars 14.65 g.
Protein 13.52 g.

387. JAMAICAN JERK CHICKEN WAFFLE
Preparation time: 15 min.
Cooking time: 4 min.
Servings: 2
Ingredients:
For the waffle:
- 2 egg
- 1 c. Mozzarella cheese (shredded)
- 1 tbsp. Butter
- 2 tbsp. Almond flour

- 1/4 tsp. Turmeric
- 1/4 tsp. Baking powder
- A pinch of xanthan gum
- A pinch of onion powder
- A pinch of garlic powder
- A pinch of salt

For the Jamaican jerk chicken:
- 1 lb. organic ground chicken
- 1 tsp. dried thyme
- 1 tsp. garlic (granulated)
- 2 tbsp. butter
- 2 tsp. dried parsley
- 1/8 tsp. black pepper
- 1 tsp. salt
- 1/2 c. chicken broth
- 2 tbsp. jerk seasoning
- 1/2 medium onion, chopped

Directions:
In a pan, melt the butter and sauté onion

Add all the remaining ingredients of chicken Jamaican jerk and sauté

Now add the chicken and chicken broth and stir

Cook on medium-low heat for 10 min.

Then cook on high heat and dry all the liquid

For the waffles, preheat a mini waffle maker if needed and grease it

In a mixing bowl, beat all the waffle ingredients

Pour the mixture to the lower plate of the waffle maker and spread it evenly to cover the plate properly and close the lid

Cook for at least 4 min. to get the desired crunch

Remove the waffle from the heat and keep aside for around 1 min.

Make as many waffles as your mixture and waffle maker allow

Add the chicken in between a waffle, fold, and enjoy

Nutrition:
Calories 991
Total Fat: 38.91 g.

Cholesterol 987 mg.
Sodium 3003 mg.
Total carbohydrate 12.58 g.
Dietary Fiber 3.1 g.
Sugars 3.67 g.
Protein: 138.66 g.

388. CHICKEN GREEN WAFFLES

Preparation time: 10 min.
Cooking time: 10 min.
Servings: 4
Ingredients:
For the waffle:

- 1/3 c. chicken, boiled and shredded
- 1/3 c. cabbage
- 1/3 c. broccoli
- 1/3 c. zucchini
- 2 egg
- 1 c. mozzarella cheese (shredded)
- 1 tbsp. butter
- 2 tbsp. almond flour
- 1/4 tsp. baking powder
- A pinch of onion powder
- A pinch of garlic powder
- A pinch of salt

Directions:
In a deep saucepan, boil cabbage, broccoli, and zucchini for 5 min. or till it tenders, strain, and blend
Mix all the remaining ingredients well together
Pour a thin layer on a preheated waffle iron
Add a layer of the blended vegetables to the mixture
Again, add more mixture over the top
Cook the waffle for around 5 min.
Serve with your favorite sauce
Nutrition:
Calories 171
Total Fat: 10.84 g.
Cholesterol 326 mg.

Sodium 286 mg.
Total carbohydrate 2.44 g.
Dietary Fiber 0.8 g.
Sugars 1.06 g.
Protein: 15.8 g.

389. PECAN PIE CAKE WAFFLE

Preparation time: 26 min.
Cooking time: 18 min.
Servings: 2
Ingredients:
For the filling:

- 2 tbsp. butter
- 2 tbsp. pecan, chopped
- 2 tbsp. maple syrup
- A pinch salt
- 1 tbsp. sukrin gold
- 2 tbsp. heavy whipping cream
- 2 large egg yolk

For the waffle:

- 1 egg
- 1/2 tbsp. maple extract
- 1 tbsp. sukrin gold
- 2 tbsp. pecan, chopped
- 2 tbsp. cream cheese
- 4 tbsp. almond flour
- 1/2 tbsp. baking powder
- 1 tbsp. heavy whipping cream

Directions:
Prepare a mix in a low heated saucepan containing heavy whipping cream, syrup, butter, and sweetener.
Mix all the ingredients together into a thick creamy paste.
Put off the heat and pour in the egg yolks, then place on heat again and mix.
Pour in the chopped pecans with a pinch of salt to taste, and then allow simmering to thicken. Put off the heat.

For the waffles, prepare the mix of all the ingredients into a blender and blend, except for the pecans. Add in the chopped pecans and stir.

Preheat and grease the waffle maker.

Pour the mixture into the lower side of the waffle maker and spread evenly. Heat the mixtures to a crunchy form for 5 min.

Repeat the process for the remaining mixture.

Put the heat off and allow the waffle to cool a bit.

Stack up the waffles into a single-row cake and garnish 1/3 of the pecan pie filling earlier prepared on the waffle.

Serve hot and enjoy the crispy taste.

Nutrition:
Calories 2189
Total Fat: 110.78 g.
Cholesterol 728 mg.
Sodium 1402 mg.
Total carbohydrate 271.38 g.
Dietary Fiber 10.4 g.
Sugars 122.22 g.
Protein: 29.7 g.

390. TIRAMISU WAFFLE CAKE

Preparation time: 41 min.
Cooking time: 21 min.
Servings: 4
Ingredients:
- 2 egg
- 2 tbsp. cream cheese
- 2 tbsp. coconut flour
- 1/2 tsp. vanilla extract
- 1/2 tsp. hazelnut extract
- 1 1/2 tbsp. organic cacao powder
- 1/2 c. mascarpone cheese
- 2 tbsp. monk fruit sweetener
- 2 tbsp. butter (melted)
- 1 tsp. baking powder
- 2 1/2 tsp. instant coffee dry mix
- 1/4 c. almond flour
- 1/8 tsp. Himalayan pink fine salt
- 1/4 c. powdered sweetener

Directions:
Prepare a butter-coffee mixture, by melting butter with the instant dry coffee added, and then stir to mix.

Prepare a mix in a bowl containing cream cheese, beaten eggs, and the butter-coffee mixture.

In another bowl, prepare a mix of mascarpone cheese with vanilla extract and sweetener.

Mix the mixture and the dry ingredients in the two bowls together.

Preheat and grease the waffle maker. Pour the egg mixture into the lower side of the waffle maker and spread evenly.

Heat the mixtures to a crunchy form for 5 min.

Repeat the process for the remaining mixture. Put the heat off and allow the waffle to cool a bit. For a two-layer cake, split the cream.

Cacao powder and instant coffee can also be separated before blending.

Place the cake, by placing the cream on one side of the waffle and top with another waffle.

Serve hot and enjoy the taste.

Nutrition:
Calories 256
Total Fat: 15.74 g.
Cholesterol 335 mg.
Sodium 352 mg.
Total carbohydrate 19.21 g.
Dietary Fiber 0.1 g.
Sugars 14.95 g.
Protein: 8.75 g.

391. CREAM COCONUT WAFFLE CAKE

Preparation time: 80 min.
Cooking time: 21 min.
Servings: 2
Ingredients:
For the filling:

- 1/4 c. coconut (shredded)
- 2 tbsp. monk fruit sweetener
- A pinch of salt
- 1/3 c. almond, unsweetened
- 2 tsp. butter
- 1/4 tsp. xanthan gum
- 2 egg yolks
- 1/3 c. coconut milk

For the waffles:

- 2 egg
- 2 tbsp. cream cheese
- 1 tbsp. butter (melted)
- 2 tbsp. coconut (shredded)
- 2 tbsp. powdered sweetener
- 1/2 tsp. vanilla extract
- 1/2 tsp. coconut extract

For garnishing:

- Whipped cream, as per your taste
- 1 tbsp. coconut (shredded)

Directions:

Prepare a mixture containing all the ingredients. Stir to mix properly.

Preheat and grease the waffle maker. Pour the mixture into the lower side of the waffle maker and spread evenly.

Heat the mixtures to a crunchy form for 5 min. Repeat the process for the remaining mixture. Put the heat off and allow the waffle to cool a bit.

For the filling, use a small pan to heat the coconut milk to steam not boil.

Using another bowl, whisk the egg yolks lightly with milk added, then heat to thicken the mixture. Add some sweetener, while whisking add xanthan gum in bits.

Mix all the ingredients properly with the heat out off.

To further thicken the mixture, refrigerate. Stack up the waffles and add the fillings in between each waffle, then garnish with coconuts and whipped cream.

Serve hot and enjoy the crispy taste.

Nutrition:
Calories 385
Total Fat: 26.66 g.
Cholesterol 834 mg.
Sodium 311 mg.
Total carbohydrate 19.59 g.
Dietary Fiber 0.6 g.
Sugars 14.65 g.
Protein: 15.57 g.

392. ALMOND CHOCOLATE WAFFLE CAKE

Preparation time: 12 min.
Cooking time: 6 min.
Servings: 2
Ingredients:
For the filling:

- 1 1/2 tbsp. melted coconut oil
- 4 tbsp. cream cheese
- 1/2 tbsp. vanilla extract
- 14 whole almonds
- 1 tbsp. heavy cream
- 1 tbsp. powdered sweetener
- 1/4 c. coconut, finely shredded

For the waffle:

- 1 egg
- 1 tbsp. powdered sweetener
- 1/4 tsp. instant coffee powder
- 1 tbsp. cocoa powder (unsweetened)
- 2 tbsp. cream cheese
- 1/2 tbsp. vanilla extract

- 1 tbsp. almond flour

Directions:

Prepare a mixture containing all the ingredients. Stir to mix properly.

Preheat and grease the waffle maker. Pour the mixture into the lower side of the waffle maker and spread evenly. Heat the mixtures to a crunchy form for 5 min.

Repeat the process for the remaining mixture.

Put the heat off and allow the waffle to cool a bit.

For the filling, except for the almond, using a small pan, prepare a mixture containing all the ingredients.

Spread the fillings on the waffle with almond to garnish, then top with another waffle. Stack up the waffles like a cake.

Serve and enjoy the crispy taste.

Nutrition:

Calories 500

Total Fat: 38.77 g.

Cholesterol 360 mg.

Sodium 390 mg.

Total carbohydrate 26.62 g.

Dietary Fiber 4.1 g.

Sugars 19.36 g.

Protein: 11.33 g.

393. VANILLA WAFFLE CAKE

Preparation time: 2 min.

Cooking time: 8 min.

Servings: 2 waffle cakes

Ingredients:

For the waffle cake:

- 1 tbsp. heavy whipping cream
- 2 tbsp. swerve granulated sweetener
- 1/4 tsp. baking powder
- 1 tbsp. coconut flour
- 1 tbsp. vanilla extract
- 1 egg

For the frosting:

- 1/8 tsp. vanilla extract
- 1 tsp. heavy cream
- 2 tsp. swerve confectioners
- 2 tbsp. cream cheese

Directions:

Reheat the mini waffle maker until hot

In a small bowl, add and whisk the waffle cake ingredients until well combined. Scoop 1/2 of the batter onto the waffle maker, spread across evenly

Cook 3–4 min., until done as desired (or crispy). Gently remove from the waffle maker and let it cool

Repeat with the remaining batter.

For the frosting:

In a small bowl add the cream cheese and microwave for 10 sec. to soften.

Add in the remaining frosting ingredients and mix until fluffy

Assembling the vanilla waffle cake:

Place each waffle on a plate, spread with a layer of frosting

Serve or refrigerate

Nutrition:

Calories 151

Net carbs 2 g.

Fat 13 g.

Protein 6 g.

394. BLUEBERRY CAKE WAFFLE

Preparation time: 4 min.

Cooking time: 12 min.

Servings: 3

Ingredients:

For the blueberry topping:

- 1/2 tbsp. swerve
- 3 fresh strawberries

For the sweet waffle:

- 1 tbsp. almond flour
- 1/2 c. mozzarella cheese

- 1 egg
- 1 tbsp. granulated swerve
- Keto Whipped Cream
- 1/4 tsp. vanilla extract

Directions:

Preheat the waffle maker until hot

Whisk the egg in a bowl, add the cheese, then mix well

In a small bowl, add the blueberries and swerve; mix until well-combined. Set aside.

In another bowl, add the sweet waffle ingredients and mix thoroughly.

Pour 1/3 of the batter into your mini waffle maker and cook for 3–4 min.

Rove gently and set aside to cool

Repeat for the remaining batter—all make 3 waffle cakes in total.

Assemble the waffle by topping with strawberries and whipped cream.

Serve and enjoy!

Nutrition:

Calories 112

Net carbs 1 g.

Fat 8 g.

Protein 7 g.

395. AVOCADO WAFFLE CAKE

Preparation time: 2 min.
Cooking time: 8 min.
Servings: 2 chocolate waffle cakes
Ingredients:
For the chocolate waffle cake:

- 1/2 tsp. vanilla extract
- 1 tbsp. almond flour
- 1 tbsp. heavy whipping cream
- 2 tbsp. swerve granulated sweetener
- 1 egg
- 2 tbsp. cocoa powder
- 1/4 tsp. baking powder

For the avocado cream frosting:

- 1/2 avocado, chopped
- 1/8 tsp. vanilla extract
- 1 tsp. almond butter
- 2 tsp. swerve confectioners
- 2 tbsp. cream cheese

Directions:

Reheat the mini waffle maker until hot

In a small bowl, add and whisk the chocolate waffle cake ingredients until well combined. Scoop 1/2 of the batter onto the waffle maker, spread across evenly

Cook 3–4 min., until done as desired (or crispy). Gently remove from the waffle maker and let it cool

Repeat with the remaining batter.

For the avocado cream frosting:

In a small bowl add the cream cheese and microwave for 10 sec. to soften.

Add in the remaining ingredients and mix until fluffy

Assembling the waffle cake:

Place each waffle on a plate, spread with a layer of frosting

Serve or refrigerate

Nutrition:

Calories 151

Net carbs 2 g.

Fat 13 g.

Protein 6 g.

396. CRANBERRY AND BRIE WAFFLE

Preparation time: 10 min.
Cooking time: 20 min.
Servings: 4 mini waffles
Ingredients:

- 4 tbsp. frozen cranberries
- 3 tbsp. swerve sweetener
- 1 c./115 g. shredded brie cheese
- 2 eggs, at room temperature

Directions:

Take a non-stick waffle iron, plug it in, select the medium or medium-high heat setting and let it preheat until ready to use; it could also be indicated with an indicator light changing its color.

Meanwhile, prepare the batter and for this, take a heatproof bowl, add the cheese in it, and microwave at a high heat setting for 15 sec. or until the cheese has softened.

Then add sweetener, berries, and egg into the cheese and whisk with an electric mixer until smooth.

Use a ladle to pour 1/4 of the prepared batter into the heated waffle iron in a spiral direction, starting from the edges, then shut the lid and cook for 4 min. or more until solid and nicely browned; the cooked waffle will look like a cake. When done, transfer the waffle to a plate with a silicone spatula and repeat with the remaining batter.

Let the waffles stand for some time until crispy and serve straight away.

Nutrition:

Cal: 336

Fat: 25.7 g.

Protein: 19.9 g.

Carb: 6 g.

Fiber: 3.1 g.

Net Carb: 2.9 g.

397. BROWNIE CHOCOLATE WAFFLE

Preparation time: 1 min.

Cooking time: 9 min.

Servings: 1

Ingredients:

- 1 egg whisked
- 1/3 c. mozzarella cheese shredded
- 1 1/2 tbsp. cocoa powder dutch processed
- 1 tbsp. almond flour
- 1 tbsp. monk fruit sweetener
- 1/4 tsp. vanilla extract
- 1/4 tsp. baking powder
- Pinch of salt

Directions:

Preheat the waffle maker

Combine all the ingredients into a bowl

Pour 1/3 of the mixture in the maker and cook for 2–4 min. and repeat

Cool and top with low-carb topping

Nutrition:

Calories: 188

Carbohydrates: 8.9 g.

Proteins: 20.5 g.

Fats: 7 g.

Saturated Fat: 3 g.

Fiber: 4 g.

Sugar: 1.3 g.

398. CAP'N CRUNCH CEREAL WAFFLE CAKE

Preparation time: 5 min.

Cooking time: 5 min.

Servings: 2

Ingredients:

- 1 egg
- 2 tbsp. almond flour
- 1/2 tsp. coconut flour
- 1 tbsp. butter
- 1 tbsp. cream cheese
- 20 drop Captain cereal flavor
- 1/4 tsp. vanilla essence
- 1/4 tsp. baking powder
- 1 tbsp. confectionery
- 1/8 tsp. xanthan gum

Directions:

Reheat the mini waffle maker.

Mix or blend all the ingredients until smooth and creamy. Let the dough rest for a few minutes until the flour has absorbed the liquid.

Add 2–3 tbsp. of the batter to the waffle maker and cook for about 2 1/2 min.
Topped with fresh whipped cream (10 drops of captain cereal flavor and syrup!)

Nutrition:
Calories 154
Total Fat: 11.2 g.
Cholesterol 113.3 mg.
Sodium 96.9 mg.
Total Carbohydrate 5.9 g.
Dietary Fiber 1.7 g.
Sugars 2.7 g.
Protein: 4.6 g.

CHAPTER 11. SANDWICH WAFFLE RECIPES

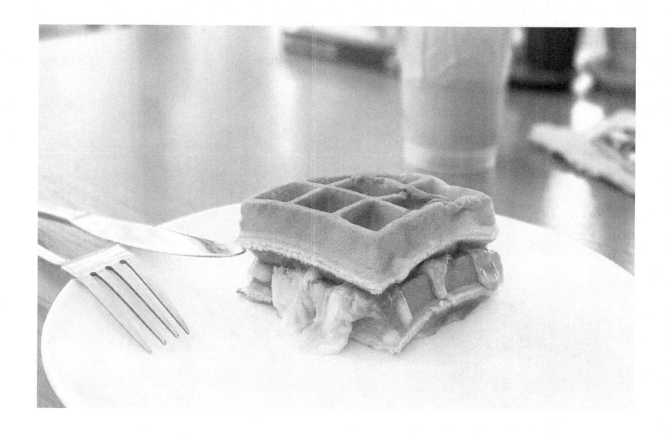

399. HOT BROWN SANDWICH WAFFLE

Preparation time: 2 min.
Cooking time: 4 min.
Servings: 2
Ingredients:

- 1 egg, beaten
- 1/4 c. cheddar cheese, shredded and divided
- 2 slices fresh tomato
- 1/2 lb roasted turkey breast
- 1/2 tsp. parmesan cheese, grated
- 2 bacon, cooked
- 2 oz. cream cheese, cubed
- 1/3 c. heavy cream
- 1/4 c. Swiss cheese, shredded
- 1/4 tsp. ground nutmeg
- White pepper

Directions:

Preheat the waffle maker.

Start by making the waffle, once heated up, sprinkle 1 tbsp. cheddar cheese onto the iron.

After 30 sec., top the cheese with a beaten egg.

Once the egg starts to cook, top the mixture with another layer of cheese.

Close the waffle maker lid and allow cooking for 3–5 min. until the waffle is crispy and golden brown.

Take out the cooked waffle and repeat the steps until you've used up all the batter.

Make the sauce by combining heavy cream and cream cheese in a small saucepan.

Place a saucepan over medium heat and whisk until the cheese completely dissolves.

Add in Swiss cheese and parmesan, then continue whisking to melt the cheese.

Add in the white pepper and nutmeg.

Continue whisking until you achieve a smooth consistency.

Remove the saucepan from the heat.

Prepare the sandwich by setting the oven for broiling.

Cover a cookie sheet with aluminum foil.

Lightly grease the foil with butter, and place two waffles on it.

Top the waffles with 4 oz. turkey and a slice of tomato each. Add some sauce and grated parmesan on top.

Broil the waffle sandwiches for 2–3 min. until you see the sauce bubble and brown spots appear on top.

Remove from the oven. Put them on a heatproof plate.

Arrange the bacon slices in a crisscrossing manner on top of the sandwich before serving.

Nutrition:

Calories: 572

Carbohydrates: 3 g.

Fat: 41 g.

Protein: 41 g.

400. KETO HAM AND CHEESE WAFFLE SANDWICH

Preparation time: 8 min.
Cooking time: 7 min.
Servings: 2
Ingredients:

- 1 egg, should be large
- 1/2 c. crushed cheddar, mozzarella, or any grated cheese
- 1/4 c. almond flour.
- 1/4 tsp. gluten-free baking powder
- 2 ham slices
- 2 (57 g.) slices of the cheese
- 4 (60 g.) tomato slices
- 2 (15 g.) small leaves of lettuce

- Optional: 1 or 2 tbsp. cream cheese, butter, or mayonnaise.

Directions:

Start making the waffles as per the directions. Either you can create 2 standard waffles or 3 thinner ones

Let the waffles all cool down. They will be soft when hot but will crisp when getting colder

Fill with ham, cheese, lettuce, and tomato croutons. Optionally, before filling, you can add 1–2 spoonsful of cream cheese and spread it over the waffles

Immediately enjoy or place the waffles in a sealed container for up to 3 days at room temperature or in the refrigerator for up to a week. Freeze for up to 3 months, for longer storage. The jar would maintain the soft texture, but if you want crispy, you should leave them untouched

Nutrition:

Calories 733
Fat 57.1 g.
Protein 45.8 g.

401. KETO BREAKFAST WAFFLE SANDWICH

Preparation time: 5 min.
Cooking time: 7 min.
Servings: 2
Ingredients:

- 1 large egg
- 1\2 of shredded cheese (cheddar)
- 2 tsp. mayonnaise
- 1–2 pcs. bacon
- 1 egg
- Sea salt and pepper to taste

Directions:

Heat up the mini waffle iron

Add the shredded cheese and the egg in a little bowl, whereas the waffle iron is heating

Pour half the batter onto the waffle maker and cook 3–4 min. or until you want waffles close

Cook the bacon in a small saucepan until crispy nicely browned, then set aside

Cook the egg to ideal doneness using the same tiny saucepan, add sea salt and pepper to fit

Put in the mayonnaise, bacon, and egg to the waffle

Nutrition:

Calories 346.6
Fat 27.9 g.
Protein 22.5 g.

402. CAJUN AND AVOCADO WAFFLE SANDWICH

Preparation time: 8 min.
Cooking time: 7 min.
Servings: 2
Ingredients:
For the waffle:

- 4 eggs, should be large
- 2 c. shredded mozzarella part-skim cheese
- 1 tsp. Cajun seasoning

For the filling:

- 1-lb. fresh shrimp peeled and deveined
- 1 tbsp. bacon (or avocado) grease
- 4 slices of bacon cooked
- 1 large sliced avocado
- 1/4 c. red onion, thinly sliced
- 1 dish bacon scallion cream cheese spread optional
- 1 tsp. Cajun seasoning
- Salt and pepper to taste

Directions:

Whisk the eggs together. Add 2 c. mozzarella cheese with low moisture, and 1 tsp. Cajun seasoning. Put 1/4 c. of the cheese and mixture of the eggs over a mini waffle pan. Cook until the waffle is browned. Repeat the process with the left egg and cheese batter

Add shrimp and combine it in a large bowl, with the remaining 1 tsp. Cajun seasoning. Garnish with salt and pepper. Fried in a pan over medium-high heat with bacon grease until the shrimp is translucent. Lift the fried shrimp and put aside. Let cool if desired

Place the bacon scallion cream cheese over a side of a waffle to create the waffle sandwich. Cover the top of the waffle with shrimp, bacon, avocado, and red onion. Cover with one more waffle. Serve as you wish

Nutrition:

Calories 488

Fat 32.2 g.

Protein 47.59 g.

403. KETO WONDER-BREAD WAFFLE SANDWICH

Preparation time: 4 min.

Cooking time: 7 min.

Servings: 2

Ingredients:

For the wonder-bread waffle:

- 2 eggs white
- 2 tbsp. almond flour
- 1 tbsp. mayonnaise
- 1 tsp. water
- 1/4 tsp. baking powder
- 1 pinch salt

For the sandwich:

- 2 tbsp. mayonnaise
- 1-piece deli ham
- 1 slice deli turkey
- 1 slice of the cheese cheddar
- 1 tomato slice
- 1 leaf green leaf lettuce

Directions:

Preheat the maker. Mix all the ingredients of the wonder-bread waffle in a tiny bowl. Combined the wonder-bread waffle ingredients in a large bowl

Place 1/2 the batter into the waffle maker and cook for about 3–5 min. until finished

Add the batter to the mini waffle maker

Remove the waffle when cooking has been completed. Repeat for the batter remaining

Made the sandwich bread in a waffle maker

Place mayonnaise on one side of each bread waffle sandwich. Place in green leaf, tomato, and cold cuts

Nutrition:

Calories 208

Fat 17.4 g.

Protein 10.3 g.

404. KETO REUBEN SANDWICH WAFFLE

Preparation time: 6 min.

Cooking time: 7 min.

Servings: 2

Ingredients:

- 1 egg
- 1/2 c. mozzarella cheese
- 2 tbsp. flour (almond)
- 2 tbsp. low-carbohydrate thousand island dressing
- 1/4 tsp. baking powder
- 1/4 tsp. seeds of caraway
- 2 corned beef slices
- 1 Swiss cheese slice
- 2 tbsp. sauerkraut

Directions:

Set the temperature to the mid-high heat of the waffle maker

In a bowl, mix together the egg, mozzarella, almond flour, 1 tbsp. low-carb dressing seeds of caraway as well as baking powder

Place the waffle batter into the waffle maker center. Shut the waffle machine and let it be cooked for 5–7 min. or till lightly browned and crisp is perfect. If a mini waffle maker is used, just spill half the mixture over the waffle machine. 2 waffles (mini) will be produced from this recipe

Take the waffle out from the waffle machine. If you are using a mini waffle machine, repeat for the residual batter

Place the corned beef on a sheet of parchment, and cover with a Swiss cheese slice. Heat for 20–30 sec in the oven, before the cheese begins to melt. Take off from the microwave. Place on each waffle the remaining tbsp. low-carbohydrate thousand island sauces spread the Swiss cheese and hot corned beef, and finish with sauerkraut as well as other waffle

Nutrition:
Calories 605
Fat 43.8 g.
Protein 45.1 g.

405. CHEESY WAFFLE SANDWICH'S WITH AVOCADO AND BACON

Preparation time: 15 min.
Cooking time: 7 min.
Servings: 2
Ingredients:

- 10 eggs
- 1 1/2 c. cheddar cheese, shredded
- 2 center-cut slices of bacon, cooked and crumbled
- 1/2 tsp. ground pepper
- 2 small, sliced avocados
- 2 little tomatoes, in slices
- 4 large lettuce leaves, torn into 3 in. parts

Directions:
In a large bowl, whisk the eggs until smooth. Stir in cheese, chopped bacon, and pepper
Preheat a 7-in. (not Belgian) round waffle iron; top it with cooking spray. Pour approximately 2/3 c. of the beaten egg into the waffle iron. Cook 4–5 min. till the eggs are set and light golden brown. Repeat with cooking spray and

the remaining mixture of the eggs (making a total of 4 waffles)

Split each of the waffles into pieces. Top half of the quarters even with slices of avocado, tomato slices, and lettuce. Also, top the remaining quarters of the waffle

Nutrition:
Calories 259
Fat 20.1 g.
Protein 14 g.

406. KETO TURKEY BRIE CRANBERRY WAFFLE SANDWICH

Preparation time: 5 min.
Cooking time: 7 min.
Servings: 2
Ingredients:

- 1/2 c. grated mozzarella
- 1 medium beaten egg
- 2 tbsp. almond flour

For the filling:

- 2 slices of turkey
- 3 slices of Brie
- 2 tbsp. chia cranberry jam

Directions:
Turn your waffle maker on and grease it gently
Add the egg, mozzarella, and almond flour to a bowl. Combine until mixed
Spoon the mixture into the waffle maker. If you want a small waffle maker, spoon half the batter in at a time)
Close the lid and cook until golden and firm for 5 min.
Use tongs to remove the cooked waffles and set them aside
Place the turkey, brie, and cranberry on a cutting board and layer on the waffle. Put the layers together with your choice
Place on top of the other waffle and sliced in half
If you just want a warm sandwich, then heat it up for 20 sec. in the microwave

Nutrition:
Calories 537
Fat 36 g.
Proteins 44 g.

407. EASY WAFFLE SANDWICH

Preparation time: 5 min.
Cooking time: 7 min.
Servings: 2
Ingredients:

- 1 large egg
- 1/2 c. mozzarella
- 1 tbsp. (standard, gluten-free, almond or coconut flour)
- 1/2 tsp. baking powder
- 1 pinch of salt

Directions:
Coat nonstick cooking spray on the interior of a waffle maker. Preheat the waffle maker
Beat the egg in a little mixing bowl or cup. Mix the flour, baking powder, salt and combine properly
Stir in the scrambled cheese
Put the batter into the waffle iron. When using a mini-waffle machine, simply add in half of the mix
Lower with the cover. If the waffle maker has indicated the waffle is finished, raise the cover and transfer the waffle gently to a cooling rack. Use tongs to protect the fingertips from burning
Repeat this step until the amount of the waffles you want is reached

Nutrition:
Calories 269
Fat 17 g.
Protein 20 g.

408. LOW-CARB KETO WAFFLE SANDWICH

Preparation time: 5 min.
Cooking time: 7 min.
Servings: 2
Ingredients:

- 10 tbsp. parmesan shredded cheese
- 1 c. mozzarella shredded
- 2 slices of bacon (chopped)
- 1/4 tsp. dry oregano
- 1 tbsp. birch benders pancake mix (can be substituted for the desired mixture)
- 2 chickens
- 2 eggs
- Mayo
- 2 tiny or 1 large, thinly cut tomato
- Salt and pepper to fit

Directions:
Put the egg, oregano, mozzarella cheese, pancake mixture, and salt and pepper into a food processor. Pulse blend until complete. Should just take a few steps
Add bacon and pulse in the mixture until bacon is uniformly dispersed
Put 1 tbsp. parmesan on the waffle maker bottom. 1 heaping waffle mixture spoonful and 1 tbsp. parmesan on top. Cover the waffle maker and finish cooking till golden brown. Repeat until the entire mix is used. It can yield about five mini waffles
Apply the mayo on the waffle side. Add sliced tomato, salt, and pepper to taste. Attach the 2nd waffle to the end, and you've got a tomato sammie waffle

Nutrition:
Calories 320
Fat 24 g.
Protein 21 g.

409. CLUB SANDWICH WAFFLE

Preparation time: 5 min.
Cooking time: 7 min.
Servings: 2
Ingredients:

- 2 batches of the waffle simple recipe
- 2 strips of sugar-free bacon
- 2 oz. free of sugar sliced deli turkey
- 2 oz. sugar-free sliced deli ham
- 1 slice of the cheese (cheddar)
- 1 tomato slice
- 3 lettuce leaves
- 1 tbsp. mayonnaise free of sugar

Directions:

Cook the waffles and put them aside, as instructed. Cover to keep warm

Cook the bacon using your chosen (oven/microwave/stovetop) cooking process. By putting them in the microwave, sealed, keep it basic for around 2–3 min. (based on how crispy you want it and the brand).

When cooked, move to a lined sheet of paper towel

Make your sandwich, start the club sandwich with one waffle, and complete with the tomato and the lettuce. Add the other waffle and the cheese, ham, turkey, and bacon on top. Smear the final waffle with mayo, then put it on top of the sandwich

Enjoy it right away

Nutrition:

Calories 178
Fat 8.6 g.
Protein 6.6 g.

410. KETO WAFFLE (CHEESE WAFFLE) PLUS OMAD SANDWICH

Preparation time: 5 min.
Cooking time: 7 min.
Servings: 2
Ingredients:
For the waffle:

- 3/4 c. (75 g) shredded cheese (any of your choice)
- 1 medium-sized egg
- 1 tsp. husk of psyllium
- Salt and pepper
- Hot sauce (optional)

For the sandwich:

- 4 bacon strips
- 4 ham slices
- 4 prosciutto slices
- 5–6 salami slices
- 5–6 small pepperoni slices
- Mustard
- Mayonnaise

Directions:

Whisk the egg, cheese, salt, pepper, psyllium husk together in a bowl, and additional hot sauce

Keep the waffle maker to heat until the batter is uniformly poured into the waffle pan

Cook 2–3 min. or more based on how crispy you like it to be

Enjoy!

Nutrition:

Calories 458
Fat 33.4 g.
Protein 26.7 g.

411. KETO WAFFLE PULLED PORK SANDWICH WITH CREAMY COLESLAW

Preparation time: 15 min.
Cooking time: 7 min.
Servings: 2
Ingredients:

- 1 pork butt, bone-in
- 8 tbsp. barbecue sauce, sugar-free
- 1 packet of coleslaw mix or chopped cabbage
- 1 c. mayo
- 2 tbsp. heavy cream
- 1 tsp. creole mustard (any mustard you want, etc.)
- 1 tbsp. erythritol
- 1 tsp. pepper (optional)
- 1 tsp. garlic powder
- 1 tsp. black chili pepper
- 1 tsp. salt

Directions:

Begins with "scoring" the roast's fat side. The scoring helps the seasoning to enter the fat and add more flavor

Use cooking oils, butter, mustard, Worcestershire sauce, or any other chosen "wet" ingredient to add a slight element of moisture to enable the seasonings or rub to stick better to the meat

Cover the whole piece of meat absolutely with your favorite rub and let it sit for around 15–20 min. until burning your Pit Barrel

Place the fat side of the pork butt on the grill so that the meat is covered, and the fat becomes crisper if you cut the pork into pieces for taste and texture pieces. Smoke exposed inside until it hits 165 °F. Put it in a foil tray, cover it and position it again in the cooker once 205 °F is achieved

Take out the pan and let it cool. To remove the fat from the liquids, dump any liquid from the pan into another dish. Then place the juices back in the pan and start cutting the pork roast into medium-sized chunks and scraping any big fat or tendon pieces

Spray the same rub you cooked over the pulled bits to provide a few extra spices and spray it with the cooking sauces

Combine all coleslaw dressing components and check taste for further changes to the seasoning. Toss the coleslaw (or cabbage mix) with the sauce. Coleslaw may appear thicker to begin with but will change for 1 hour while resting in the fridge

Heat the waffle iron. Drop one slice of the cheese onto the waffle iron or scatter grated mozzarella cheese to cover the waffle maker's rim. Place 1/2 of a deviled egg over the cheese, which might melt. Place segmented cheese slice or cover with grated cheese and cover the waffle iron. If you like it to be crunchier let it steam for 3 min. (until sides crisp) or more. When it cools, it can become crunchier, so check first to see what consistency you want and then change the period accordingly

Place the waffle sandwich together or eat in a bowl if you like to skip the waffles

Use this remaining pulled pork at lunch for the next two days

Nutrition:

Calories 100
Fat 4.8 g.
Protein 8.8 g.

412. KETO WAFFLE SAUSAGE AND EGG BREAKFAST SANDWICH

Preparation time: 5 min.
Cooking time: 7 min.
Servings: 2
Ingredients:

- 2 large raw eggs

- 2 tbsp. coconut flour
- 2 tbsp. mayo
- 1/2 tsp. baking powder
- 1 tsp. absolute substitute icing sugar by swerve
- 1 x 2 sausage patty
- 3 /4 oz. or 2 slice American cheese slices

Directions:

At medium-high temperature, preheat the waffle iron. In a big mixing dish, add 1 egg, coconut flour, mayo, baking powder, and whisk

Whisk well. Let the batter stay for around 1 min. to thicken

Spray the waffle iron with nonstick spray high heat grill. Put into the hot waffle iron and cook as directed. Take away the waffles from the iron. Slice the waffle in half

Meanwhile, use a nonstick cooking spray with a 4 oz. ramekin. Add one egg and gently scramble it with a fork. Place the completely cooked sausage patty in the middle and microwave for around 1 min. on 60% power before the egg is cooked through

Put the egg and sausage with a slice of American cheese on 1/4 of the waffle. Repeat on the other sandwich with the cooking of another egg and sausage. Right away, enjoy or freeze in plastic wrap

Nutrition:

Calories 433
Fat 28.4 g.
Protein 17.6 g.

413.   KETO BLT AVOCADO WAFFLE SANDWICH

Preparation time: 15 min.
Cooking time: 7 min.
Servings: 2
Ingredients:

- 3–4 bacon pieces
- 1 egg
- 1/2 c. mozzarella
- 1 tsp. flour of almonds
- 1 tsp. all Bagel Seasoning (or preferably a sprinkle of salt, garlic, onion powder)
- 2 lettuce slices
- 1 sliced tomato
- 1 avocado slice
- 1 tbsp. mayonnaise

Directions:
For the bacon:

Start with a cold saucepan. Put the bacon in the pan and turn on the heat to a minimum. At minimum temperature, the bacon cooks better. When the bacon warms up a little bit and loses more of its fat, it begins curling up gently. You can then use tongs to rotate the bacon and start cooking on the other side. Then proceed to turn consistently until all sides of the bacon are fried, around 10 min. for thin or up to 15 min. for thicker sliced bacon.

For the sandwich:

Plugin, the mini waffle maker, to preheat

Crack the egg into a little bowl to create the waffle and blend along with 1/2 c. mozzarella, almond flour, and all bagel seasoning. This blend produces 2 waffles

Pour 1/2 of the mix into the preheated waffle maker and permit 3–4 min. of cooking (depending on how crispy you like your waffles) When cooking your first waffle, prepare the tomato and avocado by cutting one slice of each Pick up the waffle and repeat for 3–4 min., adding the other half of the blend into the waffle machine. When done, unplug the waffle maker

In the waffle, add your fried bacon, then finish with lettuce, tomato, avocado, and mayo

Put 2 toothpicks in the waffle to tie them together and slice them in half. Your waffle BLT avocado is ready to serve now

Nutrition:

Calories 208
Fat 19.4 g.
Protein 20.3 g.

414. KETO FRENCH DIP CHAFFWICH

Preparation time: 5 min.
Cooking time: 7 min.
Servings: 2
Ingredients:

- 4 oz. roasted beef
- 2 eggs (egg whites only)
- 2 tbsp. almond flour
- 1 tbsp. sour cream
- 1–1/2 c. mozzarella
- 1/2 c. beef broth low in sodium

Directions:

To make the waffle, whip the egg white till foamy. Include the almond flour and sour cream and mix properly. Add the cheese in

Heat up the mini waffle maker according to instructions from the manufacturer. Add half the batter when heated and cook for 7–10 min. once the waffle is nicely browned and readily releases. Repeat with the batter left behind

In the meanwhile, heat the beef broth in a tiny pot or pan. Heat up the sliced beef, don't overcook it!

Put the processed beef on the waffle to be assembled, top with cheese and serve sideways with the available broth

Nutrition:

Calories 444
Fat 26 g.
Protein 45 g

415. KETO TUNA-MOZZARELLA WAFFLE SANDWICH

Preparation time: 15 min.
Cooking time: 7 min.
Servings: 2
Ingredients:

- 1 egg
- 3/4 c. almond flour
- 1/2 tsp. baking powder
- 1/8 t of salt
- 2 tbsp. melted butter
- 1/4 c. mozzarella shredded cheese
- 1/4 c. sour cream

Directions:

Mix together the ingredients and place the batter into a mini waffle iron to produce a batch of the waffles

For the tuna sandwich:

Take two waffles and bring them together to make a sandwich with your St. Jude tuna salad. Choose your unique flavor of St. Jude tuna; blend with a little bit of olive oil and pepper. Add pepperoncini, tomatoes, red onion, red peppers, and all other preferred toppings

Nutrition:

Calories 100
Fat 3.7 g.
Protein 9.6 g.

416. KETO WAFFLE CUBAN SANDWICH

Preparation time: 5 min.
Cooking time: 7 min.
Servings: 2
Ingredients:

- 1 large egg
- 1 tbsp. almond flour
- 1 tbsp. Greek full-fat yogurt
- 1/8 tsp. baking powder
- 1/4 c. swiss cheese crushed

For the filling:

- 3 oz. roast pork
- 2 once deli ham
- 1 slice of Swiss cheese
- Chips of 3–5 pickles, sliced
- 1/2 tbsp. Dijon mustard

Directions:

Preheat your waffle iron

Scourge egg, yogurt, almond flour, and baking powder together

Scatter one-fourth of the Swiss shredded straight onto the hot waffle iron. Cover with half of the mixture of the egg, then apply 1/4 more Swiss on it. Cover the iron and cook until lightly brown and crunchy for 3–5 min.

Repeat the same procedure with the remaining ingredients

For the fillings:

In a small microwaveable dish, place the pork, Swiss cheese slice, and ham in order. Microwave the cheese for 40–50 sec., before it melts

Cover with the mustard on the inner part of one waffle, then finish with pickles. Reverse the bowl, so the molten Swiss hits the pickles on top of the waffle. Put the waffle at the bottom on the roast pork and reverse the sandwich to keep the side of pork below and the side of mustard up

Nutrition:

Calories 522

Fat 33 g.

Protein 46 g.

417. OPEN-FACED FRENCH DIP KETO WAFFLE SANDWICH

Preparation time: 5 min.
Cooking time: 7 min.
Servings: 2
Ingredients:

- 1 egg white
- 1/4 c., shredded (packed) mozzarella cheese
- 1/4 c., shredded (packed) sharp cheddar cheese
- 3/4 tsp. water
- 1 tsp. coconut flour
- 1/4 tsp. baking powder
- 1 pinch salt

Directions:

Preheat the oven to 425 °F. Plugin the wall of the mini waffle maker and graze gently until it is hot

Mix all the ingredients in a dish until combine

At the waffle maker, spoon 1/2 of the batter out and cover with a lid. Set a 4-minute timer, and do not raise the lid until the cooking period is complete. Preliminary lifting can cause separation of the waffle keto sandwich recipe and stick to the waffle iron. Before you raise the lid, you have to let it cook the whole 4 min.

Take the waffle from the iron, then put it aside. Repeat for the remaining waffle batter on the same measures above

Position the waffle a few inches apart and cover a baking sheet with parchment paper

Add 1/4–1/3 c. slow cooker keto roast beef. Before applying to the top of the waffle, be sure to remove the extra broth/gravy

Cover with a slice of deli cheese or sliced cheese. Both Swiss and the provolone are fantastic choices

Put on the oven's top rack for 5 min. to allow the cheese to melt. If you want to bubble the cheese and start browning, set the oven to broil for 1 min. (Swiss cheese does not brown)

Enjoy open-faced and dipping with a tiny cup of beef broth

Nutrition:

Calories 118

Fat 8 g.

Protein 9 g.

418. CHOCOLATE SANDWICH WAFFLES

Preparation time: 10 min.
Cooking time: 10 min.
Servings: 2
Ingredients:
For the waffles:

- 1 organic egg, beaten
- 1-oz. cream cheese, softened
- 2 tbsp. almond flour

- 1 tbsp. cacao powder
- 2 tsp. Erythritol
- 1 tsp. organic vanilla extract

For the filling:
- 2 tbsp. cream cheese, softened
- 2 tbsp. Erythritol
- 1/2 tbsp. cacao powder
- 1/4 tsp. organic vanilla extract

Directions:
Preheat a mini waffle iron and then grease it.

For the waffles:
In a medium bowl, add all the ingredients and, with a fork, mix until well combined.

Place half of the mixture into the preheated waffle iron and cook for about 3–5 min.

Repeat with the remaining mixture.

For the filling:
In a medium bowl, add all the ingredients and with a hand mixer, beat until well combined.

Spread the filling mixture over 1 waffle and top with the remaining waffle.

Cut in half and serve.

Nutrition:
Calories: 192
Net Carb: 2.5 g.
Fat: 16.6 g.
Carbohydrates: 4.4 g.
Dietary Fiber: 1.9 g.
Sugar: 0.8 g.
Protein: 5.7 g.

419. CHOCOLATE OREO SANDWICH WAFFLES

Preparation time: 0 min.
Cooking time: 0 min.
Servings: 2
Ingredients:
For the waffles:
- 1 organic egg
- 1 tbsp. heavy cream
- 2 tbsp. Erythritol

- 1 1/2 tbsp. cacao powder
- 1 tsp. coconut flour
- 2 tbsp. Erythritol
- 1/2 tsp. organic baking powder
- 1/2 tsp. organic vanilla extract

For the filling:
- 3 tbsp. mascarpone cheese, softened
- 2 tbsp. heavy whipping cream
- 1/2 tsp. organic vanilla extract
- 2 tbsp. powdered Erythritol

Directions:
Preheat a mini waffle iron and then grease it.

For the waffles:
In a medium bowl, put all the ingredients and, with a fork, mix until well combined.

Place half of the mixture into the preheated waffle iron and cook for about 3–5 min.

Repeat with the remaining mixture.

For the filling:
In a bowl, add all the ingredients and mix well.

Spread filling mixture over 1 waffle and top with the remaining waffle.

Cut in half and serve.

Nutrition:
Calories: 168
Net Carb: 3.2 g.
Fat: 14.4 g.
Carbohydrates: 5 g.
Dietary Fiber: 1.7 g.
Sugar: 0.4 g.
Protein: 6.8 g.

420. PEANUT BUTTER SANDWICH WAFFLES

Preparation time: 10 min.
Cooking time: 10 min.
Servings: 2
Ingredients:
For the waffles:
- 1 organic egg, beaten
- 2 tbsp. almond flour

- 1/2 tsp. organic baking powder
- 1/2 c. Mozzarella cheese, shredded

For the filling:

- 2 tbsp. natural peanut butter
- 2 tbsp. heavy cream
- 2 tsp. powdered Erythritol

Directions:

Preheat a mini waffle iron and then grease it.

For the waffles:

In a medium bowl, add all the ingredients and, with a fork, mix until well combined.

Place half of the mixture into the preheated waffle iron and cook for about 3–5 min.

Repeat with the remaining mixture.

For the filling:

In a bowl, add all the ingredients and mix well.

Spread peanut butter mixture over 1 waffle and top with the remaining waffle.

Cut in half and serve.

Nutrition:

Calories: 243

Net Carb: 4.1 g.

Fat: 20.8 g.

Carbohydrates: 5.8 g.

Dietary Fiber: 1.7 g.

Sugar: 1.9 g.

Protein: 9.1 g.

421. PEANUT BUTTER AND JAM SANDWICH WAFFLES

Preparation time: 10 min.

Cooking time: 8 min.

Servings: 2

Ingredients:

For the waffles:

- 1 organic egg
- 1/2 c. Monterey Jack cheese, shredded
- 1 tbsp. almond flour

For the filling:

- 1 tbsp. peanut butter
- 1 tbsp. sugar-free Strawberry jam

Directions:

Preheat a mini waffle iron and then grease it.

For the waffles:

In a medium bowl, add all the ingredients and, with a fork, mix until well combined.

Place half of the mixture into the preheated waffle iron and cook for about 3–4 min.

Spread peanut butter and jam over 1 waffle and top with the remaining waffle.

Cut in half and serve.

Nutrition:

Calories: 206

Net Carb: 6.6 g.

Fat: 16.7 g.

Carbohydrates: 2.6 g.

Dietary Fiber: 0.9 g.

Sugar: 1.2 g.

Protein: 11.7 g.

422. STRAWBERRY CREAM SANDWICH WAFFLES

Preparation time: 10 min.

Cooking time: 6 min.

Servings: 2

Ingredients:

For the waffles:

- 1 large organic egg, beaten
- 1/2 c. Mozzarella cheese, shredded finely

For the filling:

- 4 tsp. heavy cream
- 2 tbsp. powdered Erythritol
- 1 tsp. fresh lemon juice
- Pinch of fresh lemon zest, grated
- 2 fresh strawberries, hulled and sliced

Directions:

Preheat a mini waffle iron and then grease it.

For the waffles:

Into a small bowl, add the egg and Mozzarella cheese and stir to combine.

Place half of the mixture into the preheated waffle iron and cook for about 2–3 min.

Repeat with the remaining mixture.

For the filling:

In a bowl, Place all the ingredients except the strawberry slices and with a hand mixer, beat until well combined.

Place the cream mixture over 1 waffle and top with strawberry slices.

Cover with the remaining waffle.

Cut in half and serve.

Nutrition:

Calories: 95

Net Carb: 1.4 g.

Fat: 7.5 g.

Carbohydrates: 1.7 g.

Dietary Fiber: 0.3 g.

Sugar: 0.9 g.

Protein: 5.5 g.

423. BLUEBERRY SANDWICH WAFFLES

Preparation time: 10 min.

Cooking time: 10 min.

Servings: 2

Ingredients:

- 1 organic egg, beaten
- 1/2 c. Cheddar cheese, shredded

For the filling:

- 2 tbsp. Erythritol
- 1 tbsp. butter, softened
- 1 tbsp. natural peanut butter
- 2 tbsp. cream cheese, softened
- 1/4 tsp. organic vanilla extract
- 2 tsp. fresh blueberries

Directions:

Preheat a mini waffle iron and then grease it.

For the waffles:

Into a small bowl, add the egg and Cheddar cheese and stir to combine.

Place half of the mixture into the preheated waffle iron and cook for about 3–5 min.

Repeat with the remaining mixture.

For the filling:

In a medium bowl, add all the ingredients and mix until well combined.

Place the filling mixture over 1 waffle and top with the remaining waffle.

Cut in half and serve.

Nutrition:

Calories: 143

Net Carb: 3.3 g.

Fat: 10.1 g.

Carbohydrates: 4.1 g.

Dietary Fiber: 0.8 g.

Sugar: 1.2 g.

Protein: 7.6 g.

424. BLACKBERRY RICOTTA WAFFLES

Preparation time: 0 min.

Cooking time: 0 min.

Servings: 4

Ingredients:

For the waffles:

- 2 large organic eggs
- 1 c. Mozzarella cheese, shredded finely

For the filling:

- 1/4 c. fresh blackberries
- 4 tsp. ricotta cheese, crumbled

Directions:

Preheat a mini waffle iron and then grease it.

For the waffles:

In a bowl, add the eggs and cheese and stir to combine.

Place 1/4 of the mixture into the preheated waffle iron and cook for about 3–4 min.

Repeat with the remaining mixture.

Place the filling ingredients over 2 waffles and top with the remaining waffles.

Cut each in half and serve.

Nutrition:

Calories: 67

Net Carb: 1.1 g.

Fat: 4.2 g.

Carbohydrates: 1.6 g.
Dietary Fiber: 0.5 g.
Sugar: 0.7 g.
Protein: 5.9 g.

425. RASPBERRY SANDWICH WAFFLES

Preparation time: 15 min.
Cooking time: 10 min.
Servings: 2
Ingredients:
For the waffles:

- 1 organic egg, beaten
- 1 tsp. organic vanilla extract
- 1 tbsp. almond flour
- 1 tsp. organic baking powder
- Pinch of ground cinnamon
- 1 c. Mozzarella cheese, shredded

For the filling:

- 2 tbsp. cream cheese, softened
- 2 tbsp. Erythritol
- 1/4 tsp. organic vanilla extract
- 4 fresh raspberries, chopped

Directions:
Preheat a mini waffle iron and then grease it.
For the waffles:
In a bowl, add the egg and vanilla extract and mix well.
Add the flour, baking powder, and cinnamon and mix until well combined.
Add the Mozzarella cheese and stir to combine.
Place half of the mixture into the preheated waffle iron and cook for about 4–5 min.
Repeat with the remaining mixture.
For the filling:
In a bowl, Place all the ingredients except the strawberry pieces and with a hand mixer, beat until well combined.
Spread cream cheese mixture over 1 waffle and top with raspberries.
Cover with the remaining waffle.
Cut in half and serve.

Nutrition:
Calories: 143
Net Carb: 6.6 g.
Fat: 10.1 g.
Carbohydrates: 4.1 g.
Dietary Fiber: 0.8 g.
Sugar: 1.2 g.
Protein: 0.8 g.

426. BERRIES SAUCE SANDWICH WAFFLES

Preparation time: 10 min.
Cooking time: 8 min.
Servings: 2
Ingredients:
For the filling:

- 3 oz. frozen mixed berries, thawed with the juice
- 1 tbsp. Erythritol
- 1 tbsp. water
- 1/4 tbsp. fresh lemon juice
- 2 tsp. cream

For the waffles:

- 1 large organic egg, beaten
- 1/2 c. Cheddar cheese, shredded
- 2 tbsp. almond flour

Directions:
For the berry sauce:
In a pan, add the berries, Erythritol, water, and lemon juice over medium heat and cook for about 8–10 min., pressing with the spoon occasionally.
Remove the pan of sauce from the heat and set it aside to cool before serving.
Preheat a mini waffle iron and then grease it.
In a bowl, add the egg, Cheddar cheese, and almond flour and beat until well combined.
Place half of the mixture into the preheated waffle iron and cook for about 3–5 min.
Repeat with the remaining mixture.
Spread berry sauce over 1 waffle and top with the remaining waffle.

Cut in half and serve.

Nutrition:
Calories: 222
Net Carb: 4.7 g.
Fat: 21.5 g.
Carbohydrates: 7 g.
Dietary Fiber: 2.3 g.
Sugar: 3.8 g.
Protein: 10.5 g.

427. GRILLED CHEESE SANDWICH WAFFLES

Preparation time: 0 min.
Cooking time: 0 min.
Servings: 2
Ingredients:
For the waffles:

- 1 organic egg
- 1/2 c. Cheddar cheese, shredded
- 1/4 tsp. garlic powder

For the filling:

- 1 tbsp. butter
- 1/4 c. Cheddar cheese, shredded

Directions:
Preheat a mini waffle iron and then grease it.
In a bowl, add the egg, Cheddar cheese, and almond flour and beat until well combined.
Place half of the mixture into the preheated waffle iron and cook for about 3–4 min.
Repeat with the remaining mixture.
In a frying pan, melt the butter over medium heat.
Cover with the second waffle and cook for about 1 min. per side.
Transfer the waffle sandwich onto a plate and cut it in half.

Serve immediately.

Nutrition:
Calories: 254
Net Carb: 1 g.
Fat: 22 g.
Carbohydrates: 1 g.
Dietary Fiber: 0 g.
Sugar: 0.5 g.
Protein: 13.4 g.

428. CHICKEN SANDWICH WAFFLES

Preparation time: 10 min.
Cooking time: 8 min.
Servings: 2
Ingredients:
For the waffles:

- 1 large organic egg, beaten
- 1/2 c. Cheddar cheese, shredded
- Pinch of salt and ground black pepper

For the filling:

- 1 (6-oz.) cooked grass-fed chicken breast, halved
- 2 lettuce leaves
- 1/4 of a small onion, sliced
- 1 small tomato, sliced

Directions:
Preheat a mini waffle iron and then grease it.
For the waffles:
In a medium bowl, add all the ingredients and, with a fork, mix until well combined.
Place half of the mixture into the preheated waffle iron and cook for about 3–4 min.
Repeat with the remaining mixture.
Place the filling ingredients over 1 waffle and top with the remaining waffle.
Cut in half and serve.

Nutrition:
Calories: 259
Net Carb: 2.5 g.
Fat: 14.1 g.
Carbohydrates: 3.3 g.

Dietary Fiber: 0.8 g.
Sugar: 2 g.
Protein: 28.7 g.

429. PORK SANDWICH WAFFLES

Preparation time: 15 min.
Cooking time: 16 min.
Servings: 4
Ingredients:
For the waffles:

- 2 large organic eggs
- 1/4 c. superfine blanched almond flour
- 3/4 tsp. organic baking powder
- 1/2 tsp. garlic powder
- 1 c. Cheddar cheese, shredded

For the filling:

- 12 oz. cooked pork, cut into slices
- 1 tomato, sliced
- 4 lettuce leaves

Directions:
Preheat a mini waffle iron and then grease it.
For the waffles:
In a bowl, add the eggs, almond flour, baking powder, and garlic powder and beat until well combined.
Add the cheese and stir to combine.
Place 1/4 of the mixture into the preheated waffle iron and cook for about 3–4 min.
Repeat with the remaining mixture.
Place the filling ingredients over 2 waffles and top with the remaining waffles.
Cut each in half and serve.
Nutrition:
Calories: 319
Net Carb: 2.5 g.
Fat: 18.2 g.
Carbohydrates: 3.5 g.
Dietary Fiber: 1 g.
Sugar: 0.9 g.
Protein: 34.2 g.

430. BACON AND EGG SANDWICH WAFFLES

Preparation time: 10 min.
Cooking time: 20 min.
Servings: 4
Ingredients:
For the waffles:

- 2 large organic eggs, beaten
- 4 tbsp. almond flour
- 1 tsp. organic baking powder
- 1 c. Mozzarella cheese, shredded

For the filling:

- 4 organic fried eggs
- 4 cooked bacon slices

Directions:
Preheat a mini waffle iron and then grease it.
For the waffles:
In a medium bowl, add all the ingredients and, with a fork, mix until well combined.
Place half of the mixture into the preheated waffle iron and cook for about 3–5 min.
Repeat with the remaining mixture.
Place the filling ingredients over 2 waffles and top with the remaining waffles.
Cut each in half and serve.
Nutrition:
Calories: 197
Net Carb: 1.9 g.
Fat: 14.5 g.
Carbohydrates: 2.7 g.
Dietary Fiber: 0.8 g.
Sugar: 0.7 g.
Protein: 15.7 g.

431. BACON AND LETTUCE SANDWICH WAFFLES

Preparation time: 10 min.
Cooking time: 8 min.
Servings: 2
Ingredients:
For the waffles:

- 1 organic egg

- 1/2 c. Mozzarella cheese, shredded
- 1 tbsp. scallion, chopped
- 1/2 tsp. Italian seasoning

For the filling:
- 2 lettuce leaves
- 2 cooked bacon slices
- 2 tomato slices

Directions:
Preheat a mini waffle iron and then grease it.

For the waffles:
In a medium bowl, add all the ingredients and, with a fork, mix until well combined.
Place half of the mixture into the preheated waffle iron and cook for about 4 min.
Repeat with the remaining mixture.
Place the lettuce, bacon, and tomato slice over the waffle and top with the remaining waffle.
Cut in half and serve.

Nutrition:
Calories: 216
Net Carb: 1.5 g.
Fat: 16 g.
Carbohydrates: 1.8 g.
Dietary Fiber: 0.3 g.
Sugar: 0.7 g.
Protein: 15.7 g.

432.　BACON AND CHEESE WAFFLES

Preparation time: 10 min.
Cooking time: 8 min.
Servings: 0
Ingredients:
For the waffles:
- 1 organic egg
- 1/2 c. Mozzarella cheese, shredded
- 2 tbsp. almond flour

For the filling:
- 2 cooked bacon slices
- 1 Cheddar cheese slice

Directions:
Preheat a mini waffle iron and then grease it.

For the waffles:
In a medium bowl, add all the ingredients and, with a fork, mix until well combined.
Place half of the mixture into the preheated waffle iron and cook for about 3–4 min.
Repeat with the remaining mixture.
Place the bacon and cheese slice over the waffle and top with the remaining waffle.
Cut in half and serve.

Nutrition:
Calories: 310
Net Carb: 1.5 g.
Fat: 24 g.
Carbohydrates: 2.3 g.
Dietary Fiber: 0.8 g.
Sugar: 0.5 g.
Protein: 19 g.

433.　HAM AND CHEESE WAFFLES

Preparation time: 10 min.
Cooking time: 8 min.
Servings: 2
Ingredients:
For the waffles:
- 1 large organic egg
- 1/2 c. cheddar cheese, shredded
- 3 tbsp. almond flour
- 1/4 tsp. organic baking powder

For the filling:
- 1–2 tbsp. mayonnaise
- 1 sugar-free ham slice
- 1 cheddar cheese slice

Directions:
Preheat a mini waffle iron and then grease it.

For the waffles:
In a medium bowl, add all the ingredients and, with a fork, mix until well combined.
Place half of the mixture into the preheated waffle iron and cook for about 3–4 min.

Repeat with the remaining mixture.

Spread mayonnaise over 1 waffle.

Place the ham and cheese slice over the waffle and top with the remaining waffle.

Cut in half and serve.

Nutrition:

Calories: 273

Net Carb: 2.7 g.

Fat: 21.2 g.

Carbohydrates: 4.1 g.

Dietary Fiber: 1.4 g.

Sugar: 0.7 g.

Protein: 14 g.

434. HAM AND TOMATO SANDWICH WAFFLES

Preparation time: 10 min.

Cooking time: 8 min.

Servings: 2

Ingredients:

For the waffles:

- 1 organic egg, beaten
- 1/2 c. Monterrey Jack cheese, shredded
- 1 tsp. coconut flour
- Pinch of garlic powder

For the filling:

- 2 sugar-free ham slices
- 1 small tomato, sliced
- 2 lettuce leaves

Directions:

Preheat a mini waffle iron and then grease it.

For the waffles:

In a medium bowl, add all the ingredients and, with a fork, mix until well combined.

Place half of the mixture into the preheated waffle iron and cook for about 3–4 min.

Repeat with the remaining mixture.

Place the filling ingredients over 1 waffle and top with the remaining waffle.

Cut in half and serve.

Nutrition:

Calories: 156

Net Carb: 2.7 g.

Fat: 8.7 g.

Carbohydrates: 5.5 g.

Dietary Fiber: 1.8 g.

Sugar: 1.5 g.

Protein: 13.9 g.

435. SMOKED SALMON AND CREAM SANDWICH WAFFLES

Preparation time: 10 min.

Cooking time: 8 min.

Servings: 2

Ingredients:

For the waffles:

- 1 organic egg, beaten
- 1/2 c. Cheddar cheese, shredded
- 1 tbsp. almond flour
- 1 tbsp. fresh rosemary, chopped

For the filling:

- 1/4 c. smoked salmon
- 1 tsp. fresh dill, chopped
- 2 tbsp. cream

Directions:

Preheat a mini waffle iron and then grease it.

For the waffles:

In a medium bowl, add all the ingredients and, with a fork, mix until well combined.

Place half of the mixture into the preheated waffle iron and cook for about 3–4 min.

Repeat with the remaining mixture.

Place the filling ingredients over 1 waffle and top with the remaining waffle.

Cut in half and serve.

Nutrition:

Calories: 202

Net Carb: 1.7 g.

Fat: 15.1 g.

Carbohydrates: 2.9 g.

Dietary Fiber: 1.2 g.

Sugar: 0.7 g.

Protein: 13.2 g.

436. SMOKED SALMON AND FETA SANDWICH WAFFLES

Preparation time: 15 min.
Cooking time: 24 min.
Servings: 4
Ingredients:
For the waffles:

- 2 organic eggs
- 1/2 oz. butter, melted
- 1 c. Mozzarella cheese, shredded
- 2 tbsp. almond flour
- Pinch of salt

For the filling:

- 1/2 c. smoked salmon
- 1/3 c. avocado, peeled, pitted, and sliced
- 2 tbsp. feta cheese, crumbled

Directions:
Preheat a mini waffle iron and then grease it.
For the waffles:
In a medium bowl, add all the ingredients and, with a fork, mix until well combined.
Place 1/4 of the mixture into the preheated waffle iron and cook for about 5–6 min.
Repeat with the remaining mixture.
Place the filling ingredients over 2 waffles and top with the remaining waffles.
Cut each in half and serve.

Nutrition:
Calories: 169
Net Carb: 1.2 g.
Fat: 13.5 g.
Carbohydrates: 2.8 g.
Dietary Fiber: 1.6 g.
Sugar: 1.6 g.

Protein: 8.9 g.

437. TUNA SANDWICH WAFFLES

Preparation time: 10 min.
Cooking time: 8 min.
Servings: 2
Ingredients:
For the waffles:

- 1 organic egg, beaten
- 1/2 c. Cheddar cheese, shredded
- 1 tbsp. almond flour
- Pinch of salt

For the filling:

- 1/4 c. water-packed tuna, flaked
- 2 lettuce leaves

Directions:
Preheat a mini waffle iron and then grease it.
For the waffles:
In a medium bowl, add all the ingredients and, with a fork, mix until well combined.
Place half of the mixture into the preheated waffle iron and cook for about 3–4 min.
Repeat with the remaining mixture.
Place the filling ingredients over 1 waffle and top with the remaining waffle.
Cut in half and serve.

Nutrition:
Calories: 186
Net Carb: 0.6 g.
Fat: 13.6 g.
Carbohydrates: 1.3 g.
Dietary Fiber: 0.4 g.
Sugar: 0.5 g.
Protein: 13.6 g.

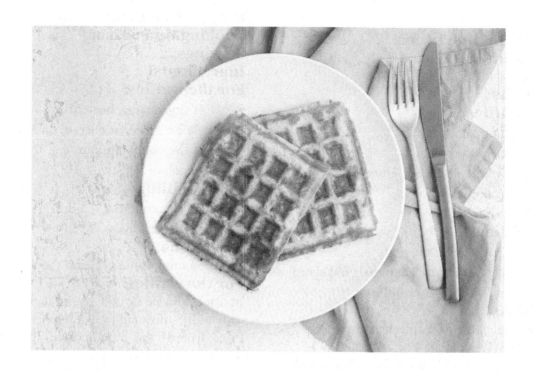

438. LAYERED CHEESE WAFFLES

Preparation time: 8 min.
Cooking time: 5 min.
Servings: 2
Ingredients:

- 1 organic egg, beaten
- 1/3 c. Cheddar cheese, shredded
- 1/2 tsp. ground flaxseed
- 1/4 tsp. organic baking powder
- 2 tbsp. Parmesan cheese, shredded

Directions:

Preheat a mini waffle iron and then grease it.
In a bowl, place all the ingredients except Parmesan and beat until well combined.
Place half the Parmesan cheese in the bottom of the preheated waffle iron.
Place half of the egg mixture over cheese and top with the remaining Parmesan cheese.
Cook for about 3-minutes or until golden brown.
Serve warm.

Nutrition:

Calories: 264
Net Carb: 1.
Fat: 20 g.
Saturated Fat: 11.1 g.
Carbohydrates: 2.1 g.
Dietary Fiber: 0.4 g.
Sugar: 0.6 g.
Protein: 18.9 g.

439. VANILLA MOZZARELLA WAFFLES

Preparation time: 10 min.
Cooking time: 12 min.
Servings: 2
Ingredients:

- 1 organic egg, beaten
- 1 tsp. organic vanilla extract
- 1 tbsp. almond flour
- 1 tsp. organic baking powder
- Pinch of ground cinnamon
- 1 c. Mozzarella cheese, shredded

Directions:

Preheat a mini waffle iron and then grease it.
In a bowl, place the egg and vanilla extract and beat until well combined.
Add the flour, baking powder, and cinnamon and mix well.
Add the Mozzarella cheese and stir to combine.
In a small bowl, place the egg and Mozzarella cheese and stir to combine.
Place half of the mixture into the preheated waffle iron and cook for about 5-minutes or until golden brown.
Repeat with the remaining mixture.
Serve warm.

Nutrition:

Calories: 103
Net Carb: 2.4 g.
Fat: 6.6 g.
Saturated Fat: 2.3 g.
Carbohydrates: 2
Dietary Fiber: 0.5 g.
Sugar: 0.6 g.
Protein: 6.8 g.

440. BRUSCHETTA WAFFLE

Preparation time: 10 min.
Cooking time: 5 min.
Servings: 2
Ingredients:

- 2 basic waffles
- 2 tbsp. sugar-free marinara sauce
- 2 tbsp. mozzarella, shredded
- 1 tbsp. olives, sliced
- 1 tomato sliced
- 1 tbsp. keto-friendly pesto sauce
- Basil leaves

Directions:

Spread marinara sauce on each waffle.

Spoon pesto and spread on top of the marinara sauce.

Top with the tomato, olives, and mozzarella.

Bake in the oven for 3 min. or until the cheese has melted.

Garnish with basil.

Serve and enjoy.

Nutrition:
Calories 182
Total Fat: 11 g.
Saturated Fat: 6.1 g.
Cholesterol 30 mg.
Sodium 508 mg.
Potassium 1 mg.
Total Carbohydrate 3.1 g.
Dietary Fiber 1.1 g.
Protein: 16.8 g.
Total Sugars 1 g.

441. EGG-FREE PSYLLIUM HUSK WAFFLES

Preparation time: 8 min.
Cooking time: 4 min.
Servings: 3
Ingredients:

- 1-oz. Mozzarella cheese, shredded
- 1 tbsp. cream cheese, softened
- 1 tbsp. psyllium husk powder

Directions:
Preheat a waffle iron and then grease it.

In a blender, place all the ingredients and pulse until a slightly crumbly mixture forms.

Place the mixture into the preheated waffle iron and cook for about 4 min. or until golden brown.

Serve warm.

Nutrition:
Calories: 137
Net Carb: 1.3 g.
Fat: 8.8 g.
Saturated Fat: 2 g.
Carbohydrates: 1.3 g.
Dietary Fiber: 0 g.
Sugar: 0 g.

Protein: 9.5 g.

442. MOZZARELLA AND ALMOND FLOUR WAFFLES

Preparation time: 10 min.
Cooking time: 8 min.
Servings: 4
Ingredients:

- 1/2 c. Mozzarella cheese, shredded
- 1 large organic egg
- 2 tbsp. blanched almond flour
- 1/4 tsp. organic baking powder

Directions:
Preheat a mini waffle iron and then grease it.

In a medium bowl, place all the ingredients and, with a fork, mix until well combined.

Place half of the mixture into the preheated waffle iron and cook for about 4 min. or until golden brown.

Repeat with the remaining mixture.

Serve warm.

Nutrition:
Calories: 98
Net Carb: 1.4 g.
Fat: 7.1 g.
Saturated Fat: 1 g.
Carbohydrates: 2.2 g.
Dietary Fiber: 0.8 g.
Sugar: 0.2 g.
Protein: 7 g.

443. PULLED PORK WAFFLE SANDWICHES

Preparation time: 9 min.
Cooking time: 28 min.
Servings: 2
Ingredients:

- 2 eggs, beaten
- 1 c. finely grated cheddar cheese
- 1/4 tsp. baking powder
- 2 c. cooked and shredded pork
- 1 tbsp. sugar-free BBQ sauce

- 2 c. shredded coleslaw mix
- 2 tbsp. apple cider vinegar
- 1/2 tsp. salt
- 1/4 c. ranch dressing

Directions:

Preheat the waffle iron.

In a medium bowl, mix the eggs, cheddar cheese, and baking powder.

Open the iron and add 1/4 of the mixture. Close and cook until crispy, 7 min.

Transfer the waffle to a plate and make 3 more waffles in the same manner.

Meanwhile, in another medium bowl, mix the pulled pork with the BBQ sauce until well combined. Set aside.

Also, mix the coleslaw mix, apple cider vinegar, salt, and ranch dressing in another medium bowl.

When the waffles are ready, on two pieces, divide the pork and then top with the ranch coleslaw. Cover with the remaining waffles and insert mini skewers to secure the sandwiches.

Enjoy afterward.

Nutrition:

Calories 374

Fats 23.61 g.

Carbs: 8.2 g.

Net Carbs: 8.2 g.

Protein: 28.05 g.

444. CHEDDAR AND EGG WHITE WAFFLES

Preparation time: 9 min.

Cooking time: 12 min.

Servings: 2

Ingredients:

- 2 egg whites
- 1 c. Cheddar cheese, shredded

Directions:

Preheat a mini waffle iron and then grease it.

In a small bowl, place the egg whites and cheese and stir to combine.

Place 1/4 of the mixture into the preheated waffle iron and cook for about 4 min. or until golden brown.

Repeat with the remaining mixture.

Serve warm.

Nutrition:

Calories: 122

Net Carb: 0.5 g.

Fat: 9.4 g.

Carbohydrates: 0.5 g.

Dietary Fiber: 0 g.

Sugar: 0.3 g.

Protein: 8.8 g.

445. SPICY SHRIMP AND WAFFLES

Preparation time: 9 min.

Cooking time: 31 min.

Servings: 4

Ingredients:

For the shrimp:

- 1 tbsp. olive oil
- 1 lb jumbo shrimp, peeled and deveined
- 1 tbsp. Creole seasoning
- Salt to taste
- 2 tbsp. hot sauce
- 3 tbsp. butter
- 2 tbsp. chopped fresh scallions to garnish

For the waffles:

- 2 eggs, beaten
- 1 c. finely grated Monterey Jack cheese

Directions:

For the shrimp:

Heat the olive oil in a medium skillet over medium heat.

Season the shrimp with the Creole seasoning and salt. Cook in the oil until pink and opaque on both sides, 2 min.

Pour in the hot sauce and butter. Mix well until the shrimp is adequately coated in the sauce, 1 min.

Turn the heat off and set it aside.

For the waffles:

Preheat the waffle iron.

In a medium bowl, mix the eggs and Monterey Jack cheese.

Open the iron and add 1/4 of the mixture. Close and cook until crispy, 7 min.

Transfer the waffle to a plate and make 3 more waffles in the same manner.

Cut the waffles into quarters and place them on a plate.

Top with the shrimp and garnish with the scallions.

Serve warm.

Nutrition:

Calories 342

Fats 19.75 g.

Carbs: 2.8 g.

Net Carbs: 2.3 g.

Protein: 36.01 g.

446. CREAMY CHICKEN WAFFLE SANDWICH

Preparation time: 10 min.

Cooking time: 10 min.

Servings: 2

Ingredients:

- Cooking spray
- 1 c. chicken breast fillet, cubed
- Salt and pepper to taste
- 1/4 c. all-purpose cream
- 4 garlic waffles
- Parsley, chopped

Directions:

Spray your pan with oil.

Put it over medium heat.

Add the chicken fillet cubes.

Season with salt and pepper.

Reduce heat and add the cream.

Spread the chicken mixture on top of the waffle.

Garnish with parsley and top with another waffle.

Nutrition:

Calories 273

Total Fat: 34 g.

Saturated Fat: 4.1 g.

Cholesterol 62 mg.

Sodium 373 mg.

Total Carbohydrate 22.5 g.

Dietary Fiber 1.1 g.

Total Sugars 3.2 g.

Protein: 17.5 g.

Potassium 177 mg.

447. STRAWBERRY SHORTCAKE WAFFLE BOWLS

Preparation time: 15 min.

Cooking time: 28 min.

Servings: 2

Ingredients:

- 1 egg, beaten
- 1/2 c. finely grated mozzarella cheese
- 1 tbsp. almond flour
- 1/4 tsp. baking powder
- 2 drops cake batter extract
- 1 c. cream cheese, softened
- 1 c. fresh strawberries, sliced
- 1 tbsp. sugar-free maple syrup

Directions:

Preheat a waffle bowl maker and grease lightly with cooking spray.

Meanwhile, in a medium bowl, whisk all the ingredients except the cream cheese and strawberries.

Open the iron, pour in half of the mixture, cover, and cook until crispy, 6–7 min.

Remove the waffle bowl onto a plate and set it aside.

Make a second waffle bowl with the remaining batter.

To serve, divide the cream cheese into the waffle bowls and top with the strawberries.

Drizzle the filling with the maple syrup and serve.

Nutrition:
Calories 235
Fats 20.62 g.
Carbs: 5.9 g.
Net Carbs: 5 g.
Protein: 7.51 g.

448. PUMPKIN AND PECAN WAFFLE

Preparation time: 10 min.
Cooking time: 10 min.
Servings: 2
Ingredients:

- 1 egg, beaten
- 1/2 c. mozzarella cheese, grated
- 1/2 tsp. pumpkin spice
- 1 tbsp. pureed pumpkin
- 2 tbsp. almond flour
- 1 tsp. sweetener
- 2 tbsp. pecans, chopped

Directions:
Turn on the waffle maker.
Beat the egg in a bowl.
Stir in the rest of the ingredients.
Pour half of the mixture into the device.
Seal the lid.
Cook for 5 min.
Remove the waffle carefully.
Repeat the steps to make the second waffle.

Nutrition:
Calories 210
Total Fat: 17 g.
Saturated Fat: 10 g.
Cholesterol 110 mg.
Sodium 250 mg.
Potassium 570 mg.
Total Carbohydrate 4.6 g.
Dietary Fiber 1.7 g.
Protein: 11 g.
Total Sugars 2 g
.

449. SPICY JALAPENO AND BACON WAFFLES

Preparation time: 10 min.
Cooking time: 3 min.
Servings: 2
Cooking time: 5 min.
Ingredients:

- 1 oz. cream cheese
- 1 large egg
- 1/2 c. cheddar cheese
- 2 tbsps. bacon bits
- 1/2 tbsp. jalapenos
- 1/4 tsp. baking powder

Directions:
Switch on your waffle maker.
Grease your waffle maker with cooking spray and let it heat up.
Mix egg and vanilla extract in a bowl first.
Add baking powder, jalapenos, and bacon bites.
Add in cheese last and mix together.
Pour the waffles batter into the maker and cook the waffles for about 2–3 min.
Once the waffles are cooked, remove them from the maker.
Serve hot and enjoy!

Nutrition:
Protein: 24% 5
Fat: 70% 175
Carbohydrates: 6% 15

450. ZUCCHINI PARMESAN WAFFLES

Preparation time: 10 min.
Cooking time: 14 min.
Servings: 2
Ingredients:

- 1 c. shredded zucchini
- 1 egg, beaten
- 1/2 c. finely grated Parmesan cheese
- Salt and freshly ground black pepper to taste

Directions:

Preheat the waffle iron.

Put all the ingredients into a medium bowl and mix well.

Open the iron and add half of the mixture. Close and cook until crispy, 7 min.

Remove the waffle onto a plate and make another with the remaining mixture.

Cut each waffle into wedges and serve afterward.

Nutrition:

Calories: 138

Fats: 9.07 g.

Carbs: 3.81 g.

Net Carbs: 3.71 g.

Protein: 10.02 g.

451.   CHEDDAR   AND ALMOND FLOUR WAFFLES

Preparation time: 10 min.

Cooking time: 10 min.

Servings: 2

Ingredients:

• 1 large organic egg, beaten

• 1/2 c. Cheddar cheese, shredded

• 2 tbsp. almond flour

Directions:

Preheat a mini waffle iron and then grease it.

In a bowl, place the egg, Cheddar cheese, and almond flour and beat until well combined.

Place half of the mixture into the preheated waffle iron and cook for about 5 min. or until golden brown.

Repeat with the remaining mixture.

Serve warm.

Nutrition:

Calories: 195

Net Carb: 1 g.

Fat: 15

Saturated Fat: 7 g.

Carbohydrates: 1.8 g.

Dietary Fiber: 0.8 g.

Sugar: 0.6 g.

Protein: 10.2 g.

452.   SIMPLE   AND BEGINNER WAFFLE

Preparation time: 10 min.

Cooking time: 5 min.

Servings: 2

Ingredients:

• 1 large egg

• 1/2 c. mozzarella cheese, shredded

• Cooking spray

Directions:

Switch on your waffle maker.

Beat the egg with a fork in a small mixing bowl.

Once the egg is beaten, add the mozzarella and mix well.

Spray the waffle maker with cooking spray.

Pour the waffles mixture into a preheated waffle maker and let it cook for about 2–3 min.

Once the waffles are cooked, carefully remove them from the maker and cook the remaining batter.

Serve hot with coffee and enjoy!

Nutrition:

Protein: 36% 42

Fat: 60% 71

Carbohydrates: 4% 5

453.   ASIAN CAULIFLOWER WAFFLES

Preparation time: 9 min.

Cooking time: 28 min.

Servings: 2

Ingredients:

For the waffles:

• 1 c. cauliflower rice, steamed

• 1 large egg, beaten

• Salt and freshly ground black pepper to taste

• 1 c. finely grated Parmesan cheese

• 1 tsp. sesame seeds

• 1/4 c. chopped fresh scallions

For the dipping sauce:
- 3 tbsp. coconut aminos
- 1 1/2 tbsp. plain vinegar
- 1 tsp. fresh ginger puree
- 1 tsp. fresh garlic paste
- 3 tbsp. sesame oil
- 1 tsp. fish sauce
- 1 tsp. red chili flakes

Directions:
Preheat the waffle iron.
In a medium bowl, mix the cauliflower rice, egg, salt, black pepper, and Parmesan cheese.
Open the iron and add 1/4 of the mixture. Close and cook until crispy, 7 min.
Transfer the waffle to a plate and make 3 more waffles in the same manner.
Meanwhile, make the dipping sauce.
In a medium bowl, mix all the ingredients for the dipping sauce.
Plate the waffles, garnish with the sesame seeds and scallions and serve with the dipping sauce.

Nutrition:
Calories 231
Fats 188 g.
Carbs: 6.32 g.
Net Carbs: 5.42 g.
Protein: 9.66 g.

454. SHARP CHEDDAR WAFFLES

Preparation time: 10 min.
Cooking time: 10 min.
Servings: 2
Ingredients:
- 1 organic egg, beaten
- 1/2 c. sharp Cheddar cheese, shredded

Directions:
Preheat a mini waffle iron and then grease it.
In a small bowl, place the egg and cheese and stir to combine.

Place half of the mixture into the preheated waffle iron and cook for about 5 min. or until golden brown.
Repeat with the remaining mixture.
Serve warm.

Nutrition:
Calories: 145
Net Carb: 0.5 g.
Fat: 11
Saturated Fat: 6.6 g.
Carbohydrates: 0.5 g.
Dietary Fiber: 0 g.
Sugar: 0.3 g.
Protein: 9.8 g.

455. CRISPY ZUCCHINI WAFFLES

Preparation time: 10 min.
Cooking time: 20 min.
Servings: 2
Ingredients:
- 1 zucchini (small)
- 1 egg
- 1/2 c. shredded mozzarella
- 1 tbsp. parmesan
- Pepper, as per your taste
- 1 tsp. basil

Directions:
Preheat your waffle iron
Grate zucchini finely
Add all the ingredients to the zucchini in a bowl and mix well
Grease your waffle iron lightly
Pour the mixture into a full-size waffle maker and spread evenly
Cook till it turns crispy
Make as many waffles as your mixture and waffle maker allow
Serve crispy and hot

Nutrition:
Calories: 118
Protein: 7.59

Fat: 5.82
Carbohydrates: 9.03

456. SIMPLE AND CRISPY WAFFLE

Preparation time: 5 min.
Cooking time: 15 min.
Servings: 2
Ingredients:

- 1/3 c. cheddar cheese
- 1 egg
- 1/4 tsp. baking powder
- 1 tsp. flaxseed (ground)
- 1/3 c. parmesan cheese

Directions:
Mix cheddar cheese, egg, baking powder, and flaxseed in a bowl
In your mini waffle iron, shred half of the parmesan cheese
Grease your waffle iron lightly
Add the mixture from step one to your mini waffle iron
Again shred the remaining cheddar cheese on the mixtures
Cook till the desired crisp is achieved
Make as many waffles as your mixture and waffle maker allow

Nutrition:
Calories: 157
Protein: 9.58 g.
Fat: 11.58 g.
Carbohydrates: 3.66 g.

457. BACON CHEDDAR WAFFLE

Preparation time: 5 min.
Cooking time: 5 min.
Servings: 2
Ingredients:

- Bacon bite, as per your taste
- 1 egg
- 1 1/2 c. cheddar cheese

Directions:
Preheat your waffle iron if needed
Mix all the above-mentioned ingredients in a bowl
Grease your waffle iron lightly
Cook in the waffle iron for about 5 min. or till the desired crisp is achieved
Serve hot
Make as many waffles as your mixture and waffle maker allow

Nutrition:
Calories: 65
Protein: 4.48 g.
Fat: 4.82 g.
Carbohydrates: 0.51 g.

458. EGGPLANT CHEDDAR WAFFLE

Preparation time: 10 min.
Cooking time: 15 min.
Servings: 2
Ingredients:

- 1 eggplant, medium-sized
- 1 egg
- 1 1/2 c. cheddar cheese

Directions:
Boil eggplant in water for 15 min.
Remove from water and blend to make a mixture
Preheat your waffle iron if needed
Mix all the above-mentioned ingredients into a bowl of the eggplants
Grease your waffle iron lightly
Cook in the waffle iron for about 5 min. or till the desired crisp is achieved
Serve hot
Make as many waffles as your mixture and waffle maker allow

Nutrition:
Calories: 174
Protein: 10.37 g.
Fat: 8.34 g.
Carbohydrates: 16.62 g.

459. CRUNCHY OLIVE WAFFLE

Preparation time: 5 min.
Cooking time: 15 min.
Servings: 2
Ingredients:

- 1/3 c. cheddar cheese
- 1 egg
- 1/4 tsp. baking powder
- 1 tsp. flaxseed (ground)
- 1/3 c. parmesan cheese
- 6–8 olive, sliced

Directions:
Mix cheddar cheese, egg, baking powder, and flaxseed together
In your mini waffle iron, shred half of the parmesan cheese
Grease your waffle iron lightly
Add the mixture from step one to your mini waffle iron
Add the sliced olives
Again shred the remaining cheddar cheese on the mixtures
Cook till the desired crisp is achieved
Make as many waffles as your mixture and waffle maker allow

Nutrition:
Calories: 157
Protein: 9.58 g.
Fat: 11.58 g.
Carbohydrates: 3.66 g.

460. HALLOUMI CHEESE WAFFLE

Preparation time: 5 min.
Cooking time: 15 min.
Servings: 2
Ingredients:

- 3 oz. halloumi cheese
- 2 tbsp. pasta sauce

Directions:
Make 1/2 in. thick slices of Halloumi cheese
Put the cheese in the unheated waffle maker and turn it on
Cook the cheese for over 4–6 min. till it turns golden brown
Remove from the heat and allow it to cool for a minute
Spread the sauce on the waffle and eat instantly

Nutrition:
Calories: 129
Protein: 7.26 g.
Fat: 9.06 g.
Carbohydrates: 4.92 g.

461. BASIC MOZZARELLA WAFFLES

Preparation time: 5 min.
Cooking time: 6 min.
Servings: 2
Ingredients:

- 1 large organic egg, beaten
- 1/2 c. Mozzarella cheese, shredded finely

Directions:
Preheat a mini waffle iron and then grease it.
In a small bowl, place the egg and Mozzarella cheese and stir to combine.
Place half of the mixture into the preheated waffle iron and cook for about 2–3 min. or until golden brown.
Repeat with the remaining mixture.
Serve warm.

Nutrition:
Calories: 56
Net Carb: 0.4 g.
Fat: 3.7 g.
Saturated Fat: 1.5 g.
Carbohydrates: 0.4 g.
Dietary Fiber: 0 g.
Sugar: 0.2 g.
Protein: 5.2 g.

462.   MOZZARELLAS AND PSYLLIUM HUSK WAFFLES

Preparation time: 10 min.
Cooking time: 8 min.
Servings: 2
Ingredients:

- 1/2 c. Mozzarella cheese, shredded
- 1 large organic egg, beaten
- 2 tbsp. blanched almond flour
- 1/2 tsp. Psyllium husk powder
- 1/4 tsp. organic baking powder

Directions:

Preheat a mini waffle iron and then grease it.

In a bowl, place all the ingredients and beat until well combined.

Place half of the mixture into the preheated waffle iron and cook for about 3–4 min. or until golden brown.

Repeat with the remaining mixture.

Serve warm.

Nutrition:
Calories: 101
Net Carb: 1.6 g.
Fat: 7.1 g.
Saturated Fat: 1.8 g.
Carbohydrates: 2.9 g.
Dietary Fiber: 1.3 g.
Sugar: 0.2 g.
Protein: 6.7 g.

463.   CHEESE   SLICES WAFFLES

Preparation time: 5 min.
Cooking time: 6 min.
Servings: 1
Ingredients:

- 2 oz. Colby Jack cheese, cut into thin triangle slices
- 1 large organic egg, beaten

Directions:

Preheat a waffle iron and then grease it.

Arrange 1 thin layer of the cheese slices in the bottom of the preheated waffle iron.

Place the beaten egg on top of the cheese.

Now, arrange another layer of the cheese slice on top to cover it evenly.

Cook for about 5–6 min. or until golden brown.

Serve warm.

Nutrition:
Calories: 292
Net Carb: 2.4 g.
Fat: 23 g.
Saturated Fat: 13.6 g.
Carbohydrates: 2.4 g.
Dietary Fiber: 0 g.
Sugar: 0.4 g.
Protein: 18.3 g.

464.   MAYONNAISE WAFFLES

Preparation time: 5 min.
Cooking time: 10 min.
Servings: 2
Ingredients:

- 1 large organic egg, beaten
- 1 tbsp. mayonnaise
- 2 tbsp. almond flour
- 1/8 tsp. organic baking powder
- 1 tsp. water

Directions:

Preheat a mini waffle iron and then grease it.

In a medium bowl, place all the ingredients and, with a fork, mix until well combined.

Place half of the mixture into the preheated waffle iron and cook for about 4–5 min. or until golden brown.

Repeat with the remaining mixture.

Serve warm.

Nutrition:
Calories: 110
Net Carb: 2.6 g.
Fat: 8.7 g.
Saturated Fat: 1.4 g.

Carbohydrates: 3.4 g.
Dietary Fiber: 0.8 g.
Sugar: 0.9 g.
Protein: 3.2 g.

465. MAYONNAISE AND CREAM CHEESE WAFFLES

Preparation time: 10 min.
Cooking time: 20 min.
Servings: 4
Ingredients:
- 4 organic eggs, large
- 4 tbsp. mayonnaise
- 1 tbsp. almond flour
- 2 tbsp. cream cheese, cut into small cubes

Directions:
Preheat a waffle iron and then grease it.
In a bowl, place the eggs, mayonnaise, and almond flour and with a hand mixer, mix until smooth.
Place about 1/4 of the mixture into the preheated waffle iron.
Place about 1/4 of the cream cheese cubes on top of the mixture evenly and cook for about 4–5 min. or until golden brown.
Repeat with the remaining mixture and cream cheese cubes.
Serve warm.

Nutrition:
Calories: 190
Net Carb: 0.6 g.
Fat: 17.7 g.
Saturated Fat: 4.2 g.
Carbohydrates: 0.8 g.
Dietary Fiber: 0.2 g.
Sugar: 0.5 g.
Protein: 6.7 g.

466. EGG-FREE COCONUT FLOUR WAFFLES

Preparation time: 10 min.
Cooking time: 10 min.
Servings: 2

Ingredients:
- 1 tbsp. flaxseed meal
- 2 1/2 tbsp. water
- 1/4 c. Mozzarella cheese, shredded
- 1 tbsp. cream cheese, softened
- 2 tbsp. coconut flour

Directions:
Preheat a waffle iron and then grease it.
In a bowl, place the flaxseed meal and water and mix well.
Set aside for about 5 min. or until thickened.
In the bowl of flaxseed mixture, add the remaining ingredients and mix until well combined.
Place half of the mixture into the preheated waffle iron and cook for about 3–5 min. or until golden brown.
Repeat with the remaining mixture.
Serve warm.

Nutrition:
Calories: 76
Net Carb: 2.3 g.
Fat: 4.2 g.
Saturated Fat: 2.1 g.
Carbohydrates: 6.3 g.
Dietary Fiber: 4 g.
Sugar: 0.1 g.
Protein: 3 g.

467. EGG-FREE ALMOND FLOUR WAFFLES

Preparation time: 15 min.
Cooking time: 10 min.
Servings: 2
Ingredients:
- 2 tbsp. cream cheese, softened
- 1 c. mozzarella cheese, shredded
- 2 tbsp. almond flour
- 1 tsp. organic baking powder

Directions:
Preheat a mini waffle iron and then grease it.

In a medium bowl, place all the ingredients and, with a fork, mix until well combined.

Place half of the mixture into the preheated waffle iron and cook for about 4–5 min. or until golden brown.

Repeat with the remaining mixture.

Serve warm.

Nutrition:
Calories: 77

Net Carb: 2.4 g.

Fat: 9.8 g.

Saturated Fat: 4 g.

Carbohydrates: 3.2 g.

Dietary Fiber: 0.8 g.

Sugar: 0.3 g.

Protein: 4.8 g.

468.   EASY KETO WAFFLE
Preparation time: 5 min.

Cooking time: 8 min.

Servings: 2

Ingredients:
• 	Half a cup of cheddar cheese (shredded)

• 	1 egg (use egg white to make the waffle crispier)

Directions:
Take a waffle maker and switch it on. This needs to be done to make the waffle iron is hot. Brush both sides of the waffle maker with butter to make them oily.

Take a small-sized bowl and an egg. Break the egg inside the bowl and combine it well with the cheddar cheese (shredded). Mix both the ingredients well to blend properly.

Take half the amount of the batter (after blending it well) and pour it into the waffle maker. Close top of the waffle maker. And allow the batter to cook.

Broil the mixture for about 3–4 min. until cooked as per your requirement.

Remove the cooked waffle from the waffle maker and allow it to settle down for some time. This will help the waffle to become crispy.

To prepare the next one, follow the same instructions.

You can make impressive sandwiches with this conventional waffle recipe.

Serve the waffle and relish it!

Nutrition:
Calories: 291

Carb: 1 g.

Protein: 20 g.

Fat: 23 g.

469.   CRANBERRY SWIRL WAFFLE
Preparation time: 15 min.

Cooking time: 10 min.

Servings: 2

Ingredients:
For the cranberry sauce:
• 	2 tablespoons of erythritol (granulated)

• 	1/2 c. water

• 	1/2 c. cranberries (frozen or fresh)

• 	1/2 tsp. vanilla extract

For the waffles:
• 	1 oz. cream cheese (must be kept at room temperature)

• 	1 egg

• 	1/4 tsp. baking powder

• 	1 tsp. coconut flour

• 	1/2 tsp. vanilla extract

• 	1 tbsp. Swerve

For the frosting:
• 	1 tbsp. swerve

• 	1 tbsp. butter (kept at room temperature)

• 	1 oz. cream cheese (kept at room temperature)

• 	Orange zest (grated)

• 	1/8 tsp. orange extract

Directions:
For the cranberry swirl:
Take a medium-sized saucepan and, in it, add water, cranberries, and erythritol. Combine all

the ingredients well and gradually bring them to a boil. Once the mixture starts to boil, allow them to simmer for a while.

Continue simmering for about 10–15 min. By this time, the sauce will start to thicken, and the cranberries will pop.

Once done, remove the saucepan from the heat and add the vanilla extract. Stir it in.

Use a spoon (specifically, the back of the spoon) to mash the cranberries properly, and this will give the sauce a chunky consistency.

When you bring the saucepan off the heat, you will notice that the sauce thickens considerably.

For the waffles:

Start by heating your waffle iron, and before you put the batter in it, you have to make sure that it is thoroughly heated.

Now, take all the ingredients of the waffle and add them to a medium-sized bowl. Whisk them well.

Take two tablespoons of the batter at a time and add them to the waffle iron.

Once you have added the batter, take half a portion of the cranberry sauce that you just prepared and add it over the batter in small dollops.

Close the iron and cook the waffle for about 5 min. Once it is done, remove the waffle and place it on a wire rack.

Do the same for the second waffle.

For the frosting:

Take all the ingredients required for the frosting apart from the orange zest and add them to a bowl. Whisk them well so that you get a smooth consistency. Now, you simply have to spread this frosting over the waffles.

Once you have applied the frosting, sprinkle the grated orange zest on top.

Nutrition:

Calories: 70
Carb: 4.9 g.
Protein: 1.8 g.

Fat: 6 g.

470. LEMON POPPY SEED WAFFLES

Preparation time: 5 min.
Cooking time: 3 min.
Servings: 2
Ingredients:
For the waffles:

- 2 tbsp. almond flour, finely ground
- 1 tsp. fresh lemon zest
- One-eighth of tsp. poppy seeds
- An egg (large-sized)
- 1/4 cup of part-skim ricotta cheese
- 1 tsp. sugar or any other sweetener you prefer

For the toppings (optional):

- Fresh berries
- Ricotta cheese

Directions:

Take the waffle iron and preheat it.

Add ricotta cheese, almond flour, lemon zest, poppy seeds, egg, and sugar into a small bowl. Whisk everything together and let them combine fully.

In the preheated waffle iron, drop half a spoon of this mixture. Spread evenly and well.

Cook for 2–3 min., or till the smoke starts subsiding

Repeat the process with the rest of the batter

While serving top with fresh berries and ricotta cheese.

Notes:

The waffles will be mildly sweet and add additional sweetener if required. Or, dust the waffles with the confectioner's sugar, just before serving. This adds to the sweetness.

Compared with granulated sugar, artificial sweeteners are sweeter. So, use the artificial sweetener in lesser quantity, if using.

Almond flour can be substituted with coconut flour. For 2 tbsp. almond flour, 2 tsps. coconut flour should be used. After mixing, let the batter sit for 10 min. This lets the flour absorb the liquid.

Refrigerate the waffles in an airtight container after wrapping them properly.

Nutrition:
Calories: 231
Carb: 1.56 g.
Protein: 15.2 g.
Fat: 16.7 g.
Fiber: 3 g.

471. SWEET POTATO CRANBERRY WAFFLES

Preparation time: 15 min.
Cooking time: 10 min.
Servings: 5
Ingredients:
- For the waffles:
- 1 1/2 c. sweet potato puree
- 2 tbsp. shredded mozzarella
- 2 tbsp. brown sugar
- 1 egg (slightly beaten)
- 1/8 tsp. ground cloves
- 1/4 tsp. ground nutmeg
- 1 tsp. ground cinnamon
- 1 1/2 c. all-purpose flour
- 1 1/2 tbsp. baking powder
- 1/4 tsp. ground ginger
- 1/8 tsp. salt

For the syrup:
- 1/2 c. cranberry sauce
- 1 c. maple syrup
- 1/2 tsp. ground cinnamon

Directions:
Start with preheating the waffle iron. Stick to the instruction manual from the manufacturer for this process.

In a bowl, add sweet potato puree, egg, and shredded mozzarella. Stir and mix together. In another large bowl, add baking powder, brown sugar, 1 tsp. cinnamon, flour, ginger, cloves, nutmeg powder, and salt. Whisk everything together. Now mix the contents of both bowls. Combine the batter together by stirring.

Now, in the waffle iron, drop the batter with a ladle. The waffles should completely turn crisp and golden. Cook for 3 min. to get this result.

In a saucepan, mix maple syrup, 1/2 tsp. cinnamon, and cranberry sauce, and heat in medium flame. Stir the content occasionally. They should be well heated and combined thoroughly. This can take around 5–10 min. Take off the cooked waffles and transfer them to a plate. Pour the syrup on the waffles.

Use aluminum foil for cooking the waffles evenly, and for keeping them moist. It can also help in making the cleaning process easy.

Nutrition:
Calories: 517
Carbs: 108.2 g.
Protein: 7.9 g.
Fat: 7 g.
Fiber: 3 g.

472. KETO WONDERBREAD WAFFLE

Preparation time: 2 min.
Cooking time: 3 min.
Servings: 2 Waffles
Ingredients:
- 1 tsp. water
- 1 tbsp. almond flour
- 1/8 tsp. baking powder
- 1 egg
- 1 tbsp. mayonnaise
- A pinch of Himalayan pink salt

Directions:
In a small bowl, mix water, egg, almond flour, mayonnaise, salt, and baking powder together.

Use a mini-dash waffle maker or any other waffle maker of your choice to make these waffles.

Place half of the batter into the waffle maker. Cook until the batter turns golden brown or for 3 1/2–4 min.

Notes:
The almond flour waffles take 3–4 min. to cook. Compared with the coconut flour waffles, the almond flour version tastes eggy.

Compared with the coconut wonderbread recipe, the almond flour waffles are also thinner.

These waffles can be reheated in the air fryer, toaster, or in the toaster oven.

If you need to store these waffles, then pack them between parchment papers. Then place in the Ziploc cover that is freezer friendly, or in an air-tight container. These can be stored later in the freezer. Reheat when you want to serve them in the air fryer or toaster.

Nutrition:
Calories: 108
Carbs: 3.2 g.
Protein: 3.7 g.
Fat: 8.2 g.
Fiber: 0.2 g.

473. JICAMA LOADED BAKED POTATO WAFFLE

Preparation time: 5 min.
Cooking time: 5 min.
Servings: 2
Ingredients:
- 1 big jicama root
- 1/2 medium onion minced
- 2 garlic cloves pressed
- 1 c. cheese of choice I used Halloumi
- 2 eggs whisked
- Salt and pepper

Directions:
Put jicama shredded in a large colander, sprinkle with 1–2 tsp. salt. Mix well and drain well.

Microwave for 5–8 min.

Mix all the ingredients.

Sprinkle a little cheese on the waffle iron before adding 3 tbsp. the mixture, sprinkle a little more cheese on top of the Cook mixture for 5 min.

2 more flip and fry.

Top with a dollop of sour cream, pieces of bacon, cheese, and peppers!

Nutrition:
Calories 168
Total Fat: 11.8 g.
Cholesterol 121 mg.
Sodium 221.8 mg.
Total Carbohydrate 5.1 g.
Dietary Fiber 1.7 g.
Sugars 1.2 g.
Protein: 10 g.

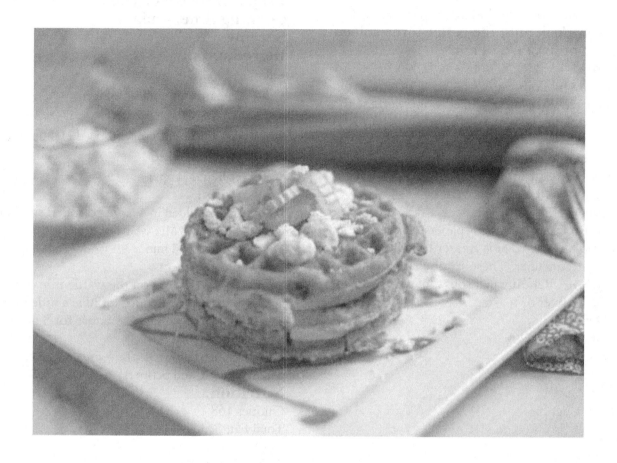

474. CRISPY WAFFLES WITH EGG AND ASPARAGUS

Preparation time: 5 min.
Cooking time: 10 min.
Servings: 1
Ingredients:

- 1 egg
- 1/4 c. cheddar cheese
- 2 tbsps. almond flour
- 1/2 tsp. baking powder

For the topping:

- 1 egg
- 4–5 stalks of asparagus
- 1 tsp. avocado oil

Directions:

Preheat the waffle maker to medium-high heat.
Whisk together egg, mozzarella cheese, almond flour, and baking powder
Pour the waffles mixture into the center of the waffle iron. Close the waffle maker and let cook for 5 min. or until the waffle is golden brown and set.
Remove the waffles from the waffle maker and serve.
Meanwhile, heat oil in a nonstick pan.
Once the pan is hot, fry asparagus for about 4–5 min. until golden brown.
Poach the egg in boil water for about 2–3 min.
Once the waffles are cooked, remove them from the maker.
Serve waffles with the poached egg and asparagus.

Nutrition:

Protein: 85 g.
Fat: 226 g.
Carbohydrates: 16 g.

475. GARLIC AND PARSLEY WAFFLES

Preparation time: 4 min.
Cooking time: 5 min.
Servings: 1
Ingredients:

- 1 large egg
- 1/4 c. cheese mozzarella
- 1 tsp. coconut flour
- 1/4 tsp. baking powder
- 1/2 tsp. garlic powder
- 1 tbsp. parsley

For serving:s:

- 1 poach egg
- 4 oz. smoked salmon

Directions:

Switch on your Dash mini waffle maker and let it preheat.
Grease the waffle maker with cooking spray.
Mix together egg, mozzarella, coconut flour, baking powder, and garlic powder, parsley to a mixing bowl until combined well.
Pour the batter into a circle waffle maker.
Close the lid.
Cook for about 2–3 min. or until the waffles are cooked.
Serve with smoked salmon and poached egg.
Enjoy!

Nutrition:

Protein: 140 g.
Fat: 160 g.
Carbohydrates: 14 g.

476. SCRAMBLED EGGS ON A SPRING ONION WAFFLE

Preparation time: 4 min.
Cooking time: 7–9 min.
Servings: 4
Ingredients:
For the batter::

- 4 eggs
- 2 c. grated mozzarella cheese
- 2 spring onions, finely chopped
- Salt and pepper to taste
- 1/2 tsp. dried garlic powder
- 2 tbsp. almond flour
- 2 tbsp. coconut flour

Other:

- 2 tbsp. butter for brushing the waffle maker
- 6–8 eggs
- Salt and pepper
- 1 tsp. Italian spice mix
- 1 tbsp. olive oil
- 1 tbsp. freshly chopped parsley

Directions:
Preheat the waffle maker.
Crack the eggs into a bowl and add the grated cheese.
Mix until just combined, then add the chopped spring onions and season with salt and pepper and dried garlic powder.
Stir in the almond flour and mix until everything is combined.
Brush the heated waffle maker with butter and add a few tablespoons of the batter.
Close the lid and cook for about 7–8 min. depending on your waffle maker.
While the waffles are cooking, prepare the scrambled eggs by whisking the eggs in a bowl until frothy, about 2 min. Season with salt and black pepper to taste and add the Italian spice mix. Whisk to blend in the spices.
Warm the oil in a non-stick pan over medium heat.
Pour the eggs in the pan and cook until the eggs are set to your liking.
Serve each waffle and top with some scrambled eggs. Top with freshly chopped parsley.

Nutrition:
Calories 194
Fat 14.7 g.
Carbs 5 g.
Protein: 1 g.

477. EGG ON A CHEDDAR CHEESE WAFFLE

Preparation time: 5 min.
Cooking time: 7–9 min.
Servings: 4
Ingredients:
For the batter::

- 4 eggs
- 2 c. shredded white cheddar cheese
- Salt and pepper to taste

Other:

- 2 tbsp. butter for brushing the waffle maker
- 4 large eggs
- 2 tbsp. olive oil

Directions:
Preheat the waffle maker.
Crack the eggs into a bowl and whisk them with a fork.
Stir in the grated cheddar cheese and season with salt and pepper.
Brush the heated waffle maker with butter and add a few tablespoons of the batter.
Close the lid and cook for about 7–8 min. depending on your waffle maker.
While waffles are cooking, cook the eggs.
Warm the oil in a large non-stick pan that has a lid over medium-low heat for 2–3 min.

Crack an egg in a small ramekin and gently add it to the pan. Repeat the same way for the other 3 eggs.

Cover and let cook for 2–2 1/2 min. for set eggs but with runny yolks.

Remove from the heat.

To serve, place a waffle on each plate and top with an egg. Season with salt and black pepper to taste.

Nutrition:
Calories 4
Fat 34 g.
Carbs 2 g.
Sugar 0.6 g.
Protein: 26 g.

478. AVOCADO WAFFLE TOAST

Preparation time: 4 min.
Cooking time: 10 min.
Servings: 3
Ingredients:
- 4 tbsps. avocado mash
- 1/2 tsp. lemon juice
- 1/8 tsp. salt
- 1/8 tsp. black pepper
- 2 eggs
- 1/2 c. shredded cheese

For servings:
- 3 eggs
- 1/2 avocado thinly sliced
- 1 tomato, sliced

Directions:
Mash avocado mash with lemon juice, salt, and black pepper in a mixing bowl, until well combined.

In a small bowl beat the egg and pour eggs in avocado mixture and mix well.

Switch on Waffle Maker to pre-heat.

Pour 1/8 of shredded cheese in a waffle maker and then pour 1/2 of the egg and avocado mixture and then 1/8 shredded cheese.

Close the lid and cook the waffles for about 3–4 min.

Repeat with the remaining mixture.

Meanwhile, fry eggs in a pan for about 1–2 min.

For serving, arrange fried egg on the waffle toast with avocado slice and tomatoes.

Sprinkle salt and pepper on top and enjoy!

Nutrition:
Protein: 66 g.
Fat: 169 g.
Carbohydrates: 15 g.

479. CAJUN AND FETA WAFFLES

Preparation time: 4 min.
Cooking time: 10 min.
Servings: 1
Ingredients:
- 1 egg white
- 1/4 c. shredded mozzarella cheese
- 2 tbsps. almond flour
- 1 tsp. Cajun Seasoning

For serving:s:
- 1 egg
- 4 oz. feta cheese
- 1 tomato, sliced

Directions:
Whisk together egg, cheese, and seasoning in a bowl.

Switch on and grease the waffle maker with cooking spray.

Pour the batter into a preheated waffle maker.

Cook the waffles for about 2–3 min. until the waffle is cooked through.

Meanwhile, fry the egg in a non-stick pan for about 1–2 min.

For serving set fried egg on the waffles with feta cheese and tomatoes slice.

Nutrition:
Protein: 119 g.
Fat: 2 g.
Carbohydrates: 31 g.

480. CRISPY WAFFLES WITH SAUSAGE

Preparation time: 5 min.
Cooking time: 10 min.
Servings: 2
Ingredients:

- 1/2 c. cheddar cheese
- 1/2 tsp. baking powder
- 1/4 c. egg whites
- 2 tsp. pumpkin spice
- 1 egg, whole
- 2 chicken sausage
- 2 slice bacon
- Salt and pepper to taste
- 1 tsp. avocado oil

Directions:

Mix together all the ingredients into a bowl.

Allow the batter to sit while the waffle iron warms.

Spray the waffle iron with nonstick spray.

Pour the batter into the waffle maker and cook according to the directions of the manufacturer.

Meanwhile, heat oil in a pan and fry the egg, according to your choice, and transfer it to a plate.

In the same pan, fry bacon slice and sausage on medium heat for about 2–3 min. until cooked.

Once the waffles are cooked thoroughly, remove them from the maker.

Serve with fried egg, bacon slice, sausages, and enjoy!

Nutrition:

Calories 208
Fat: 13.5 g.
Carbohydrate 0.7 g.
Protein: 8.2 g.
Sugars 0.6 g.

481. CHILI WAFFLE

Preparation time: 4 min.
Cooking time: 7–9 min.
Servings: 4
Ingredients:
For the batter::

- 4 eggs
- 1/2 c. grated parmesan cheese
- 1 1/2 c. grated yellow cheddar cheese
- 1 hot red chili pepper
- Salt and pepper to taste
- 1/2 tsp. dried garlic powder
- 1 tsp. dried basil
- 2 tbsp. almond flour

Other:

- 2 tbsp. olive oil for brushing the waffle maker

Directions:

Preheat the waffle maker.

Crack the eggs into a bowl and add the grated parmesan and cheddar cheese.

Mix until just combined and add the chopped chili pepper. Season with salt and pepper, dried garlic powder and dried basil. Stir in the almond flour.

Mix until everything is combined.

Brush the heated waffle maker with olive oil and add a few tablespoons of the batter.

Close the lid and cook for about 7–8 min. depending on your waffle maker.

Nutrition:

Calories 36
Fat 30.4 g.
Carbs 3.1 g.

482. SIMPLE SAVORY WAFFLE

Preparation time: 4 min.
Cooking time: 7–9 min.
Servings: 4
Ingredients:
For the batter::

- 4 eggs
- 1 c. grated mozzarella cheese
- 1 c. grated provolone cheese
- 1/2 c. almond flour
- 2 tbsp. coconut flour
- 2 1/2 tsp.s baking powder
- Salt and pepper to taste

Other:

- 2 tbsp. butter to brush the waffle maker

Directions:
Preheat the waffle maker.
Add the grated mozzarella and provolone cheese to a bowl and mix.
Add the almond and coconut flour and baking powder and season with salt and pepper.
Mix with a wire whisk and crack in the eggs.
Stir everything together until the batter forms.
Brush the heated waffle maker with butter and add a few tablespoons of the batter.
Close the lid and cook for about 8 min. depending on your waffle maker.
Serve and enjoy.

Nutrition:
Calories 352
Fat 27.2 g.
Carbs 8.3 g.
Protein: 15 g.

483. PIZZA WAFFLE

Preparation time: 3 min.
Cooking time: 7–9 min.
Servings: 4
Ingredients:
For the batter::

- 4 eggs
- 1 1/2 c. grated mozzarella cheese
- 1/2 c. grated parmesan cheese
- 2 tbsp. tomato sauce
- 1/4 c. almond flour
- 1 1/2 tsp.s baking powder
- Salt and pepper to taste
- 1 tsp. dried oregano
- 1/4 c. sliced salami

Other:

- 2 tbsp. olive oil for brushing the waffle maker
- 1/4 c. tomato sauce for serving

Directions:
Preheat the waffle maker.
Add the grated mozzarella and grated parmesan to a bowl and mix.
Add the almond flour and baking powder and season with salt and pepper and dried oregano.
Mix with a wooden spoon or wire whisk and crack in the eggs.
Stir everything together until the batter forms.
Stir in the chopped salami.
Brush the heated waffle maker with olive oil and add a few tablespoons of the batter.
Close the lid and cook for about 7-minutes depending on your waffle maker.
Serve with extra tomato sauce on top and enjoy.

Nutrition:
Calories 319
Fat 25.2 g.
Carbs 5.9 g.
Protein: 19.3 g.

484. BACON WAFFLE

Preparation time: 3 min.
Cooking time: 7–9 min.
Servings: 4
Ingredients:
For the batter::

- 4 eggs
- 2 c. shredded mozzarella
- 2 oz. finely chopped bacon
- Salt and pepper to taste
- 1 tsp. dried oregano

Other:

- 2 tbsp. olive oil for brushing the waffle maker

Directions:
Preheat the waffle maker.
Crack the eggs into a bowl and add the grated mozzarella cheese.
Mix until just combined and stir in the chopped bacon.
Season with salt and pepper and dried oregano.
Brush the heated waffle maker with olive oil and add a few tablespoons of the batter.
Close the lid and cook for about 7–8 min. depending on your waffle maker.
Nutrition:
Calories 241
Fat 19.8 g.
Carbs 1.3 g.
Protein: 14.8 g.

485. WAFFLES BREAKFAST BOWL

Preparation time: 4 min.
Cooking time: 5 min.
Servings: 2
Ingredients:

- 1 egg
- 1/2 c. cheddar cheese shredded pinch of Italian seasoning
- 1 tbsp. pizza sauce

For the topping::

- 1/2 avocado sliced
- 2 eggs boiled
- 1 tomato, halves
- 4 oz. fresh spinach leaves

Directions:
Preheat your waffle maker and grease it with cooking spray.
Crack an egg into a small bowl and beat it with Italian seasoning and pizza sauce.
Add the shredded cheese to the egg and spices mixture.
Pour 1 tbsp. shredded cheese in a waffle maker and cook for 30 sec.
Pour Waffles batter into the waffle maker and close the lid.
Cook the waffles for about 4 min. until crispy and brown.
Carefully remove the waffles from the maker.
Serve on the bed of spinach with boil egg, avocado slice, and tomatoes.
Enjoy!
Nutrition:
Protein: 77 g.
Fat: 222 g.
Carbohydrates: 39 g.

486. KETO WAFFLE BREAKFAST SANDWICH

Preparation time: 3 min.
Cooking time: 6 min.
Servings: 1
Ingredients:

- 1 egg
- 1/2 c. Monterey Jack Cheese
- 1 tbsp. almond flour
- 2 tbsp. butter

Directions:
In a small bowl, mix the egg, almond flour, and Monterey Jack Cheese.

Pour half of the batter into your mini waffle maker and cook for 3–4 min. Then cook the rest of the batter to make a second waffle.

In a small pan, melt 2 tbsp. butter. Add the waffles and cook on each side for 2 min. Pressing down while they are cooking lightly on the top of them, so they crisp up better.

Remove from the pan and let sit for 2 min.

Nutrition:
Calories: 514
Carbohydrates: 2 g.
Protein: 21 g.
Fat: 47 g.

487. KETO WAFFLE TACO SHELLS

Preparation time: 5 min.
Cooking time: 20 min.
Servings: 5
Ingredients:
- 1 tbsp. almond flour
- 1 c. taco blend cheese
- 2 eggs
- 1/4 tsp. taco seasoning

Directions:
In a bowl, mix almond flour, taco blend cheese, eggs, and taco seasoning. I find it easiest to mix everything using a fork.

Add 1.5 tbsp. taco waffle batter to the waffle maker at a time—Cook waffle batter in the waffle maker for 4 min.

Remove the taco waffle shell from the waffle maker and drape it over the side of a bowl. I used my pie pan because it was what I had on hand, but just about any bowl will work.

Continue making waffle taco shells until you are out of the batter. Then fill your taco shells with taco meat, your favorite toppings, and enjoy!

Nutrition:
Calories: 113
Carbohydrates: 1 g.
Protein: 8 g.

Fat: 9 g.

488. FRENCH DIP KETO WAFFLE SANDWICH

Preparation time: 5 min.
Cooking time: 12 min.
Servings: 2
Ingredients:
- 1 egg white
- 1/4 c. mozzarella cheese, shredded (packed)
- 1/4 c. sharp cheddar cheese, shredded (packed) 3/4 tsp. water
- 1 tsp. coconut flour
- 1/4 tsp. baking powder
- Pinch of salt

Directions:
Preheat the oven to 425 °F. Plug the Dash Mini Waffle Maker in the wall and grease lightly once it is hot.

Combine all of the ingredients into a bowl and stir to combine.

Spoon out 1/2 of the batter on the waffle maker and close the lid. Set a timer for 4 min. and do not lift the lid until the cooking time is complete. Lifting beforehand can cause the Waffle keto sandwich recipe to separate and stick to the waffle iron. You have to let it cook the entire 4 min. before lifting the lid.

Remove the waffle from the waffle iron and set it aside. Repeat the same steps above with the rest of the waffle batter.

Cover a cookie sheet with parchment paper and place waffles a few inches apart.

Add 1/4–1/3 c. the slow cooker keto roast beef from the following recipe. Make sure to drain the excess broth/gravy before adding it to the top of the waffle.

Add a slice of deli cheese or shredded cheese on top. Swiss and provolone are both great options. Place on the top rack of the oven for 5 min. so that the cheese can melt. If you'd like the cheese to bubble and begin to brown, turn the oven to broil for 1 min. (The swiss cheese may not brown.) Enjoy open-faced with a small bowl of beef broth for dipping.

Nutrition:
Calories: 118
Carbohydrates: 2 g.
Protein: 9 g.
Fat: 8 g.

489. KETO WAFFLE STUFFING

Preparation time: 5 min.
Cooking time: 12 min.
Servings: 2
Ingredients:
For the batter::
- 1/2 c. cheese mozzarella, cheddar, or a combo of both
- 2 eggs
- 1/4 tsp. garlic powder
- 1/2 tsp. onion powder
- 1/2 tsp. dried poultry seasoning
- 1/4 tsp. salt
- 1/4 tsp. pepper

For stuffing:
- 1 small onion diced
- 2 celery stalks
- 4 oz. mushrooms diced
- 4 tbsp. butter for sautéing
- 3 eggs

Directions:
First, make your waffles.
Preheat the mini waffle iron.
Preheat the oven to 350 °F
In a medium-size bowl, combine the waffle ingredients.

Pour 1/4 of the mixture into a mini waffle maker and cook each waffle for about 4 min. each.
Once they are all cooked, set them aside.
In a small frying pan, sauté the onion, celery, and mushrooms until they are soft.
In a separate bowl, tear up the waffles into small pieces, add the sautéed veggies, and 3 eggs. Mix until the ingredients are fully combined.
Add the stuffing mixture to a small casserole dish (about a 4 x 4) and bake it at 350 °F for about 30–40 min.
Combine the waffles with the other ingredients and Serve!

Nutrition:
Calories: 170
Carbohydrates: 2 g.
Protein: 11 g.
Fat: 13 g.

490. CRISPY BAGEL WAFFLE CHIPS

Preparation time: 5 min.
Cooking time: 10 min.
Servings: 1
Ingredients:
- 3 tbsp. Parmesan cheese shredded
- 1 tsp. Everything Bagel Seasoning

Directions:
Preheat the mini waffle maker.
Place the Parmesan cheese on the griddle and allow it to bubble. About 3 min. Be sure to leave it long enough, or else it won't turn crispy when it cools. Important step!
Sprinkle the melted cheese with about 1 tsp. Everything Bagel Seasoning. Leave the waffle iron open when it cooks!
Unplug the mini waffle maker and allow it to cool for a few minutes. This will allow the cheese to cool enough to bind together and get crispy.
After about 2 min. of it cooling off, it will still be warm.
Use a mini spatula to peel the warm (but not hot) cheese from the mini waffle iron.

Allow it to cool completely for crispy chips! These chips pack a powerful crunch, which is something I tend to miss on Keto!

Nutrition:
Total Fat: 5.6 g.
Total Carbohydrate 1.2 g.
Protein: 6.2 g.

491. TOASTED ALMOND FLOUR WAFFLES

Preparation time: 10 min.
Cooking time: 20 min.
Servings: 2
Ingredients:
- 1 large egg
- 1 tbsp. toasted almond flour
- 1/4 tsp. baking powder
- Pinch of Salt
- 1/2 c. shredded mozzarella cheese

Directions:
Whisk the egg, almond flour, and baking powder together. Stir in mozzarella and set batter aside.
Turn on the waffle maker to heat and oil it with cooking spray.
Pour half of the batter onto the waffle maker and spread it evenly with a spoon. Cook for 3 min., or until it reaches desired doneness.
Transfer to a plate and repeat with the remaining batter. Let waffles cool for 2–3 min. to crisp up.

Nutrition:
Carbs 2 g.
Fat 13 g.
Protein 10 g.
Calories 131

492. CHICKEN JALAPENO POPPER WAFFLE

Preparation time: 5 min.
Cooking time: 5 min.
Servings: 2
Ingredients:
- 1/2 c. canned chicken breast
- 1/4 c. cheddar cheese

- 1/8 c. parmesan cheese
- 1 egg
- 1 diced jalapeno (raw or pickled)
- 1/8 tsp. onion powder
- 1/8 tsp. garlic powder
- 1 tsp. cream cheese

Directions:
Reheat the mini waffle maker.
In an average bowl, add all the ingredients and stir together till it's completely incorporated.
Half this mixture and Pour a part of the mixture into a mini waffle maker and cook for a minimum of 5 min.

Note:
Optional toppings: sour cream, ranch dressing, hot sauce, coriander, leek, feta cheese, jalapeno!

Nutrition:
Calories 224
Total Fat: 21.8 g.
Cholesterol 134.6 mg.
Sodium 871 mg.
Total Carbohydrate 9.2 g.
Dietary Fiber 2.3 g.
Sugars 4.7 g.
Protein: 18.5 g.
Vitamin A 163.1µg
Vitamin C 0 mg.

493. BURGER WAFFLE

Preparation time: 12 min.
Cooking time: 10 min.
Servings: 1
Ingredients:
For the cheeseburgers:
- 1/3 lb beef, ground
- 1/2 tsp. garlic salt
- 3 slices American cheese

For the waffles:
- 1 large egg
- 1/2 c. mozzarella, finely shredded
- Salt and ground pepper to taste

For the big mac sauce:
- 2 tsp. mayonnaise
- 1 tsp. ketchup
- To Assemble:
- 2 tbsp. lettuce, shredded
- 4 dill pickles
- 2 tsp. onion, minced

Directions:

For the cheeseburgers:

Heat a pan over medium-high heat.

Divide your ground beef into 2 equal balls. Press them to form patties and sprinkle salt and pepper on top. Place balls on the heated griddle and cook for 3 min. each side.

Place the cheese slices on top of each patty. Proceed to stack them on top of each other and set them aside.

For the waffles:

Heat your waffle iron and spray with cooking spray.

Add the egg, cheese, and salt to a small mixing bowl. Whisk together until well combined.

Pour half of the egg mixture into the waffle iron. Cook for 3 min.

Set aside and repeat the process with the remaining batter.

For the big mac sauce:

Mix together all the ingredients and whisk properly until combined.

To assemble the burgers:

Take your burger patties and place them on one waffle. Top with the shredded lettuce, onions, and pickles.

Spread the sauce over the other waffle and place it on top of the veggies, sauce side down.

Enjoy.

Nutrition:

Calories: 850

Fats: 56 g.

Carbs: 8 g.

Protein: 67 g.

494. CORNBREAD WAFFLE

Preparation time: 4 min.

Cooking time: 10 min.

Servings: 4

Ingredients:
- 4 eggs
- 1 c. cheddar cheese, shredded
- 8 slices jalapeno, optional
- 1 tsp. red hot sauce
- 1/4 tsp. low-carb corn extract
- Pinch salt

Directions:

Preheat the waffle maker.

Crack the eggs into a small bowl and whip. Add all the other ingredients and mix thoroughly.

Add a pinch of shredded cheese to the hot waffle maker. Cook for 30 sec.

Pour half the egg mixture into the preheated waffle maker.

Cook for 5 min.

Remove, allow cooling, and enjoy.

Nutrition:

Calories: 155

Fats: 12 g.

Carbs: 1.2 g.

Protein: 10 g.

495. TACO WAFFLE

Preparation time: 10 min.

Cooking time: 8 min.

Servings: 2

Ingredients:

For the waffle:
- 1/2 c. mozzarella, shredded
- 1 egg
- 1/4 tsp. Italian seasoning

For the taco meat:
- 1 lb turkey, ground

- 1 tsp. chili powder
- 1 tsp. cumin, ground
- 1/2 tsp. garlic powder
- 1/4 tsp. onion powder
- 1/4 tsp. salt
- 1/2 tsp. paprika, smoked

Directions:

Cook your ground turkey and add all the taco meat seasonings.

As the meat cooks, start preparing the waffles.

Preheat your mini waffle maker.

Whip the egg in a mixing bowl, add in the cheese and sprinkle with seasoning.

Place half of the waffle mixture into the waffle maker. Cook for 4 min.

Repeat the process with the second half of the egg mixture.

Remove from the waffle maker and add the taco meat on top. To get the perfect taco form you'd better use a taco stand.

Top with lettuce, tomatoes, and cheese.

Enjoy warm!

Nutrition:

Calories: 120

Fats: 10

Carbs: 1 g.

Protein: 8 g.

496.   WAFFLE SANDWICH

Preparation time: 5 min.

Cooking time: 8 min.

Servings: 2

Ingredients:

For the waffle bread:

- 1/2 c. mozzarella cheese, shredded
- 1 egg
- 1 tbsp. green onion, diced
- 1/2 tsp. Italian seasoning

For the sandwich:

- 1/2 lb bacon, pre-cooked

- 1 small lettuce
- 1 medium tomato sliced
- 1 tbsp. mayo

Directions:

Preheat your mini waffle maker.

Whip the egg in a small mixing bowl.

Add the seasonings, cheese, and onion. Mix thoroughly until it's well incorporated. Add 1 tsp. shredded cheese to the waffle maker and cook for 30 sec.

Place half the batter in the waffle pan and cook for 4 min.

Once the first waffle is done, repeat the process with the remaining mixture.

Once ready remove and place on a plate.

Top with mayo, lettuce, bacon, and tomato. Place the second waffle on top, slice into 2 and enjoy!

Nutrition:

Calories: 240

Fats: 18 g.

Carbs: 2 g.

Protein: 17 g.

497.   CAULIFLOWER RICE WAFFLE

Preparation time: 9 minutes

Cooking Time: 8 Minutes

Ingredients:

- 1 cup cauliflower rice
- ¼ tsp salt or to taste
- 1 tbsp melted butter
- 1 egg
- ¼ tsp nutmeg
- ¼ tsp cinnamon
- ¼ tsp garlic powder
- 1/8 tsp ground black pepper or to taste
- 1/8 tsp white pepper or to taste
- ¼ tsp Italian seasoning
- ½ cup shredded parmesan cheese

- ½ cup shredded mozzarella cheese
- Garnish:
- Chopped green onions

Directions:

1. Pour ¼ of the parmesan cheese into a blender, add the mozzarella cheese, egg, salt, nutmeg, butter, cinnamon, garlic powder, black pepper, white pepper, Italian seasoning and cauliflower.
2. Add the egg and blend until you form a smooth batter.
3. Plug the waffle maker and preheat it. Spray the waffle maker with a non-stick spray.
4. Sprinkle about tbsp of the remaining parmesan cheese on top of the waffle maker.
5. Fill the waffle maker with ¼ of the batter and spread out the batter to cover all the holes on the waffle maker. Sprinkle some shredded parmesan over the batter.
6. Close the lid of the waffle maker and cook for about 4 to 5 minutes or according to your waffle maker's settings.
7. After the cooking cycle, remove the waffle with a rubber or silicone utensil.
8. Repeat step 4 to 7 until you have cooked all the batter into chaffles.
9. Serve and enjoy.

Nutrition: Fat 15.8g 20% .Carbohydrate 6.2g 2% .Sugars 2.4g. Protein 15g

498.   TUNA WAFFLES

Preparation time: 5 min.
Cooking time: 8 min.
Servings: 2
Ingredients:

- 1 packet tuna, drained
- 1/2 c. mozzarella cheese
- 1 egg
- A pinch of salt

Directions:
Preheat the waffle maker
Whip the egg in a small mixing bowl.
Add the tuna, cheese, and season with the salt. Mix well.
For a crispy crust, add 1 tsp. shredded cheese to the waffle maker and cook for 30 sec.
Pour half the mixture into the mini waffle maker and cook for 4 min.
Remove it and repeat the process with the remaining tuna waffle mixture.
Once ready, remove and enjoy warm.
Nutrition:
Calories: 650
Fats: 39 g.
Carbs: 6 g.
Protein: 63 g.

499.   GARLIC   WAFFLE   STICKS

Preparation time: 10 min.
Cooking time: 15 min.
Servings: 4
Ingredients:

- 2 eggs
- 1 c. mozzarella cheese, grated
- 4 tbsp. almond flour
- 1 tsp. garlic powder
- 1 tsp. oregano
- 1/2 tsp. salt

For the toppings::
4 tbsp. butter, unsalted softened
1/2 tsp. garlic powder
1/2 c. mozzarella cheese, grated
Directions:
Preheat your waffle maker.
Whisk the eggs into a small bowl.
Add the almond flour, mozzarella, oregano, garlic powder, and salt. Mix well.
Spoon half the egg mixture into your waffle maker. Cook for 5 min. and remove.

Repeat the process with the remaining batter and cook for 5 min.

Remove from the waffle maker and cut into 4 strips out of each waffle.

Place the waffle sticks on a tray and pre-heat your grill.

Add the butter and garlic powder to a small mixing bowl. Mix properly.

Using a brush spread the garlic mixture over the sticks.

Sprinkle the shredded mozzarella over the sticks. Place under the grill for 3 min. or until the cheese starts to melt and bubble. Eat immediately!

Nutrition:
Calories: 109
Fats: 19 g.
Carbs: 7 g.
Protein: 27 g.

500.   CRAB WAFFLES
Preparation time: 10 min.
Cooking time: 25 min.
Servings: 6
Ingredients:

- 1 lb crab meat
- 1/3 c. Panko breadcrumbs
- 1 egg
- 2 tbsp. fat greek yogurt
- 1 tsp. Dijon mustard
- 2 tbsp. parsley and chives, fresh
- 1 tsp. Italian seasoning
- 1 lemon, juiced
- Salt, pepper to taste

Directions:
Preheat the waffle maker
Mix all the ingredients in a small mixing bowl, except crab meat.
Add the meat. Mix well.
Form the mixture into round patties.
Cook 1 patty for 3 min.

Remove it and repeat the process with the remaining crab waffle mixture.

Once ready, remove and enjoy warm.

Nutrition:
Calories: 99
Fats: 8 g.
Carbs: 4 g.
Protein: 16 g.

501.   PROTEIN WAFFLES
Preparation time: 3 min.
Cooking time: 4 min.
Servings: 1
Ingredients:

- 1/4 c. almond milk
- 1/4 c. plant-based protein powder
- 2 tbsp. almond butter
- 1 tbsp. psyllium husk

Directions:
Preheat the waffle maker.
Combine almond milk, protein powder, psyllium husk, and mix thoroughly until the mixture gets the form of a paste.
Add in butter, combine well and form round balls
Place the ball in the center of the preheated waffle maker.
Cook for 4 min.
Remove, top as prefer and enjoy.

Nutrition:
Calories: 310
Fats: 19 g.
Carbs: 5 g.
Protein: 25 g.

502.   CHICKEN WAFFLES
Preparation time: 5 min.
Cooking time: 15 min.
Servings: 4
Ingredients:

- 2 oz. chicken breasts, cooked, shredded
- 1/2 c. mozzarella cheese, finely shredded

- 2 eggs
- 6 tbsp. parmesan cheese, finely shredded
- 1 c. zucchini, grated
- 1/2 c. almond flour
- 1tsp baking powder
- 1/4 tsp. garlic powder
- 1/4 tsp. black pepper, ground
- 1/2 tsp. Italian seasoning
- 1/4 tsp. salt

Directions:
Sprinkle the zucchini with a pinch of salt and set it aside for a few minutes. Squeeze out the excess water.
Warm-up your mini waffle maker.
Mix chicken, almond flour, baking powder, cheeses, garlic powder, salt, pepper, and seasonings in a bowl.
Use another small bow for beating eggs. Add them to squeezed zucchini, mix well.
Combine the chicken and egg mixture, and mix.
For a crispy crust, add 1 tsp. shredded cheese to the waffle maker and cook for 30 sec.
Then, pour the mixture into the waffle maker and cook for 5 min. or until crispy.
Carefully remove. Repeat with the remaining batter the same steps.
Enjoy!

Nutrition:
Calories: 135
Fats: 10 g.
Carbs: 3 g.
Protein: 11 g.

503. BROCCOLI WAFFLES

Preparation time: 3 min.
Cooking time: 8 min.
Servings: 2
Ingredients:
- 1/2 c. cheddar cheese, finely shredded
- 1 egg

- 1/3 c. broccoli, fresh chopped
- 1 tbsp. almond flour
- 1/3 tsp. garlic powder

Directions:
Warm-up your mini waffle maker.
Mix the egg, almond flour, garlic powder with cheese into a small bowl.
Add half broccoli to the cheese mixture.
For a crispy crust, add 1 tsp. shredded cheese to the waffle maker and cook for 30 sec.
Then, pour the mixture into the waffle maker and cook for 5 min. or until crispy.
Repeat with the remaining batter. Serve with a fried slice of bacon and enjoy!

Nutrition:
Calories: 180
Fats: 13 g.
Carbs: 2 g.
Protein: 11 g.

504. CAULIFLOWER WAFFLES

Preparation time: 6 min.
Cooking time: 5 min.
Servings: 1
Ingredients:
- 1/2 c. almond milk ricotta, finely shredded
- 1 egg
- 1 c. cauliflower, riced
- 1/4 tsp. garlic powder
- 1/4 tsp. black pepper, ground
- 1/2 tsp. Italian seasoning
- 1/4 tsp. salt

Directions:
Add all the ingredients into a blender. Blend until you have a smooth batter.
Evenly spread a spoon of shredded almond milk ricotta into the waffle maker.

Pour the cauliflower mixture into the waffle maker.

Add another sprinkle of almond milk ricotta on top of the mixture.

Cook for 5 min. or until crispy.

Carefully remove and enjoy warm.

Nutrition:

Calories 270

Fats: 16 g.

Carbs: 8 g.

Protein: 22 g.

505. KETO PROTEIN WAFFLE WITH SALTED CARAMEL COLLAGEN SYRUP

Preparation time: 3mins

Cooking time: 10mins

Servings: 2

Ingredients:

- 1 egg
- 1/2 c. mozzarella cheese
- 1 scoop Keto Whey Protein
- 1/4 tsp. baking powder

For syrup:

- 2 tbsp. unsalted butter
- 1 tbsp. powdered erythritol
- 1 scoop collagen powder
- 1/4 c. heavy cream
- 1/8 tsp. salt

Directions:

Mix all the ingredients well

Pour it on a preheat waffle maker and close until done

For the syrup, melt the butter and let it get brown on medium flame

Whisk in powdered erythritol and collagen powder on low heat

Add cream and remove from flame. Then add salt.

Nutrition:

Calories: 607

Carbohydrates: 5.2 g.

Proteins: 48 g.

Fats: 44.9 g.

Saturated Fat: 17 g.

Fiber: 4 g.

Sugar: 5 g.

506. BLUEBERRY WAFFLES WITH COCONUT FLOUR

Preparation time: 5 min.

Cooking time: 8 min.

Servings: 2

Ingredients:

- 1 egg
- 1/3 c. mozzarella cheese, shredded
- 1 tbsp. blueberries
- 1 tsp. cream cheese
- 1 tsp. coconut flour
- 1/4 tsp. baking powder
- 1/4 tsp. vanilla extract
- 2 squirts liquid Pyure Sweetener
- 1/4 tsp. cinnamon
- A pinch of salt

Directions:

Mix all the ingredients well except blueberries

Preheat the waffle maker

Pour half a mixture and cook for 2–4 min. and remove

Repeat with the other half of the mixture

Serve with sugar-free maple syrup, whipped cream, or keto ice cream.

Nutrition:

Calories: 113

Carbohydrates: 3 g.

Proteins: 7 g.

Fats: 7 g.

Saturated Fat: 4 g.

Fiber: 1 g.

Sugar: 1 g.

507. KETO WAFFLE CHURROS

Preparation time: 2 min.
Cooking time: 2 min.
Servings: 2
Ingredients:

- 1 egg
- 1/2 c. mozzarella cheese shredded
- 2 tbsp. Swerve Brown Sweetener
- 1/2 tsp. cinnamon

Directions:
Mix cheese and egg well
Pour half a mixture into the preheated waffle maker and cook for 2–4 min. and remove
Repeat with the other half of the mixture
Combine sweetener and cinnamon in a bowl
Slice the waffles and soak in cinnamon mixture

Nutrition:
Calories: 76
Carbohydrates: 4.1 g.
Proteins: 5.5 g.
Fats: 4.3 g.
Saturated Fat: 1.3 g.
Fiber: 1.2 g.
Sugar: 1.9 g.

508. PEANUT BUTTER CUP WAFFLES

Preparation time: 10 min.
Cooking time: 6mins
Servings: 1
Ingredients:

- 1 large egg
- 2 tbsp. cocoa powder
- 1 tbsp. sweetener
- 1 tbsp. sugar-free chocolate chips
- 1/4 tsp. espresso powder
- 1/2 c. finely shredded mozzarella

For filling:
3 tbsp. creamy peanut butter

2 tbsp. powdered sweetener
1 tbsp. butter, softened

Directions:
Mix all the waffle ingredients
Pour 2 tbsp. batter on the preheated iron and cook for 4 min.
Repeat the above step
For the filling, mix all the ingredients into a small bowl and stir well until smooth and creamy.
Spread peanut butter on the waffles and close to form a sandwich

Nutrition:
Calories: 210
Carbohydrates: 5 g.
Proteins: 8 g.
Fats: 14 g.
Saturated Fat: 5 g.
Fiber: 1 g.
Sugar: 2 g.

509. FUDGY CHOCOLATE WAFFLES

Preparation time: 5 min.
Cooking time: 8 min.
Servings: 2
Ingredients:

- 1 egg
- 2 tbsp. mozzarella cheese, shredded
- 2 tbsp. cocoa
- 2 tbsp. Lakanto monk fruit powdered
- 1 tsp. coconut flour
- 1 tsp. heavy whipping cream
- 1/4 tsp. baking powder
- 1/4 tsp. vanilla extract
- pinch of salt

Directions:
Mix all the ingredients well except blueberries
Preheat the waffle maker
Pour half a mixture and cook for 2–4 min. and remove
Repeat with the other half of the mixture
Serve with sugar-free whipped topping.

Nutrition:
Calories: 109
Carbohydrates: 5 g.
Proteins: 7 g.
Fats: 7 g.
Saturated Fat: 4 g.
Fiber: 3 g.
Sugar: 1 g.

510.   FUNFETTI WAFFLE

Preparation time: 5 min.
Cooking time: 10 min.
Servings: 1
Ingredients:

- 1 Egg
- 1 tbsp. Almond flour
- 1 1/2 tbsp. Heavy whipping cream
- 1/2 tsp. Vanilla extract
- 1 tbsp. Sugar-free sprinkles
- 1/3 c. Mozzarella cheese shredded
- 2 tbsp. Swerve confectioners' sugar substitute

Directions:
Mix all the ingredients well
Preheat the waffle maker
Pour half a mixture and cook for 2–5 min. and remove
Repeat with the other half of the mixture
Serve with sugar-free whipped topping and sprinkles

Nutrition:
Calories: 165
Carbohydrates: 4 g.
Proteins: 11 g.
Fats: 12 g.
Saturated Fat: 5 g.
Fiber: 1 g.
Sugar: 1 g.

511.   PROTEIN   VANILLA WAFFLE

Preparation time: 2 min.
Cooking time: 15mins
Servings: 2
Ingredients:

- 2 eggs
- 1/2 c. shredded mozzarella cheese
- 1 tbsp. vanilla protein powder.

Directions:
Mix all the ingredients well
Preheat the waffle maker
Pour 1/4 of the mixture and cook for 2–4 min. and remove
Repeat with the other half of the mixture

Nutrition:
Calories: 120
Carbohydrates: 4 g.
Proteins: 16 g.
Fats: 6 g.
Saturated Fat: 2.1 g.
Fiber: 1 g.
Sugar: 2 g.

512.   BAKED   POTATO WAFFLE USING JICAMA

Preparation time: 15 min.
Cooking time: 5 min.
Servings: 1
Ingredients:

- 1 jicama root
- 1/2 onion, medium, minced
- 2 cloves garlic, pressed
- 1 c. cheese
- 1 egg, whisked
- Salt and pepper

Directions:
Peel the jicama root and shred it using a food processor.
Place the shredded jicama root in a colander to allow the water to drain. Mix in 2 tsp. salt as well.

Squeeze out the remaining liquid.

Microwave the shredded jicama for 5–8 min. This step pre-cooks it.

Mix all the remaining ingredients with the jicama. Start preheating the waffle maker.

Once preheated, sprinkle a bit of the cheese on the waffle maker, allowing it to toast for a few seconds.

Place 3 tbsp. the jicama mixture onto the waffle maker. Sprinkle more cheese on top before closing the lid.

Cook for 5 min. Flip the waffle and let it cook for 2 more minutes.

Servings your baked jicama by topping it with sour cream, cheese, bacon pieces, and chives.

Nutrition:

Calories: 168

Carbohydrates: 5.1 g.

Fat: 11.8 g. Protein: 10 g.

513. SWEET WAFFLE

Preparation time: 1 Minute
Cooking time: 3 min.
Servings: 1
Ingredients:

- 2 oz. cream cheese
- 1 egg
- 1 tbsp. coconut powder
- 2 tsp. cocoa
- 1.5 c. sweetener (can be used between 2–3, but 2.5 is preferred)
- 1 tsp. vanilla
- 1/2 tsp. baking soda
- 1 tsp. cinnamon (optional)
- Coconut oil spray
- 1 tsp. butter (optional)

Directions:

Place cream cheese for 20 sec. in a microwave-safe bowl and microwave. (If your cream cheese is at room temperature, this move is not required.) Combine the rest of your sweet ingredients with the cream cheese in the tub.

Plug in your coconut oil waffle maker and spray.

Only spoon enough of the combined ingredients of the delicious waffle onto the waffle maker.

Open your waffle maker and wait patiently, yes-it's going to be difficult.

Depending on your waffle maker, the exact cooking time varies. We notice that in about 2 min. most waffle makers cook delicious waffles.

Take your sweet, cooked waffle and put it on a plate.

Top with a buttered slice.

Enjoy!

Notes:

If you're not an individual with cinnamon, you should take the ingredient absolutely out of your delicious waffles. We hope this recipe for keto dessert will be your new favorite! If you like it as much as we do, please share it with your friends on social media.

Nutrition:

Calories 170

Calories from Fat 141

Fat 15.7 g. 24%

Sodium 209 mg. 9%

Potassium 128 mg. 4%

Carbohydrates 9.9 g. 3%

514. LOW-CARB KETO BROCCOLI CHEESE WAFFLES

Preparation time: 5 min.
Cooking time: 5 min.
Servings: 2
Ingredients:

- 1 c. broccoli, processed
- 1 c. shredded cheddar cheese
- 1/3 c. grated parmesan cheese
- 2 eggs, beats

Directions:

Spray the cooking spray on the waffle iron and preheat.

Use a powerful blender or food processor to process the broccoli until rice consistency.

Mix all the ingredients into a medium bowl. Add 1/3 of the mixture to the waffle iron and cook for 4–5 min. until golden.

Nutrition:

Calories 160
Total Fat: 11.8 g. 18%
Cholesterol 121 mg. 40%
Sodium 221.8 mg. 9%
Total Carbohydrate 5.1 g. 2%
Dietary Fiber 1.7 g. 7%
Sugars 1.2 g.
Protein: 10 g. 20%

515. BROCCOLI AND CHEDDAR KETO WAFFLES

Preparation time: 5 min.
Cooking time: 5 min.
Servings: 1
Ingredients:

- 1/3 raw broccoli, finely chopped 20 g.
- 1/4 c. cheddar cheese, shredded 28 g.
- 1 egg
- 1/2 tsp. garlic powder
- 1/2 tsp. dried onion
- Salt and pepper flavor
- Cooking spray

Directions:

To reach the temperature, insert a waffle iron.

Beat the egg with a fork into a small bowl.

Fold in broccoli, cheese, powdered garlic, onions, salt, pepper.

Use cooking spray as soon as the waffle iron is ready (if needed) and add the egg mixture. Cover well waffle iron and apply heat till the light indicates that one cycle is complete.

Close the lid again and cook for another period.

When finished, gently remove the waffle iron with a tongue or fork.

Enjoy! Enjoy! Serve with honey, sour cream, pasture, and other sauces.

Note:

This recipe makes one or two mini waffles at full size.

Sprinkle with crushed cheddar cheese before and after spreading the egg mixture.

Nutrition

Calories: 125
Carbohydrates: 4 g.
Protein: 7 g.
Fat: 9 g.
Fiber: 1 g.

516. MAPLE CREAM CHEESE ICING

Preparation time: 5 min.
Cooking time: 10 min.
Servings: 5
Ingredients:

- 4 oz. cream cheese
- 1/2 c. heavy cream
- 1/4 c. lakanto maple flavor syrup
- 1 tsp. vanilla essence
- 1/4 tsp. cinnamon

Directions:
Combine the cream cheese and all the other ingredients in a blender
Start with a pulse to combine before blending until smooth
Nutrition:
Calories 70
Carbohydrates 1 g.
Protein: 1 g.
Fat: 7 g.
Saturated Fat: 4 g.
Cholesterol 24 mg.
Sodium 34 mg.
Potassium 20 mg.
Fiber: 1 g.

517. PUMPKIN WAFFLE CHURROS

Preparation time: 5 min.
Cooking time: 20 min.
Servings: 3
Ingredients:

- 1 egg
- 1 c. mozzarella cheese
- 1/4 c. pumpkin puree
- 1/4 c. coconut flour
- 2 tbsp. lakanto golden monk fruit sweetener
- 1 tsp. vanilla essence
- 1 tsp. baking powder
- 1/2 tsp. pumpkin spice seasoning
- 1/8 tsp. real salt

For the topping:

- 1 tbsp. cinnamon ground
- 1 tbsp. Lakanto Golden Monk Fruit Sweetener

Directions:
Put all the ingredients in a mixing bowl, then pour the mixture into a piping bag
Cut the chips from the piping bag and pipe the pumpkin waffle mixture into each slot of the churro maker
Cook until brown (about 4 min.)
Nutrition
Calories 98
Carbohydrates 6 g.
Protein: 6 g.
Fat: 6 g.
Saturated Fat: 3 g.
Cholesterol 42 mg.
Sodium 188 mg.
Potassium 130 mg.
Fiber 3 g

518. CINNAMON ROLL WAFFLES WITH CREAM CHEESE FROSTING

Preparation time: 5 min.
Cooking time: 5 min.
Servings: 1
Ingredients:

- 1 tbsp. cream cheese, tender (or an alternative to sour cream or ricotta cheese)
- 1 large egg
- 1 tsp. melted butter
- 2 tbsp. almond flour (or 1 tbsp. coconut powder)
- 1/4 tsp. baking powder
- 1 tsp. ground cinnamon
- 1/2 tsp. vanilla extract
- 1/4 tsp. cinnamon extract (or add 1/2 tsp. cinnamon)
- 6–8 drops of LaKanto Monkfruit extract to taste (or 2 tsp. granular erythritol)

For the frosting:

- 1 oz. cream cheese, softened
- 2 tsp. powdered erythritol or taste
- 1 tsp. vanilla essence
- 1–2 tbsp. heavy cream

Directions:

Preheat a waffle maker with a mini 4. (If you use a regular size waffle maker, double or triple the recipe.) Mix all the ingredients until a smooth batter forms. (If necessary, microwave the cold cream cheese for about 5–8 sec. to soften before adding the remaining ingredients.) Divide the batter into two and cook each cake for 4 min. until well browned and crispy. 2 mini 4 in. waffles are made from this recipe.

Whisk together the whole frosting components into a small bowl and add enough heavy cream to achieve the desired consistency of spreading. Spread the frosting on the warm waffles and add extra cinnamon to sprinkle. Enjoy! Enjoy!

Nutrition:

Calories 408
Carbohydrate 2.8 g.
Dietary Fiber 2.3 g.
Sugars 34.8 g.
Total Fat 16.8 g.
Saturated Fat 0 g.
Trans fat 271 mg.
Cholesterol 352 mg.
Sodium 202 mg.

519. KETO PUMPKIN CHEESECAKE WAFFLE

Preparation time: 2 min.
Cooking time: 4 min.
Servings: 2
Ingredients:
For the waffle:

- 1 egg
- 1/2 c. mozzarella cheese
- 1 1/2 tbsp. pumpkin puree (100% pumpkin)
- 1 tbsp. almond flour
- 1 tbsp. La Canto Golden Sweetener or Sweetener Choice
- 2 tsp. heavy cream
- 1 tsp. cream cheese
- 1/2 tsp. pumpkin spice
- 1/2 tsp. baking powder
- 1/2 tsp. vanilla
- 1 tsp. chocolate zero maple syrup or 1/8 tsp. maple extract

For the filling:

- 2 tbsp. cream cheese
- 1 tbsp. Lakanto powder sweetener
- 1/4 tsp. vanilla essence

Directions:

Preheating mini waffle maker

In a small bowl, mix all the waffle ingredients.

Pour half of the waffle mixture into the center of the waffle iron. Cook for 3–5 min. Carefully remove and repeat the second waffle. While making the filling, set it to the crunchy side.

With a whisk or fork, mix all the matte ingredients together. Add a frost between the two waffles. pleasant!

Optional: add a whipped cream top, crushed pecans, chocolate zero maple syrup, and more.

Nutrition:

Calories: 204.25,
Total Fat: 15.25 g.
Carbohydrates: 3.3 g.
Net Carbohydrates: 2.65 g.
Fiber: 0.65 g.
Protein: 12.05 g.

520. CINNAMON APPLE WAFFLE

Preparation time: 10 min.
Cooking time: 5 min.
Servings: 4
Ingredients:
For the sauce:

- 1/2 tsp. monk fruit sweetener
- 1/2 tsp. vanilla essence
- 1 egg yolk
- 1 c. whipped cream
- 1 tbsp. ghee or butter
- 2 oz. cream cheese softened
- Whole vanilla bean

For the waffle:

- 2 tbsp. coconut powder
- 1 tsp. baking powder
- 2 tsp. cinnamon
- 1/2 tsp. monk fruit sweetener
- 3 large eggs
- 1/4 c. Granny Smith Apple Skin + Dice (or 1 tbsp. natural erythritol apple flavor)
- 3/4 c. mozzarella cheese shredded
- 1/4 c. mild cheddar cheese shredded

Directions:
For the sauce:

Add heavy cream, ghee, and vanilla bean to a mild sauce.

Heat over medium-high heat, then add sweetener and lower heat and cook for 10 min. Remove the vanilla bean into whipping cream and scrape the remaining vanilla seeds, then discard the bean.

Remove from the heat and stir vigorously in egg yolk.

Apply cream cheese until the cheese is melted.

Put the vanilla sauce in a heat-safe container and cool in the refrigerator.

For the waffle:

Preheat the waffle maker with low-carb non-stick spray and spray generously.

Add the egg and beat in a large mixing bowl until frothy.

Add vanilla and cheese and beat until thoroughly combined.

Whisk flour, baking powder, sweetener, and cinnamon in a small mixing bowl.

To the egg mixture, add dry ingredients and mix until combined.

Fold gently in the diced apples.

Fluid the cooking spray from the waffle maker

Pour the batter on low, high heat into the waffle maker and cook until the outside starts to brown—about 4 min.

Slightly cool "hole" and then top with vanilla sauce.

Nutrition

Calories 185
Carbohydrates 7 g.
Protein: 12 g.
Fat: 10 g.

521. PEANUT BUTTER AND JELLY SAMMICH WAFFLE

Preparation time: 5 min.
Cooking time: 5 min.
Servings: 2
Ingredients:
For the waffle:

- 2 eggs
- 1/4 c. mozzarella cheese
- 1 tsp. cinnamon
- 1 tbsp. confectionery
- 2 tsp. coconut flour
- 1/8 tsp. baking powder
- 1 tsp. vanilla essence

For the blueberry compote:

- 1 c. washed blueberries
- 1/2 lemon peel

- 1 tbsp. lemon juice, freshly squeezed
- 1 tbsp. confectionery
- 1/8 tsp. xanthan gum
- 2 tbsp. water

Directions:
Add everything except xanthan gum to a small pot.
Bring to a boil, lower the heat and cook for 5–10 min. until it starts to thicken.
Sprinkle xanthan gum and stir well.
Remove from the heat and cool.
Keep in the refrigerator until ready to use.

Nutrition:
Calories 168
Total Fat: 11.8 g. 18%
Cholesterol 121 mg. 40%
Sodium 221.8 mg. 9%
Total Carbohydrate 5.1 g. 2%
Dietary Fiber 1.7 g. 7%
Sugars 1.2 g.

522. KETO SNICKERDOODLE WAFFLE

Preparation time: 5 min.
Cooking time: 10 min.
Servings: 2
Ingredients:
- 1 egg
- 1/2 c. mozzarella cheese
- 2 tbsp. almond flour
- 1 tbsp. Lakanto Golden Sweetener
- 1/2 tsp. vanilla essence
- 1/4 tsp. cinnamon
- 1/2 tsp. baking powder
- 1/4 tsp. tartare cream, optional

For coating:
- 1 tbsp. butter
- 2 tbsp. Lakanto Classic Sweetener
- 1/2 tsp. cinnamon

Directions:
Reheat the mini waffle maker.

In a small bowl, mix all the waffle ingredients.
Pour half of the waffle mixture into the center of the waffle iron. Cook for 3–5 min. Carefully remove and repeat the second waffle. Cool the waffle just as the waffle cools.
In a small bowl, mix sweetener and cinnamon and coat.
Melt the butter in a small microwave-safe bowl and polish the waffle with butter.
After brushing with butter, sprinkle a mixture of sweetener and cinnamon on both sides of the waffle.

Nutrition
Calories 182
Total Fat: 13.75 g.
Carbs: 2 g.
Carbs: 1.5 g.
Fiber 0.5 g.
Protein: 11.5 g.

523. CHERRY CHOCOLATE WAFFLE

Preparation time: 5 min.
Cooking time: 5 min.
Servings: 1
Ingredients:
- 1 tbsp. almond powder
- 1 tbsp. cocoa powder
- 1 tbsp. sugar-free sweetener
- 1/2 t baking powder
- 1 whole egg
- 1/2 c. mozzarella cheese shredded
- 2 tbsp. heavy whip cream whip
- 2 tbsp. sugar-free cherry pie filling
- 1 tbsp. releases chocolate chip

Directions:
Preheat the waffle maker.
In a small bowl, mix all the dry ingredients.
Crack the egg and combine well in the cup.
Add the cheese and mix it together.

Spoon into a hot waffle maker in the center Heat for about 5 min. until the waffle stops steaming.

Top with cream whipping, cherries, and chocolate chips from Lilly.

Enjoy!

Nutrition:

Calorie 193

Total Fats 12 g.

Sodium 325 mg.

Carbohydrate 9 g.

Net Carbs: 3 g.

Fiber 2 g.

Sugar Alcohol 4 g.

Protein: 13 g.

524. EASY DOUBLE CHOCOLATE WAFFLES

Preparation time: 5 min.

Cooking time: 4 min.

Servings: 4

Ingredients:

- 1 egg
- 1/2 c. mozzarella cheese finely cut
- 1 tbsp. granulated sweetener, if desired
- 1 tsp. vanilla
- 2 tbsp. almond meal/flour
- 1 tbsp. unsweetened chocolate chips or cocoa nibs
- 2 tbsp. sugar-free cocoa powder
- 1 tsp. heavy/double cream

Directions:

Put the ingredients of the selected flavor into a bowl.

Preheat the waffle maker. If it's hot, spray olive oil and put half of the dough in a mini waffle maker (or put the whole dough in a large waffle maker).

After cooking for 2–4 min., remove and repeat. You should be able to create two mini-waffles or one large waffle per recipe. Top, serve, enjoy.

Nutrition:

Calories 215.8

Calories from Fat: 141

Fat: 15.7 g. 24%

Sodium 209 mg. 9%

Potassium 128 mg. 4%

Carbohydrates 9.9 g. 3%

Fiber 2.9 g. 12%

Sugar 0.9 g. 1%

Protein: 11.5 g. 23%

525. BACON AND HAM WAFFLE SANDWICH

Preparation time: 10 min.

Cooking time: 5 min.

Servings: 2

Ingredients:

- 3 egg
- 1/2 c. grated Cheddar cheese
- 1 tbsp. almond flour
- 1/2 tsp. baking powder

For the topping:

- 4 strips cooked bacon
- 2 pieces Bibb lettuce
- 2 slices preferable ham
- 2 slices tomato

Directions:

Turn on the waffle maker to heat and oil it with cooking spray.

Combine all waffle components into a small bowl.

Add around 1/4 of the total batter to the waffle maker and spread to fill the edges. Close and cook for 4 min.

Remove and let it cool on a rack.

Repeat for the second waffle.

Top one waffle with a tomato slice, a piece of lettuce, and bacon strips, then cover it with a second waffle.

Plate and enjoy.

Nutrition:

Carbs 5 g.

Fat 60 g.
Protein 31 g.
Calories 631

526. CHICKEN AND HOT SAUCE WAFFLES

Preparation time: 5 min.
Cooking time: 5 min.
Servings: 4
Ingredients:

- 1/4 c. almond flour
- 1 tsp. baking powder
- 2 large eggs
- 1/2 c. chicken, shredded
- 3/4 c. sharp cheddar cheese, shredded
- 1/4 c. mozzarella cheese, shredded
- 1/4 c. Red-Hot Sauce + 1 tbsp.for topping
- 1/4 c. feta cheese, crumbled
- 1/4 c. celery, diced

Directions:

Whisk baking powder and almond flour into a small bowl and set aside.
Turn on the waffle maker to heat and oil it with cooking spray.
Beat the eggs in a large bowl until frothy.
Add hot sauce and beat until combined.
Mix in the flour mixture.
Add the cheeses and mix until well combined.
Fold in the chicken.
Pour the batter into the waffle maker and cook for 4 min.
Remove and repeat until all batter is used up.
Top with celery, feta, and hot sauce.

Nutrition:

Carbs: 4 g.
Fat: 26 g.
Protein: 22 g.
Calories: 337

527. GARLIC CHEESE WAFFLE BREAD STICKS

Preparation time: 5 min.
Cooking time: 5 min.
Servings: 8
Ingredients:

- 1 medium egg
- 1/2 c. mozzarella cheese, grated
- 2 tbsp.almond flour
- 1/2 tsp. garlic powder
- 1/2 tsp. oregano
- 1/2 tsp. salt

For the topping:

- 2 tbsp.butter, unsalted softened
- 1/2 tsp. garlic powder
- 1/4 c. grated mozzarella cheese
- 2 tsp. dried oregano for sprinkling

Directions:

Turn on the waffle maker to heat and oil it with cooking spray.
Beat the egg in a bowl.
Add mozzarella, garlic powder, flour, oregano, and salt, and mix.
Spoon half of the batter into the waffle maker.
Close and cook for 5 min. Remove cooked waffle.
Repeat with the remaining batter.
Place waffles on a tray and preheat the grill.
Mix butter with garlic powder and spread over the waffles.
Sprinkle mozzarella over top and cook under the broiler for 2–3 min., until cheese has melted.

Nutrition:

Carbs: 1 g.
Fat: 7 g.
Protein: 4 g.
Calories: 74

528. EGGS BENEDICT WAFFLE

Preparation time: 20 min.
Cooking time: 10 min.
Servings: 2
Ingredients:
For the chaffle:

- 2 egg whites
- 2 tbsp.almond flour
- 1 tbsp.sour cream
- 1/2 c. mozzarella cheese

For the hollandaise:

- 1/2 c. salted butter
- 4 egg yolks
- 2 tbsp.lemon juice

For the poached eggs:

- 2 eggs
- 1 tbsp.white vinegar
- 3 oz. deli ham

Directions:

Whip the egg white until frothy, then mix in the remaining ingredients.

Turn on the waffle maker to heat and oil it with cooking spray.

Cook for 7 min. until golden brown.

Remove the waffle and repeat with the remaining batter.

Fill half the pot with water and bring to a boil.

Place a heat-safe bowl on top of the pot, ensuring the bottom doesn't touch the boiling water.

Heat butter to boiling in a microwave.

Add yolks to double boiler bowl and bring to boil.

Add hot butter to the bowl and whisk briskly.

Cook until the egg yolk mixture has thickened.

Remove the bowl from the pot and add lemon juice. Set aside.

Add more water to the pot if needed to make the poached eggs (water should completely cover the eggs). Bring to a simmer. Add white vinegar to the water.

Crack the eggs into simmering water and cook for 1 min. 30 sec. Remove using a slotted spoon. Warm waffles in the toaster for 2–3 min. Top with ham, poached eggs, and hollandaise sauce.

Nutrition:

Carbs 4 g.
Fat 26 g.
Protein 26 g.
Calories 365

529. FRIED PICKLE WAFFLE STICKS

Preparation time: 10 min.
Cooking time: 4 min.
Servings: 1
Ingredients:

- 1 egg
- 1/2 c. mozzarella cheese
- 1/4 c. pork panko
- 6–8 pickle slices, thinly sliced
- 1 tbsp. pickle juice

Directions:

Mix all the ingredients, except the pickle slices, into a small bowl.

Use a paper towel to blot out excess liquid from the pickle slices.

Add a thin layer of the mixture to a preheated waffle iron.

Add some pickle slices before adding another thin layer of the mixture.

Close the waffle maker's lid and allow the mixture to cook for 4 min.

Optional: combine hot sauce with ranch to create a great-tasting dip.

Nutrition:

Calories: 465
Carbohydrate: 3.3 g.
Fat: 22.7 g.
Protein: 59.2 g.

530. PEANUT BUTTER AND JELLY WAFFLES

Preparation time: 10 min.
Cooking time: 4 min.
Servings: 1
Ingredients:

- 1 egg
- 2 slices cheese, thinly sliced
- 1 tsp. natural peanut butter
- 1 tsp. sugar-free raspberry preserves
- Cooking spray

Directions:

Crack and whisk the egg into a small bowl or a measuring cup.

Lightly grease the waffle maker with cooking spray.

Preheat the waffle maker.

Once it is heated up, place a slice of the cheese on the waffle maker and wait for it to melt.

Once melted, pour the egg mixture onto the melted cheese.

Once the egg starts cooking, carefully place another slice of the cheese on the waffle maker.

Close the lid. Cook for 3–4 min.

Take out the waffles and place them on a plate.

Top the waffles with whipped cream.

Drizzle some natural peanut butter and raspberry preserves on top.

Nutrition:

Calories: 337

Carbohydrates: 3 g.

Fat: 27 g.

Protein: 21 g.

CHAPTER 14. SPICY WAFFLE RECIPES

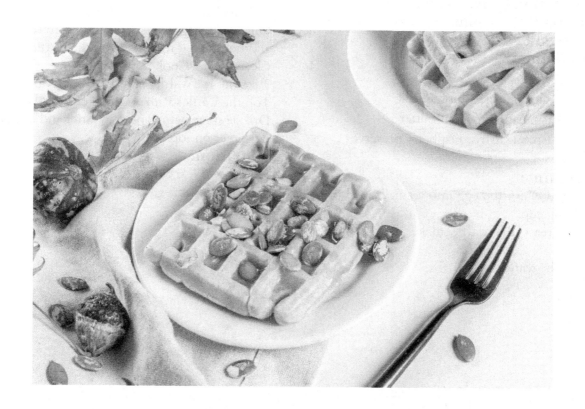

531.   JALAPENO WAFFLE

Preparation time: 5 min.
Cooking time: 10 min.
Servings: 6
Ingredients:

- 2 eggs, whisked
- 2 c. almond milk
- 2 tbsp. avocado oil
- 1/2 c. cheddar, shredded
- 1 c. almond flour
- 1 tbsp. baking powder
- A pinch of salt and black pepper
- 1/2 tsp. garlic powder
- 2 jalapenos, minced

Directions:

In a bowl, mix the eggs with the milk, oil, and the other ingredients and whisk well.

Preheat the waffle iron, pour 1/6 of the batter, cook for 8 min. and transfer to a plate.

Repeat with the rest of the batter and serve.

Nutrition:

Calories 381
Fat 14 g.
Fiber 3.6 g.
Carbs 13 g.
Protein 13 g.

532.   GREEN   CHILI WAFFLE

Preparation time: 10 min.
Cooking time: 10 min.
Servings: 6
Ingredients:

- 2 eggs, whisked
- 1 and 1/2 c. almond flour
- 1/2 c. cream cheese, soft
- 1/2 c. almond milk
- 1 tsp. baking soda
- A pinch of salt and black pepper
- 1/2 c. green chilies, minced
- 1 tbsp. chives, chopped

Directions:

In a bowl, mix the eggs with the flour, cream cheese, and the other ingredients and whisk.

Preheat the waffle iron, pour 1/6 of the batter, close the waffle maker, cook for 8 min. and transfer to a plate.

Repeat with the rest of the batter and serve.

Nutrition:

Calories 265
Fat 7 g.
Fiber 3 g.
Carbs 5.4 g.
Protein 6 g.

533.   HOT PORK WAFFLES

Preparation time: 10 min.
Cooking time: 10 min.
Servings: 4
Ingredients:

- 1 c. pulled pork, cooked
- 2 tbsp. parmesan, grated
- 2 eggs, whisked
- 2 red chilies, minced
- 1 c. almond milk
- 1 c. almond flour
- 2 tbsp. coconut oil, melted
- 1 tsp. baking powder

Directions:

In a bowl, mix the pulled pork with the eggs, parmesan, and the other ingredients and whisk well.

Heat up the waffle maker, pour 1/4 of the waffle mix, cook for 8 min. and transfer to a plate.

Repeat with the rest of the mix and serve.

Nutrition:

Calories 300
Fat 13 g.
Fiber 4 g.
Carbs 7.2 g.
Protein 15 g.

534. SPICY CHICKEN WAFFLES

Preparation time: 10 min.
Cooking time: 10 min.
Servings: 4
Ingredients:

- 2 eggs, whisked
- 1 c. rotisserie chicken, skinless, boneless, and shredded
- 1 c. mozzarella, shredded
- 1/2 c. milk
- 2 tsp. chili powder
- 1 tsp. sriracha sauce
- 1 tbsp. chives, chopped
- 1/2 tsp. baking powder

Directions:

In a bowl, mix the eggs with the chicken, mozzarella, and the other ingredients and whisk. Preheat the waffle maker, pour 1/4 of the batter, cook for 10 min. and transfer to a plate.
Repeat with the rest of the batter and serve.

Nutrition:

Calories 320
Fat 8 g.
Fiber 2 g.
Carbs 5.3 g.
Protein 12 g.

535. SPICY RICOTTA WAFFLES

Preparation time: 10 min.
Cooking time: 10 min.
Servings: 4
Ingredients:

- 2 c. coconut flour
- 1 and 1/2 c. coconut milk
- 2 tbsp. olive oil
- A pinch of salt and black pepper
- 1/2 c. ricotta cheese
- 1 tsp. baking powder
- 2 eggs, whisked

- 1/2 c. chives, chopped
- 1 red chili pepper, minced
- 1 jalapeno, chopped

Directions:

In a bowl, mix the flour with the milk, oil, and the other ingredients and whisk well.
Heat up the waffle iron, pour 1/4 of the batter, cook for 10 min. and transfer to a plate.
Repeat with the rest of the waffle mix and serve.

Nutrition:

Calories 262
Fat 8 g.
Fiber 2.4 g.
Carbs 3.2 g.
Protein 8 g.

536. SPICY BLACK SESAME WAFFLES

Preparation time: 10 min.
Cooking time: 10 min.
Servings: 4
Ingredients:

- 2 c. almond flour
- 2 c. almond milk
- Juice of 1/2 lemon
- 1/3 c. black sesame seeds
- A pinch of salt and black pepper
- 2 eggs, whisked
- 1 tsp. chili powder
- 1 tsp. hot paprika

Directions:

In a bowl mix the almond flour with the almond milk and the other ingredients and whisk well.
Heat up the waffle iron, pour 1/4 of the batter and cook for 10 min.
Repeat with the rest of the mix and serve.

Nutrition:

Calories 252
Fat 8 g.
Fiber 2.3 g.
Carbs 4 g.
Protein 4.5 g.

537. SPICY ZUCCHINI WAFFLES

Preparation time: 10 min.
Cooking time: 8 min.
Servings: 6
Ingredients:

- 1 and 1/2 c. almond flour
- 2 tsp. baking powder
- 2 eggs, whisked
- 1 and 1/2 c. coconut milk
- 2 zucchinis, grated
- 1 tsp. chili powder
- 1 tsp. cayenne pepper
- 1 c. cheddar cheese, shredded

Directions:

In a bowl, mix the almond flour with the eggs, milk, and the other ingredients and whisk well. Preheat the waffle iron, pour 1/6 of the batter, cook the waffle for 8 min. and transfer to a plate. Repeat with the rest of the batter and serve.

Nutrition:

Calories 252
Fat 7 g.
Fiber 2.3 g.
Carbs 5 g.
Protein 8.4 g.

538. TABASCO WAFFLE

Preparation time: 5 min.
Cooking time: 8 min.
Servings: 4
Ingredients:

- 1 c. coconut milk
- 1 c. coconut flour
- 2 tsp. Tabasco sauce
- 2 eggs, whisked
- 2 tbsp. ghee, melted
- 1/2 c. mozzarella, shredded
- 1 tsp. cayenne pepper
- 1 tbsp. chives, chopped
- 1 tbsp. baking powder

- A pinch of salt and black pepper

Directions:

In a bowl, mix the milk with the flour, Tabasco sauce, and the other ingredients and whisk well. Preheat the waffle iron, pour 1/4 of the batter, cook for 8 min. and transfer to a plate. Repeat with the rest of the batter and serve.

Nutrition:

Calories 301
Fat 11 g.
Fiber 3.6 g.
Carbs 10 g.
Protein 8.3 g.

539. GREEN CAYENNE WAFFLE

Preparation time: 10 min.
Cooking time: 10 min.
Servings: 4
Ingredients:

- 1 c. coconut flour
- 1/2 c. cream cheese, soft
- 1/2 c. coconut milk
- 1 tbsp. chives, chopped
- 1 tbsp. parsley, chopped
- 1 green chili pepper, minced
- 1/2 tsp. cayenne pepper
- 1 tsp. baking soda

Directions:

In a bowl, mix the eggs with the cream cheese, milk, and the other ingredients and whisk well. Preheat the waffle iron, pour 1/4 of the batter, close the waffle maker, cook for 10 min. and transfer to a plate. Repeat with the rest of the batter and serve.

Nutrition:

Calories 273
Fat 11.2 g.
Fiber 3 g.
Carbs 5.4 g.
Protein 6 g.

540. HOT PESTO WAFFLES

Preparation time: 10 min.
Cooking time: 7 min.
Servings: 4
Ingredients:

- 1 c. almond milk
- 1 c. mozzarella, shredded
- 1 c. coconut flour
- 3 tbsp. basil pesto
- 1 tsp. hot paprika
- 1 tsp. chili powder
- 2 eggs, whisked
- 1 tbsp. ghee, melted
- 1 tsp. baking soda

Directions:

In a bowl, mix the milk with the cheese, pesto, and the other ingredients and whisk.

Heat up the waffle maker, pour 1/4 of the mix, cook for 7 min. and transfer to a plate.

Repeat with the rest of the mix and serve.

Nutrition:

Calories 250
Fat 13 g.
Fiber 4 g.
Carbs 7.2 g.
Protein 15 g.

541. HABANERO WAFFLES

Preparation time: 10 min.
Cooking time: 6 min.
Servings: 4
Ingredients:

- 2 eggs, whisked
- 1 c. roasted red peppers, chopped
- 1 habanero pepper, minced
- 1 c. mozzarella, shredded
- 1/2 c. almond milk
- 1 tsp. smoked paprika
- 1 tbsp. cilantro, chopped
- 1/2 tsp. baking powder

Directions:

In a bowl, mix the eggs with the roasted peppers, habanero, and the other ingredients and whisk well.

Preheat the waffle maker, pour 1/4 of the batter, cook for 6 min. and transfer to a plate.

Repeat with the rest of the batter and serve.

Nutrition:

Calories 220
Fat 4 g.
Fiber 2 g.
Carbs 5.3 g.
Protein 5.6 g.

542. HOT SALSA WAFFLES

Preparation time: 10 min.
Cooking time: 7 min.
Servings: 4
Ingredients:

- 1 c. almond milk
- 1 c. almond flour
- 1/2 c. hot salsa
- 2 tbsp. ghee, melted
- 2 eggs, whisked
- 1 tsp. baking soda
- 1/2 c. mozzarella, shredded
- A pinch of salt and black pepper
- 1/2 c. chives, chopped

Directions:

In a bowl, mix the milk with the flour, salsa, and the other ingredients and whisk really well.

Heat up the waffle iron, pour 1/4 of the batter, cook for 7 min. and transfer to a plate.

Repeat with the rest of the salsa waffle mix and serve.

Nutrition:

Calories 262
Fat 8 g.
Fiber 2.4 g.
Carbs 3.2 g.
Protein 8 g.

543. CHILI PASTE WAFFLES

Preparation time: 10 min.
Cooking time: 8 min.
Servings: 4
Ingredients:

- 1 c. coconut flour
- 1 c. water
- 1 tbsp. chili paste
- 2 eggs, whisked
- ½ c. parmesan, grated
- 1 tsp. chili powder
- A pinch of salt and black pepper
- 1 tsp. baking soda

Directions:

In a bowl mix the flour with the water, chili paste, and the other ingredients and whisk well.
Heat up the waffle iron, pour 1/4 of the batter, cook for 8 min., transfer to a platter, repeat with the rest of the mix and serve.

Nutrition:

Calories 272
Fat 9.4 g.
Fiber 2.3 g.
Carbs 4 g.
Protein 4 g.

544. HOT BBQ WAFFLES

Preparation time: 10 min.
Cooking time: 10 min.
Servings: 6
Ingredients:

- 1 c. coconut flour
- 1 c. warm water
- 1/2 c. cheddar cheese, shredded
- 1/2 c. BBQ sauce
- 1 tsp. chili powder
- 1 tsp. hot paprika
- 1 tbsp. spring onions, chopped
- 2 scallions, chopped
- 2 tsp. baking powder
- 2 eggs, whisked
- 1 tsp. cayenne pepper

Directions:

In a bowl, mix the flour with the water, BBQ sauce, and the other ingredients and whisk well.
Preheat the waffle iron, pour 1/6 of the batter, cook for 10 min. and transfer to a plate.
Repeat with the rest of the batter and serve.

Nutrition:

Calories 292
Fat 7 g.
Fiber 2.3 g.
Carbs 5 g.
Protein 8 g.

545. CHILI OIL WAFFLES

Preparation time: 10 min.
Cooking time: 8 min.
Servings: 4
Ingredients:

- 2 eggs, whisked
- 1 c. spring onions, chopped
- 1 c. mozzarella, shredded
- 1/2 c. coconut milk
- 1 tbsp. chili olive oil
- 1 tsp. chili powder
- 1/2 tsp. parsley flakes, ground

Directions:

In a bowl, mix the eggs with the spring onions, mozzarella, and the other ingredients and whisk well.
Preheat the waffle iron, pour 1/4 of the batter, cook for 8 min. and transfer to a plate.
Repeat with the rest of the batter and serve.

Nutrition:

Calories 260
Fat 8.2 g.
Fiber 2.2 g.
Carbs 5.3 g.
Protein 12 g.

546. RED PEPPER WAFFLES

Preparation time: 10 min.
Cooking time: 6 min.
Servings: 4
Ingredients:

- 1 c. almond flour
- 1/2 c. cream cheese, soft
- 1/2 c. coconut milk
- 1 tsp. red pepper, crushed
- 2 green chilies, minced
- 1 tbsp. ghee, melted
- A pinch of salt and black pepper
- 1 tsp. baking powder
- 2 eggs, whisked
- 1/2 c. chives, chopped

Directions:

In a bowl, mix the almond flour with the cream cheese, milk, and the other ingredients and whisk well.

Heat up the waffle iron, pour 1/4 of the batter, cook for 6 min. and transfer to a plate.

Repeat with the rest of the mix and serve.

Nutrition:

Calories 273
Fat 8 g.
Fiber 3.4 g.
Carbs 4.2 g.
Protein 8 g.

547. HOT MANGO CHUTNEY WAFFLES

Preparation time: 10 min.
Cooking time: 10 min.
Servings: 6
Ingredients:

- 2 c. coconut flour
- 1 c. mango chutney
- 1/2 c. coconut milk
- 1 tsp. hot paprika
- 1 tsp. chili powder
- 1 tsp. rosemary, dried
- 1/2 tsp. cayenne pepper
- A pinch of salt and black pepper
- 2 eggs, whisked

Directions:

In a bowl mix the flour with the milk, chutney, and the other ingredients and whisk really well.

Heat up the waffle iron, pour 1/6 of the batter and cook for 10 min.

Repeat with the rest of the waffle mix and serve.

Nutrition:

Calories: 262
Fat: 4.5 g.
Fiber: 2.3 g.
Carbs: 3.4 g.
Protein: 7 g.

548. SPICY CURRY WAFFLES

Preparation time: 10 min.
Cooking time: 8 min.
Servings: 4
Ingredients:

- 1/2 c. almond flour
- 1/2 c. coconut flour
- 1 tbsp. red curry paste
- 1 tsp. hot paprika
- 1 red chili, minced
- 2 eggs, whisked
- 1 and 1/2 c. coconut milk
- 1/2 c. mozzarella, shredded

Directions:

In a bowl, mix the flour with the curry paste, eggs, and the other ingredients and whisk well.

Preheat the waffle iron, pour 1/4 of the batter, cook for 8 min. and transfer to a plate.

Repeat with the rest of the batter and serve.

Nutrition:

Calories: 263
Fat: 4.3 g.

Fiber: 2.3 g.
Carbs: 4 g.
Protein: 8 g.

549.   SPICY SALSA VERDE WAFFLES

Preparation time: 10 min.
Cooking time: 8 min.
Servings: 4
Ingredients:

- 1 c. coconut flour
- 1 c. coconut cream
- 2 tbsp. Salsa Verde
- 1 tsp. cayenne pepper
- 1/4 c. shallots, chopped
- 1/3 c. chives, chopped
- 1/2 c. mozzarella, shredded
- 2 eggs, whisked
- A pinch of salt and black pepper

Directions:

In a bowl mix the flour with the cream, salsa Verde, and the other ingredients and whisk well. Heat up the waffle iron, pour 1/4 of the batter and cook for 8 min.

Repeat with the rest of the salsa Verde waffle mix and serve.

Nutrition:

Calories 263
Fat 5.3 g.
Fiber 2.3 g.
Carbs 4 g.
Protein 4 g.

550.   HOT ARTICHOKE WAFFLES

Preparation time: 10 min.
Cooking time: 10 min.
Servings: 6
Ingredients:

- 1 c. coconut flour
- 1 c. cream cheese, soft
- 1/2 c. canned artichoke hearts, drained and chopped
- 2 red chilies, minced
- 1 tsp. hot chili powder
- 1 tsp. baking soda
- 2 eggs, whisked
- 1/2 c. coconut milk
- 2 zucchinis, grated

Directions:

In a bowl, mix the flour with the cheese, artichokes, and the other ingredients and whisk well.

Preheat the waffle iron, pour 1/6 of the batter, cook for 10 min. and transfer to a plate.

Repeat with the rest of the waffle batter and serve them warm.

Nutrition:

Calories 282
Fat 8.6 g.
Fiber 2.3 g.
Carbs 5 g.
Protein 8 g.

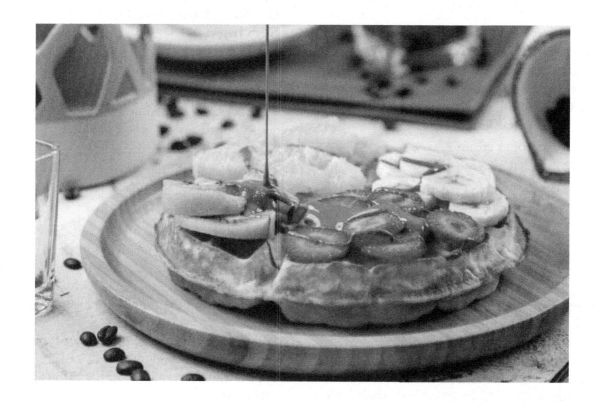

551. RICH AND CREAMY MINI WAFFLES

Preparation time: 5 min.
Cooking time: 10 min.
Servings: 2
Ingredients:

- 2 eggs
- 1 c. shredded mozzarella
- 2 tbsp. cream cheese
- 2 tbsp. almond flour
- 3/4 tbsp. baking powder
- 2 tbsp. water (optional)

Directions:

Preheat your mini waffle iron if needed
Mix all the above-mentioned ingredients into a bowl
Grease your waffle iron lightly
Cooking in your mini waffle iron for at least 4 min. or till the desired crisp is achieved and serve hot
Make as many waffles as your mixture and waffle maker allow

Nutrition:

Calories: 220
Protein: 19 g.
Carbohydrates: 20 g.
Fat: 7 g.
Cholesterol: 36 mg.
Sodium: 168 mg.
Potassium: 374 mg.
Phosphorus: 162 mg.
Fiber: 1.3 g.

552. JALAPENO CHEDDAR WAFFLES

Preparation time: 4 min.
Cooking time: 10 min.
Servings: 2
Ingredients:

- 2 egg
- 1 1/2 c. cheddar cheese
- 16 slices deli jalapeno

Directions:

Preheat a mini waffle maker if needed
In a mixing bowl, beat the eggs and add half cheddar cheese to them
Mix them all well
Shred some of the remaining cheddar cheese to the lower plate of the waffle maker
Now pour the mixture into the shredded cheese
Add the cheese again on the top with around 4 slices of jalapeno and close the lid
Cooking for at least 4 min. to get the desired crunch and serve hot
Make as many waffles as your mixture allows

Nutrition:

Calories: 363
Protein: 18 g.
Carbohydrates: 30 g.
Fat: 19 g.
Cholesterol: 40 mg.
Sodium: 194 mg.
Potassium: 507 mg.
Phosphorus: 327 mg.
Fiber: 4.3 g.

553. COCONUT CRISPY WAFFLES

Preparation time: 5 min.
Cooking time: 20 min.
Servings: 4
Ingredients:

- 1/3 c. cheddar cheese
- 1 egg
- 2 tbsp. coconut flour
- 1/4 tsp. baking powder
- 2 tbsp. coconut flakes
- 1/3 c. mozzarella cheese

Directions:

Mix cheddar cheese, egg, coconut flour, coconut flakes, and baking powder together in a bowl
Preheat your waffle iron and grease it

In your mini waffle iron, shred half of the Mozzarella cheese

Add the mixture to your mini waffle iron

Again, shred the remaining Mozzarella cheese on the mixture

Cooking till the desired crisp is achieved

Make as many waffles as your mixture and waffle maker allow

Nutrition:
Calories: 294
Protein: 20 g.
Carbohydrates: 31 g.
Fat: 10 g.
Cholesterol: 137 mg.
Sodium: 186 mg.
Potassium: 300 mg.
Phosphorus: 197 mg.
Fiber: 0.8 g.

554. YOGURT PARMESAN WAFFLES

Preparation time: 5 min.
Cooking time: 10 min.
Servings: 2
Ingredients:

- 1/3 c. cheddar cheese
- 1 egg
- 1/4 tsp. baking powder
- 2 tbsp. yogurt
- 1/3 c. parmesan cheese

Directions:

Mix cheddar cheese, egg, yogurt, and baking powder together

Preheat your waffle iron and grease it

In your mini waffle iron, shred half of the parmesan cheese

Add the mixture to your mini waffle iron

Again, shred the remaining parmesan cheese on the mixtures

Cooking till the desired crisp is achieved

Make as many waffles as your mixture and waffle maker allow

Nutrition:
Calories: 415
Protein: 22 g.
Carbohydrates: 39 g.
Fat: 19 g.
Cholesterol: 88 mg.
Sodium: 266 mg.
Potassium: 400 mg.
Phosphorus: 306 mg.
Fiber: 3.2 g.

555. ALMONDS AND COCONUT WAFFLES

Preparation time: 15 min.
Cooking time: 20 min.
Servings: 4
Ingredients:

- 1/3 c. cheddar cheese
- 1 egg
- 3 tbsp. almond flour
- 2 tbsp. coconut flakes
- 1/4 tsp. baking powder
- 2 tbsp. ground almonds
- 1/3 c.mozzarella cheese

Directions:

Mix cheddar cheese, egg, almond flour, almond ground, coconut flakes, and baking powder together in a bowl

Preheat your waffle iron and grease it

In your mini waffle iron, shred half of the Mozzarella cheese

Add the mixture to your mini waffle iron

Again, shred the remaining Mozzarella cheese on the mixture

Cooking till the desired crisp is achieved

Make as many waffles as your mixture and waffle maker allow

Nutrition:
Calories: 250
Protein: 22 g.
Carbohydrates: 19 g.
Fat: 10 g.

Cholesterol: 53 mg.
Sodium: 124 mg.
Potassium: 401 mg.
Phosphorus: 262 mg.
Fiber: 1.2 g.
Sugar: 2 g.

556.   CREAMY JALAPEÑO MINI WAFFLE

Preparation time: 5 min.
Cooking time: 10 min.
Servings: 2
Ingredients:

- 2 eggs
- 1 c. shredded mozzarella
- 16 slices deli jalapeno
- 2 tbsp. cream cheese
- 2 tbsp. almond flour
- 3/4 tbsp. baking powder
- 2 tbsp. water (optional)

Directions:
Preheat your mini waffle iron if needed
Mix all the above-mentioned ingredients into a bowl
Grease your waffle iron lightly
Adds the mixture to the waffle iron and add at least 4 jalapeños on top
Close the lid and cook for 4-minutes
Make as many waffles as your mixture and waffle maker allow

Nutrition:
Calories: 292
Protein: 20 g.
Carbohydrates: 1 g.
Fat: 23 g.
Cholesterol: 57 mg.
Sodium: 228 mg.
Potassium: 237 mg.
Phosphorus: 128 mg.
Calcium: 14 mg.

557.   CHEESE WAFFLES

Preparation time: 5 min.
Cooking time: 20 min.
Servings: 2
Ingredients:

- 1 egg:
- 1 1/2 c. cheddar cheese:
- 1/2 tsp. butter:
- 1 per two waffles cheese slices

Directions:
Preheat your waffle iron if needed
Mix all egg and cheddar cheese and whisk well
Grease your waffle iron lightly
Cooking in the waffle iron for about 5 min. or till the desired crisp is achieved
Make as many waffles as your mixture and waffle maker allow
Heat the pan and grease it with butter
Place one waffle on the pan and top with the slice and then add another waffle
Grill this waffle sandwich from both sides and serve hot

Nutrition:
Calories 391
Total Fat: 27 g.
Cholesterol 94 mg.
Sodium 320 mg.
Carbohydrates 39 mg.
Dietary Fiber 7 g.
Protein: 37 g.

558.   SEASONED MUSHROOM WAFFLES

Preparation time: 5 min.
Cooking time: 15 min.
Servings: 2
Ingredients:

- 1 egg
- 1/2 c. mozzarella cheese, shredded
- 1 tbsp. Chinese five-spice
- 1 c. mushrooms, finely sliced
- 1 garlic clove, minced

- 1 tbsp. onion powder
- 1/2 tsp. salt

Directions:

Add all the ingredients together and whisk well

Preheat your mini waffle iron if needed and grease it

Cooking your mixture in the mini waffle iron for at least 4 min.

Make as many waffles as you can

Nutrition:

Calories 201;

Total Fat: 5 g.

Saturated Fat: 1 g.

Cholesterol 101 mg.

Sodium 121 mg.

Total Carbohydrates 1 g.

Dietary Fiber 1 g.

Protein: 39 g.

Sugars 1 g.

559. SPICY WAFFLES WITH SPECIAL SAUCE

Preparation time: 5 min.

Cooking time: 10 min.

Servings: 2

Ingredients:

- 1 egg
- 1/2 c. mozzarella cheese, shredded
- 1/2 tsp. dried basil
- 1/2 tsp. smoked paprika
- 1/2 tsp. salt

For the sauce:

- 1/4 c. mayonnaise
- 1 tsp. vinegar
- 3 tbsp. sweet chili sauce
- 1 tbsp. hot sauce

Directions:

Add the egg, dried basil, smoked paprika, salt, and cheese to a bowl and whisk

Preheat your mini waffle iron if needed and grease it

Cooking your mixture in the mini waffle iron for at least 4 min.

Make as many waffles as you can

Combine the sauce ingredient well together

Serve spicy waffles with the sauce

Nutrition:

Saturated Fat: 3 g.

Cholesterol 207 mg.

Sodium 313 mg.

Total Carbohydrates 16 g.

Dietary Fiber 5 g.

Protein: 22 g.

Sugars 2 g.

Calories 155;

Total Fat: 5 g.

560. GARLIC SWISS WAFFLES

Preparation time: 5 min.

Cooking time: 10 min.

Servings: 2

Ingredients:

- 1 egg
- 1 c. swiss cheese, shredded
- 2 garlic cloves, finely chopped
- 1 tsp. garlic salt

Directions:

Preheat your mini waffle iron if needed and grease it

Add the egg, cheese, garlic salt, and garlic to a bowl and whisk

Cooking your mixture in the mini waffle iron for at least 4 min.

Make as many waffles as your mixture and waffle maker allow

Nutrition:

Calories 391

Total Fat: 18 g.

Saturated Fat: 9 g.

Cholesterol 94 mg.

Sodium 320 mg. Total

Carbohydrates 39 g.

Dietary Fiber 7 g.
Protein: 37 g.
Sugars 17 g.

561. CRISPY BACON WAFFLE

Preparation time: 5 min.
Cooking time: 10 min.
Servings: 2
Ingredients:
1/3 c. cheddar cheese
1 egg
1/4 tsp. baking powder
1 tsp. flaxseed (ground)
1/3 c. parmesan cheese
2 tbsp. bacon piece

Directions:
Cooking the bacon pieces separately in the pan
Mix cheddar cheese, egg, baking powder, and flaxseed to it
In your mini waffle iron, shred half of the parmesan cheese
Grease your waffle iron lightly
Add the mixture from step one to your mini waffle iron
Again, shred the remaining cheddar cheese on the mixtures
Cooking till the desired crisp is achieved
Make as many waffles as your mixture and waffle maker allow

Nutrition:
Calories 207;
Total Fat: 4 g.
Saturated Fat: 0 g.
Cholesterol 168 mg.
Sodium 536 mg.
Total Carbohydrates 5 g.
Dietary Fiber 1 g.
Protein: 32 g.
Sugars 0 g.

562. ALMONDS CRISPY WAFFLE

Preparation time: 15 min.
Cooking time: 20 min.
Servings: 4
Ingredients:
- 1/3 c. cheddar cheese
- 1 egg
- 2 tbsp. almond flour
- 1/4 tsp. baking powder
- 2 tbsp. ground almonds
- 1/3 c. mozzarella cheese

Directions:
Mix cheddar cheese, egg, almond flour, almond ground, and baking powder together in a bowl
Preheat your waffle iron and grease it
In your mini waffle iron, shred half of the Mozzarella cheese
Add the mixture to your mini waffle iron
Again, shred the remaining Mozzarella cheese on the mixture
Cooking till the desired crisp is achieved
Make as many waffles as your mixture and waffle maker allow

Nutrition:
Calories 107
Total Fat: 3 g.
Saturated Fat: 0 g.
Cholesterol 8 mg.
Sodium 200 mg.
Total Carbohydrates 15 g.
Dietary Fiber 2 g.
Protein: 5 g.
Sugars 0 g.

563. OLIVES LAYERED WAFFLE

Preparation time: 15 min.
Cooking time: 20 min.
Servings: 4
Ingredients:
For the waffle:

- 3 egg
- 1 1/2 c. mozzarella cheese (shredded)
- 1/2 tsp. garlic powder
- 1 tsp. Italian seasoning

For the vegetable:

- 1 c. mushrooms
- 1/2 tsp. garlic powder
- 1/2 tsp. Italian seasoning
- 1 tbsp. butter

For layering:

- 1/2 c. mozzarella cheese (shredded)
- 1/2 c. olives
- 1 tbsp. parsley
- 1 tbsp. oregano

Directions:

Preheat a mini waffle maker if needed and grease it

In a mixing bowl, add all the ingredients of the waffle and mix well

Pour the mixture into the waffle maker

Cooking for at least 4 min. to get the desired crunch and make as many waffles as your batter allows

In the meanwhile, melt the butter and add all mushrooms ingredients and cooking

Remove the waffles from the heat and spread on the baking sheet

Spread the cooked mushrooms on the top and sprinkle cheese and olives

Top again with waffles, then mushrooms, then cheese and olives, then again waffles and make as many layers as you want using this layering technique

Bake for 5 min. in an oven at 350 °F to melt the cheese

Sprinkle parsley and oregano on the top and serve hot

Nutrition:

Calories 395
Fat: 2 g.
Carbs: 61 g.
Protein: 33 g.
Fiber 5 g.
Potassium 796 mg.
Sodium 215 mg.

564. CIN-CHEESE WAFFLES WITH THE SAUCE

Preparation time: 5 min.
Cooking time: 15 min.
Servings: 2
Ingredients:
For the waffle:

- 1 egg
- 1/2 c. mozzarella cheese, shredded
- 1/2 tsp. cinnamon

For the sauce:

- 1/4 c. mayonnaise
- 1 tsp. vinegar
- 3 tbsp. sweet chili sauce
- 1 tbsp. hot sauce

Directions:

Add the egg, cinnamon, and cheese to a bowl and whisk

Preheat your mini waffle iron if needed and grease it

Cooking your mixture in the mini waffle iron for at least 4 min.

Make as many waffles as you can

Combine the sauce ingredient well together

Nutrition:

Calories 215
Fat: 11 g.
Carbs: 7 g.

Protein: 24 g.
Fiber 2 g.
Potassium 520 mg.
Sodium 200 mg.

565. FRIED PICKLE WAFFLE

Preparation time: 5 min.
Cooking time: 10 min.
Servings: 2
Ingredients:

- 1 egg
- 1/2 c. mozzarella cheese (shredded)
- 1/2 c. pork panko
- 6–8 pickle slices, thin
- 1 tbsp. pickle juice

Directions:

Mix all the ingredients well together
Pour a thin layer on a preheated waffle iron
Remove any excess juice from pickles
Add pickle slices and pour again more mixture over the top
Cooking the waffle for around 5 min.
Make as many waffles as your mixture and waffle maker allow
Serve hot!

Nutrition:

Calories 509
Fat: 5 g.
Carbs: 69 g.
Protein: 48 g.
Fiber 7 g.
Potassium 629 mg.
Sodium 400 mg.

566. PLAIN BBQ CRISPY WAFFLE

Preparation time: 5 min.
Cooking time: 10 min.
Servings: 2
Ingredients:

- 1/3 c. cheddar cheese
- 1 egg
- 1 tbsp. BBQ sauce
- 1/4 tsp. baking powder
- 1 tsp. flaxseed (ground)
- 1/3 c. parmesan cheese

Directions:

Mix cheddar cheese, egg, baking powder, BBQ sauce, and flaxseed in a bowl
In your mini waffle iron, shred half of the parmesan cheese
Grease your waffle iron lightly
Add the cheese mixture to the mini waffle iron
Again, shred the remaining parmesan cheese on the mixture
Cooking till the desired crisp is achieved
Make as many waffles as your mixture and waffle maker allow

Nutrition:

Calories 434
Fat: 16 g.
Carbs: 27 g.
Protein: 39 g.
Fiber 4 g.
Potassium 714 mg.
Sodium 378 mg.

567. BAGEL WAFFLES

Preparation time: 5 min.
Cooking time: 10 min.
Servings: 2
Ingredients:

- 1 egg:
- 1/2 c. mozzarella cheese, shredded
- 1 tsp. coconut flour
- 1 tsp. everything bagel seasoning
- 2 tbsp. cream cheese, for serving

Directions:

Add all the ingredients into a bowl and whisk

Preheat your mini waffle iron if needed and grease it

Cooking your mixture in the mini waffle iron for at least 4 min.

Make as many waffles as you can and spread cream cheese on top

Nutrition:

Calories: 311

Fat: 13 g.

Carbs: 27 g.

Protein: 14 g.

Fiber: 12 g.

Potassium: 911 mg.

Sodium: 600 mg.

568. WAFFLE WITH CREAM AND SALMON

Preparation time: 8 min.

Cooking time: 20 min.

Servings: 2

Ingredients:

- 1/2 medium onion sliced
- 2 tbsps. parsley chopped
- 4 oz. smoked salmon
- 4 tbsp. heavy cream

For the waffle:

1 egg

1/2 c. mozzarella cheese

1 tsp. stevia

1 tsp. vanilla

2 tbsps. almond flour

Directions:

Make 4 heart-shaped waffles with the waffle ingredients

Arrange smoked salmon and heavy cream on each waffle.

Top with onion slice and parsley.

Serve as it is and enjoy!

Nutrition:

Calories 388

Fat: 3 g.

Carbs: 42 g.

Protein: 52 g.

Fiber: 8 g.

Potassium: 874 mg.

Sodium: 600 mg.

CHAPTER 16. FESTIVE WAFFLE RECIPES

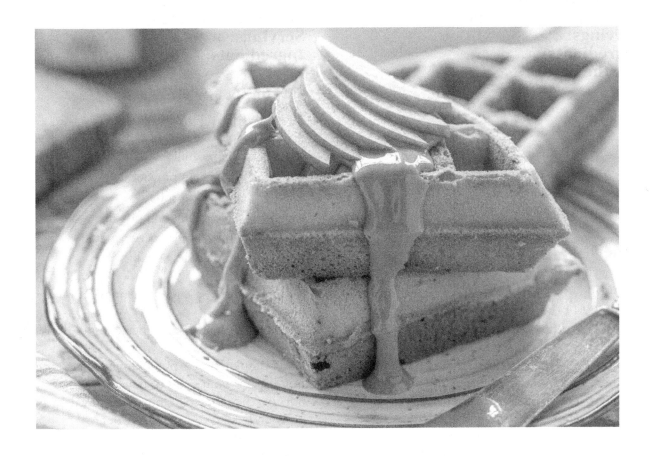

569. COOKIE DOUGH WAFFLE

Preparation time: 10 min.
Cooking time: 7–9 min.
Servings: 4
Ingredients:
For the batter:

- 4 eggs
- 1/4 c. heavy cream
- 1 tsp. vanilla extract
- 1/4 c. stevia
- 6 tbsp. coconut flour
- 1 tsp. baking powder
- Pinch of salt
- 1/4 c. unsweetened chocolate chips

Other:

- 2 tbsp. cooking spray to brush the waffle maker
- 1/4 c. heavy cream, whipped

Directions:
Preheat the waffle maker.

Add the eggs and heavy cream to a bowl and stir in the vanilla extract, stevia, coconut flour, baking powder, and salt. Mix until just combined. Stir in the chocolate chips and combine.

Brush the heated waffle maker with cooking spray and add a few tablespoons of the batter.

Close the lid and cook for about 7–8 min. depending on your waffle maker.

Serve with whipped cream on top.

Nutrition:
Calories 3
Fat 32.3 g.
Carbs 12.6 g.
Sugar 0.5 g.
Protein: 9 g.
Sodium 117 mg

570. THANKSGIVING PUMPKIN SPICE WAFFLE

Preparation time: 5 min.
Cooking time: 5 min.
Servings: 4
Ingredients:

- 1 c. egg whites
- 1/4 c. pumpkin puree
- 2 tsps. pumpkin pie spice
- 2 tsps. coconut flour
- 1/2 tsp. vanilla
- 1 tsp. baking powder
- 1 tsp. baking soda
- 1/8 tsp. cinnamon powder
- 1 c. mozzarella cheese, grated
- 1/2 tsp. garlic powder

Directions:
Switch on your square waffle maker. Spray with non-stick spray.

Beat the egg whites with a beater, until fluffy and white.

Add pumpkin puree, pumpkin pie spice, coconut flour in egg whites and beat again.

Stir in the cheese, cinnamon powder, garlic powder, baking soda, and powder.

Pour 1/2 of the batter into the waffle maker.

Close the maker and cook for about 3 min.

Repeat with the remaining batter.

Remove the waffles from the maker.

Serve hot and enjoy!

Nutrition:
Protein: 51% 66 g.
Fat: 41% 53 g.
Carbohydrates: 8%

571. WAFFLE FRUIT SNACKS

Preparation time: 10 min.
Cooking time: 14 min.
Servings: 2
Ingredients:

- 1 egg, beaten
- 1/2 c. finely grated cheddar cheese
- 1/2 c. Greek yogurt for topping
- 8 raspberries and blackberries for topping

Directions:

Preheat the waffle iron.

Mix the egg and cheddar cheese in a medium bowl.

Open the iron and add half of the mixture. Close and cook until crispy, 7 min.

Remove the waffle onto a plate and make another with the remaining mixture.

Cut each waffle into wedges and arrange it on a plate.

Top each waffle with a tablespoon of yogurt and then two berries.

Serve afterward.

Nutrition:

Calories 207
Fats 15.29 g.
Carbs: 4.36 g.
Net Carbs: 3.g
Protein: 12.91 g.

572. OPEN-FACED HAM AND GREEN BELL PEPPER WAFFLE SANDWICH

Preparation time: 10 min.
Cooking time: 10 min.
Servings: 2
Ingredients:

- 2 slices ham
- Cooking spray
- 1 green bell pepper, sliced into strips
- 2 slices cheese
- 1 tbsp. black olives, pitted and sliced
- 2 basic waffles

Directions:

Cook the ham in a pan coated with oil over medium heat.

Next, cook the bell pepper.

Assemble the open-faced sandwich by topping each waffle with ham and cheese, bell pepper, and olives.

Toast in the oven until the cheese has melted a little.

Nutrition:

Calories 36
Total Fat: 24.6 g.
Saturated Fat: 13.6 g.
Cholesterol 91 mg.
Sodium 1154 mg.
Potassium 440 mg.
Total Carbohydrate 8 g.
Dietary Fiber 2.6 g.
Protein: 24.5 g.
Total Sugars 6.3 g.

573. CHRISTMAS MORNING CHOCO WAFFLE CAKE

Preparation time: 10 min.
Cooking time: 5 min.
Servings: 8
Ingredients:

- 8 keto chocolate square waffles
- 2 c. peanut butter
- 16 oz. raspberries

Directions:

Assemble waffles in layers.

Spread peanut butter in each layer.

Top with raspberries.

Enjoy cake on Christmas morning with keto coffee!

Nutrition:

Protein: 3% 1 g.

Fat: 94% 207 g.
Carbohydrates: 3% 15 g.

574. LT WAFFLE SANDWICH

Preparation time: 5 min.
Cooking time: 15 min.
Servings: 2
Ingredients:

- Cooking spray
- 4 slices bacon
- 1 tbsp. mayonnaise
- 4 basic waffles
- 2 lettuce leaves
- 2 tomato slices

Directions:

Coat your pan with foil and place it over medium heat.
Cook the bacon until golden and crispy.
Spread mayo on top of the waffle.
Top with lettuce, bacon, and tomato.
Top with another waffle.

Nutrition:

Calories 238
Total Fat: 18.4 g.
Saturated Fat: 5.
Cholesterol: 44 mg.
Sodium: 931 mg.
Potassium: 258 mg.
Total Carbohydrate: 3 g.
Dietary Fiber: 0.2 g.
Protein: 14.3 g.
Total Sugars: 0.9 g.

575. MOZZARELLA PEANUT BUTTER WAFFLE

Preparation time: 10 min.
Cooking time: 15 min.
Servings: 2
Ingredients:

- 1 egg, lightly beaten
- 2 tbsp. peanut butter
- 2 tbsp. Swerve
- 1/2 c. mozzarella cheese, shredded

Directions:

Preheat your waffle maker.
In a bowl, mix egg, cheese, Swerve, and peanut butter until well combined.
Spray the waffle maker with cooking spray.
Pour half batter into the hot waffle maker and cook for 4–5 min. or until golden brown. Repeat with the remaining batter.
Serve and enjoy.

Nutrition:

Calories: 150
Fat: 11.5 g
Carbohydrates: 5.g
Sugar: 1.7 g
Protein: 8.8 g
Cholesterol: 86 mg.

576. CINNAMON AND VANILLA WAFFLE

Preparation time: 10 min.
Cooking time: 7–9 min.
Servings: 4
Ingredients:
For the batter:

- 4 eggs
- 4 oz. sour cream
- 1 tsp. vanilla extract
- 1 tsp. cinnamon
- 1/4 c. stevia
- 5 tbsp. coconut flour

Other:

- 2 tbsp. coconut oil to brush the waffle maker
- 1/2 tsp. cinnamon for garnishing the waffles

Directions:

Preheat the waffle maker.
Add the eggs and sour cream to a bowl and stir with a wire whisk until just combined.

Add the vanilla extract, cinnamon, and stevia and mix until combined.

Stir in the coconut flour and stir until combined.

Brush the heated waffle maker with coconut oil and add a few tablespoons of the batter.

Close the lid and cook for about 7–8 min. depending on your waffle maker.

Serve and enjoy.

Nutrition:
Calories: 224

Fat: 11 g.

Carbs: 8.4 g.

Sugar: 0.5 g.

Protein: 7.7 g.

Sodium: 77 mg.

577. NEW YEAR CINNAMON WAFFLE WITH COCONUT CREAM

Preparation time: 10 min.

Cooking time: 5 min.

Servings: 2

Ingredients:

- 2 large eggs
- 1/8 c. almond flour
- 1 tsp. cinnamon powder
- 1 tsp. sea salt
- 1/2 tsp. baking soda
- 1 c. shredded mozzarella

For the topping:

- 2 tbsps. coconut cream
- 1 tbsp. unsweetened chocolate sauce

Directions:
Preheat the waffle maker according to the manufacturer's directions.

Mix together recipe ingredients in a mixing bowl.

Add the cheese and mix well.

Pour about 1/2 c. mixture into the center of the waffle maker and cook for about 2–3 min. until golden and crispy.

Repeat with the remaining batter.

For serving, coat coconut cream over the waffles.

Drizzle chocolate sauce over the waffle.

Freeze waffle in the freezer for about 10 min.

Serve on Christmas morning and enjoy!

Nutrition:
Protein: 3 100 g.

Fat: 56% 145 g.

Carbohydrates: 5% 13 g.

578. CHOCO CHIP PUMPKIN WAFFLE

Preparation time: 10 min.

Cooking time: 15 min.

Servings: 2

Ingredients:

- 1 egg, lightly beaten
- 1 tbsp. almond flour
- 1 tbsp. unsweetened chocolate chips
- 1/4 tsp. pumpkin pie spice
- 2 tbsp. Swerve
- 1 tbsp. pumpkin puree
- 1/2 c. mozzarella cheese, shredded

Directions:
Preheat your waffle maker.

In a small bowl, mix egg and pumpkin puree.

Add pumpkin pie spice, Swerve, almond flour, and cheese and mix well.

Stir in chocolate chips.

Spray the waffle maker with cooking spray.

Pour half batter into the hot waffle maker and cook for 4 min. Repeat with the remaining batter.

Serve and enjoy.

Nutrition:
Calories: 130

Fat: 9.2 g.

Carbohydrates: 5.9 g.

Sugar 0.6 g.

Protein: 6.6 g.

Cholesterol mg.

579. SAUSAGE AND PEPPERONI WAFFLE SANDWICH

Preparation time: 20 min.
Cooking time: 10 min.
Servings: 4
Ingredients:

- Cooking spray
- 2 cervelat sausage, sliced into rounds
- 12 pieces pepperoni
- 6 mushroom slices
- 4 tsp. mayonnaise
- 4 big white onion rings
- 4 basic waffles

Directions:

Spray your skillet with oil.

Place over medium heat.

Cook the sausage until brown on both sides.

Transfer on a plate.

Cook the pepperoni and mushrooms for 2 min.

Spread mayo on top of the waffle.

Top with the sausage, pepperoni, mushrooms, and onion rings.

Top with another waffle.

Nutrition:

Calories 373
Total Fat: 24.4 g.
Saturated Fat: 6 g.
Cholesterol: 27 mg.
Sodium: 717 mg.
Potassium: 105 mg.
Total Carbohydrate: 28 g.
Dietary Fiber: 1.1 g.
Protein: 8.1 g.
Total Sugars: 4.5 g.

580. PIZZA FLAVORED WAFFLE

Preparation time: 15 min.
Cooking time: 12 min.
Servings: 3
Ingredients:

- 1 egg, beaten
- 1/2 c. cheddar cheese, shredded
- 2 tbsp. pepperoni, chopped
- 1 tbsp. keto marinara sauce
- 4 tbsp. almond flour
- 1 tsp. baking powder
- 1/2 tsp. dried Italian seasoning
- Parmesan cheese, grated

Directions:

Preheat your waffle maker.

In a bowl, mix the egg, cheddar cheese, pepperoni, marinara sauce, almond flour, baking powder, and Italian seasoning.

Add the mixture to the waffle maker.

Close the device and cook for 4–5 min.

Open it and transfer the waffle to a plate.

Let cool for 2 min.

Repeat the steps with the remaining batter.

Top with the grated parmesan and serve.

Nutrition:

Calories: 17
Total Fat: 14.3 g.
Saturated Fat: 7.5 g.
Cholesterol: 118 mg.
Sodium: 300 mg.
Potassium: 326 mg.
Total Carbohydrate: 1.8 g.
Dietary Fiber: 0.1 g.
Protein: 11.1 g.
Total Sugars: 0.4 g.

581.   MAPLE WAFFLE

Preparation time: 10 min.
Cooking time: 15 min.
Servings: 2
Ingredients:

- 1 egg, lightly beaten
- 2 egg whites
- 1/2 tsp. maple extract
- 2 tsp. Swerve
- 1/2 tsp. baking powder, gluten-free
- 2 tbsp. almond milk
- 2 tbsp. coconut flour

Directions:

Preheat your waffle maker.
In a bowl, whip egg whites until stiff peaks form.
Stir in maple extract, Swerve, baking powder, almond milk, coconut flour, and egg.
Spray the waffle maker with cooking spray.
Pour half batter into the hot waffle maker and cook for 3-minutes or until golden brown.
Repeat with the remaining batter.
Serve and enjoy.

Nutrition:

Calories 122
Fat: 6.6 g
Carbohydrates 9 g
Sugar 1 g
Protein: 7 g
Cholesterol 82 mg.

582.   CINNAMON WAFFLE

Preparation time: 10 min.
Cooking time: 8 min.
Servings: 2
Ingredients:

- 1 egg
- 1/2 c. mozzarella cheese, shredded
- 2 tbsp. almond flour
- 1 tsp. baking powder
- 1 tsp. vanilla
- 2 tsp. cinnamon

- 1 tsp. sweetener

Directions:

Preheat your waffle maker.
Beat the egg in a bowl.
Stir in the rest of the ingredients.
Transfer half of the batter into the waffle maker.
Close and cook for 4 min.
Open and put the waffle on a plate. Let cool for 2 min.
Do the same steps for the remaining batter.

Nutrition:

Calories 136
Total Fat: 7.4 g.
Saturated Fat: 2.9 g.
Cholesterol 171 mg.
Sodium 152 mg.
Potassium 590 mg.
Total Carbohydrate 9.6 g.
Dietary Fiber 3.6 g.
Protein: 9.9 g.
Total Sugars 1 g.

583.   CREAMY WAFFLES

Preparation time: 10 min.
Cooking time: 5 min.
Servings: 4
Ingredients:

- 1 c. egg whites
- 1 c. cheddar cheese, shredded
- 2 oz. cocoa powder.
- 1 pinch salt

For the topping:

- 4 oz. cream cheese
- Strawberries
- Blueberries
- Coconut flour

Directions:

Beat the eggs whites with beater until fluffy and white
Chop Italian cheese with a knife and beat with egg whites.

Add cocoa powder and salt in the mixture and again beat.

Spray round waffle maker non-stick cooking spray.

Pour the batter into a round waffle maker.

Cook the waffle for about 5 min.

Once cooked carefully remove the waffle from the maker.

For serving, spread cream cheese on the waffle. Top with strawberries, blueberries, and coconut flour.

Serve and enjoy!

Nutrition:
Protein: 26% 68 g.
Fat: 71% 187 g.
Carbohydrates: 3% 9 g.

584. PUMPKIN WAFFLES WITH CHOCO CHIPS

Preparation time: 15 min.
Cooking time: 12 min.
Servings: 3
Ingredients:
- 1 egg
- 1/2 c. shredded mozzarella cheese
- 4 tsp. pureed pumpkin
- 1/4 tsp. pumpkin pie spice
- 2 tbsp. sweetener
- 1 tbsp. almond flour
- 4 tsp. chocolate chips (sugar-free)

Directions:
Turn your waffle maker on.

In a bowl, beat the egg and stir in the pureed pumpkin.

Mix well.

Add the rest of the ingredients one by one.

Pour 1/3 of the mixture into your waffle maker.

Cook for 4 min.

Repeat the same steps with the remaining mixture.

Nutrition:
Calories: 93
Total Fat: 7 g.
Saturated Fat: 3 g.
Cholesterol: 69 mg.
Sodium: 13 mg.
Potassium: 48 mg.
Total Carbohydrate: 2 g.
Dietary Fiber: 1 g.
Protein: 7 g.
Total Sugars: 1 g.

585. WALNUTS LOWCARB WAFFLES

Preparation time: 10 min.
Cooking time: 5 min.
Servings: 2
Ingredients:
- 2 tbsps. cream cheese
- 1/2 tsp. almonds flour
- 1/4 tsp. baking powder
- 1 large egg
- 1/4 c. chopped walnuts
- Pinch of stevia extract powder

Directions:
Preheat your waffle maker.

Spray the waffle maker with cooking spray.

In a bowl, add cream cheese, almond flour, baking powder, egg, walnuts, and stevia.

Mix all the ingredients.

Spoon walnut batter in the waffle maker and cook for about 2–3 min.

Let waffles cool at room temperature before serving.

Nutrition:
Protein: 12% 11 g.
Fat: 80%
Carbohydrates: 8% 8 g.

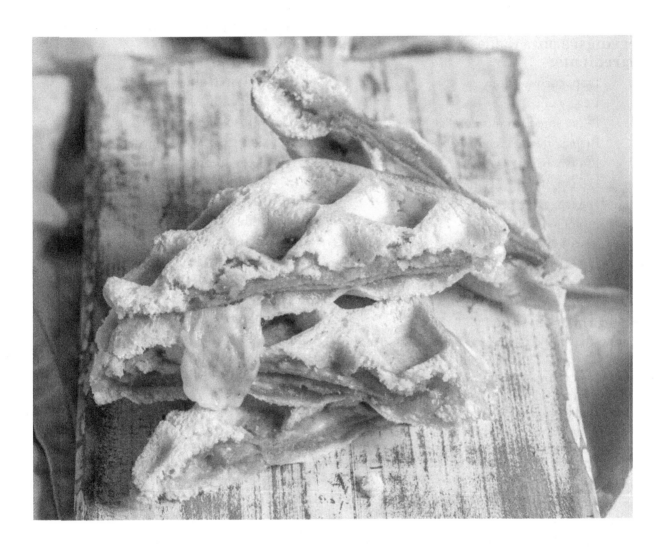

586. ITALIAN PIZZA WAFFLE

Preparation time: 5 min.
Cooking time: 10 min.
Servings: 2 pizza waffles
Ingredients:

- 1 tsp. coconut flour
- 1 egg white
- 1/2 c. shredded mozzarella cheese
- 1 tsp. softened cream cheese
- 1/4 tsp. baking powder
- 1/8 tsp. Italian seasoning
- 1/8 tsp. garlic powder
- A pinch of salt
- 3 tsp. low-carb tomato sauce
- 1/2 c. mozzarella cheese
- 1 tbsp. shredded parmesan cheese
- 1/4 tsp. basil

Directions:

Heat up the waffle maker and preheat the oven to 400°F.

Mix coconut flour, egg white, mozzarella cheese, softened cream cheese, baking powder, garlic powder, Italian seasonings, and a pinch of salt in a small mixing bowl.

Pour half of the batter into the waffle maker and cook for about 4 min. Repeat with the rest of the batter to make another waffle.

Top each waffle with tomato sauce, mozzarella cheese, and parmesan cheese.

Place in the oven on a baking sheet and broil the pizza for approx. 2 min. so that cheese begins to bubble and brown.

Remove from oven, sprinkle basil on top.

Serve and enjoy!

Nutrition:
Calories: 111
Fats: 1.48 g.
Carbs: 3.65 g.
Protein: 20.77 g.

587. HAM AND OLIVES PIZZA WAFFLE

Preparation time: 5 min.
Cooking time: 13 min.
Servings: 2 waffles
Ingredients:
For the waffles:

- 1/2 c. shredded mozzarella cheese
- 1 tbsp. almond flour
- 1/2 tsp. baking powder
- 1 egg, beaten
- A pinch of salt

For topping:

- 2 tbsp. low-carb pasta sauce
- 2 tbsp. mozzarella cheese, shredded
- 2 slices of ham
- 2 tsp. olives, pitted and chopped

Directions:

Heat up the waffle maker.

Add all the waffle ingredients to a small mixing bowl and combine well.

Pour half of the batter into the waffle maker and cook for about 4 min. until golden brown. Repeat with the rest of the batter to make another waffle.

Once both waffles are cooked, place them on the baking sheet of the toaster oven.

Put 1 tbsp. low-carb pasta sauce on top of each waffle.

Sprinkle 1 tbsp. shredded mozzarella cheese on top of each one.

Top with a slice of ham and sprinkle with olives. Bake at 350° F in the toaster oven for about 5 min., until the cheese is melted.

Serve and enjoy!

Nutrition:
Calories: 303
Fats: 6.44 g.
Carbs: 7.86 g.
Protein: 53.52 g.

588. PEPPERONI PIZZA WAFFLE

Preparation time: 5 min.
Cooking time: 10 min.
Servings: 2 pizza waffles
Ingredients:
For the waffles:

- 1 egg
- 1/2 c. shredded mozzarella cheese
- 1/2 tsp. Italian seasoning
- A pinch of garlic powder

For the toppings::

- 2 tbsp. tomato sauce
- 1/2 c. shredded mozzarella cheese
- 6 slices of pepperoni salami

Directions:

Heat up the waffle maker and preheat the oven to 400° F.

Mix egg, cheese, garlic, and herbs in a small mixing bowl. Stir until well combined.

Pour 1/2 of the batter in the waffle maker and cook for about 4 min. Repeat with the rest of the batter to make another waffle.

Top the waffle with tomato sauce, cheese, and pepperoni. Place in the oven on a baking sheet for 2 min.

Serve and enjoy!

Nutrition:
Calories: 276
Fats: 14.18 g.
Carbs: 6.48 g.
Protein: 29.05 g.

589. CHICKEN PIZZA WAFFLE

Preparation time: 5 min.
Cooking time: 10 min.
Servings: 2 pizza waffles
Ingredients:

- 1/3 c. chicken, cooked
- 1 egg
- 1/3 c. mozzarella cheese
- 1/4 tsp. basil
- 1/4 tsp. garlic powder
- 2 tbsp. tomato sauce
- 2 tbsp. mozzarella cheese

Directions:

Heat up the mini waffle maker and preheat the oven to 400° F.

Add the egg, chicken, basil, garlic, and mozzarella cheese to a small mixing bowl and combine well.

Pour 1/2 of the batter in the waffle maker and cook for about 4 min. Repeat with the rest of the batter to make another waffle.

Top each waffle with tomato sauce and mozzarella cheese.

Place in the oven on a baking sheet and broil the pizza for approx. 2 min. so that cheese begins to bubble and brown.

Remove from oven, sprinkle basil on top.
Serve and enjoy!

Nutrition:
Calories: 285
Fats 9.13 g.
Carbs: 4.87 g.
Protein: 42.91 g.

590. MUSHROOM AND BACON PIZZA WAFFLE

Preparation time: 5 min.
Cooking time: 13 min.
Servings: 2 pizza waffles
Ingredients:
For the waffles:

- 1/2 c. shredded mozzarella cheese
- 1 tbsp. almond flour
- 1/2 tsp. baking powder
- 1 egg
- 1/4 tsp. garlic powder
- 1/4 tsp. basil

For topping:
- 2 tbsp. low-carb pasta sauce
- 2 tbsp. mozzarella cheese
- 2 slices of bacon
- 2 tbsp. mushrooms, chopped

Directions:
Heat up the waffle maker.

Add mozzarella cheese, baking powder, garlic, basil, egg, and almond flour to a medium mixing bowl and combine well.

Pour half of the batter into the waffle maker and cook for about 4 min. Repeat with the rest of the batter to make another waffle.

Once both waffles are cooked, place them on the baking sheet of the toaster oven.

Put 1 tbsp. low-carb pasta sauce on top of each waffle.

Sprinkle 1 tbsp. shredded mozzarella cheese on top of each one.

Top with a slice of bacon and 1 tbsp. mushrooms.

Bake at 350° F in the toaster oven for about 5 min., until the cheese is melted.

Serve and enjoy!

Nutrition:
Calories: 226
Fats 15.6 g.
Carbs: 4.27 g.
Protein: 17.27 g.

591. TURKEY PIZZA WAFFLE
Preparation time: 5 min.
Cooking time: 10 min.
Servings: 2 pizza waffles
Ingredients:
- 1/2 c. turkey breast, cooked and chopped
- 1 egg, beaten
- 1/2 c. mozzarella cheese, shredded
- 1/4 tsp. basil
- 2 tbsp. tomato sauce

- 2 tbsp. mozzarella cheese

Directions:
Heat up the mini waffle maker and preheat the oven to 400° F.

Add the egg, turkey, basil, and mozzarella cheese to a small mixing bowl and combine well.

Pour half of the batter into the waffle maker and cook for about 4 min. Repeat with the rest of the batter to make another waffle.

Top each waffle with tomato sauce and mozzarella cheese.

Place in the oven on a baking sheet and broil the pizza for approx. 2 min. so that cheese begins to bubble and brown.

Remove from oven, sprinkle basil on top.

Serve and enjoy!

Nutrition:
Calories: 667
Fats 19.82 g.
Carbs: 4.92 g.
Protein: 109.62 g.

592. TUNA PIZZA WAFFLE
Preparation time: 5 min.
Cooking time: 10 min.
Servings: 2 waffles
Ingredients:
For the waffles:
- 1/2 c. shredded mozzarella cheese
- 1 tbsp. almond flour
- 1/2 tsp. baking powder
- 1 egg, beaten
- A pinch of salt

For topping:
- 2 tbsp. low-carb pasta sauce
- 2 tbsp. mozzarella cheese, shredded
- 1 can tuna, drained
- 1 tsp. dried oregano

Directions:
Heat up the waffle maker.

Add all the waffle ingredients to a small mixing bowl and combine well.

Pour half of the batter into the waffle maker and cook for about 4 min. until golden brown. Repeat with the rest of the batter to make another waffle.

Once both waffles are cooked, place them on the baking sheet of the toaster oven.

Put 1 tbsp. low-carb pasta sauce on top of each waffle.

Sprinkle 1 tbsp. shredded mozzarella cheese on top of each one.

Top with tuna and sprinkle with oregano.

Bake at 350° in the toaster oven for about 2 min., until the cheese is melted.

Serve and enjoy!

Nutrition:
Calories: 349
Fats 6.18 g.
Carbs: 7.81 g.
Protein: 65.7 g.

593.   HAM PIZZA WAFFLE
Preparation time: 5 min.
Cooking time: 10 min.
Servings: 2 waffles
Ingredients:
For the waffles:
- 1/2 c. shredded mozzarella cheese
- 1 tbsp. almond flour
- 1/2 tsp. baking powder
- 1 egg, beaten
- A pinch of salt

For topping:
- 2 tbsp. low-carb pasta sauce
- 2 tbsp. mozzarella cheese, shredded
- 2 slices of ham
- 1 tsp. dried oregano

Directions:
Heat up the waffle maker.

Add all the waffle ingredients to a small mixing bowl and combine well.

Pour half of the batter into the waffle maker and cook for about 4 min. until golden brown.

Repeat with the rest of the batter to make another waffle.

Once both waffles are cooked, place them on the baking sheet of the toaster oven.

Put 1 tbsp. low-carb pasta sauce on top of each waffle.

Sprinkle 1 tbsp. shredded mozzarella cheese on top of each one.

Top with a slice of ham and sprinkle with oregano.

Bake at 350° F in the toaster oven for about 2 min., until the cheese is melted.

Serve and enjoy!

Nutrition:
Calories: 302
Fats 6.17 g.
Carbs: 8.03 g.
Protein: 53.55 g.

594.   BACON   PIZZA   WAFFLE
Preparation time: 5 min.
Cooking time: 10 min.
Servings: 2 waffles
Ingredients:
For the waffles:
- 1/2 c. shredded mozzarella cheese
- 1 tbsp. almond flour
- 1/2 tsp. baking powder
- 1 egg, beaten
- A pinch of salt

For topping:
- 2 tbsp. low-carb pasta sauce
- 2 tbsp. mozzarella cheese, shredded
- 2 tbsp. bacon bits

Directions:
Heat up the waffle maker.

Add all the waffle ingredients to a small mixing bowl and combine well.

Pour half of the batter into the waffle maker and cook for about 4 min. until golden brown.

Repeat with the rest of the batter to make another waffle.

Once both waffles are cooked, place them on the baking sheet of the toaster oven.

Put 1 tbsp. low-carb pasta sauce on top of each waffle.

Sprinkle 1 tbsp. shredded mozzarella cheese on top of each one.

Top with bacon bits.

Bake at 350° F in the toaster oven for about 2 min., until the cheese is melted.

Serve and enjoy!

Nutrition:
Calories: 310
Fats 7.17 g.
Carbs: 9.46 g.
Protein: 51.85 g.

595. ZUCCHINI AND BRIE PIZZA WAFFLE

Preparation time: 5 min.
Cooking time: 10 min.
Servings: 2 pizza waffles
Ingredients:
- 1 egg
- 1/3 c. mozzarella cheese
- 1/4 tsp. garlic powder
- 1/2 c. zucchini, grated
- 2 tbsp. tomato sauce
- 2 tbsp. mozzarella cheese
- 2 tsp. Brie cheese

Directions:
Heat up the mini waffle maker and preheat the oven to 400° F.

Add the egg, garlic, zucchini, and mozzarella cheese to a small mixing bowl and combine well.

Pour 1/2 of the batter in the waffle maker and cook for about 4 min. until golden brown. Repeat with the rest of the batter to make another waffle.

Top each waffle with tomato sauce, mozzarella cheese, and Brie cheese.

Place in the oven on a baking sheet and broil the pizza for approx. 2 min. so that cheese begins to bubble and brown.

Remove from oven.

Serve and enjoy!

Nutrition:
Calories: 111
Fats 4.88 g.
Carbs: 4.91 g.
Protein: 10.96 g.

596. MUSHROOMS PIZZA WAFFLE

Preparation time: 5 min.
Cooking time: 10 min.
Servings: 2 waffles
Ingredients:
For the waffles:
- 1/2 c. shredded mozzarella cheese
- 1 tbsp. almond flour
- 1/2 tsp. baking powder
- 1 egg, beaten
- A pinch of salt

For topping:
2 tbsp. low-carb pasta sauce
2 tbsp. mozzarella cheese, shredded
1 can of mushrooms, drained
1 tsp. dried oregano

Directions:
Heat up the waffle maker.

Add all the waffle ingredients to a small mixing bowl and combine well.

Pour half of the batter into the waffle maker and cook for about 4 min. until golden brown. Repeat with the rest of the batter to make another waffle.

Once both waffles are cooked, place them on the baking sheet of the toaster oven.

Put 1 tbsp. low-carb pasta sauce on top of each waffle.

Sprinkle 1 tbsp. shredded mozzarella cheese on top of each one.

Top with mushrooms and sprinkle with oregano. Bake at 350° F in the toaster oven for about 2 min., until the cheese is melted.

Serve and enjoy!

Nutrition:
Calories: 283
Fats 5.4 g.
Carbs: 9.16 g.
Protein: 49.83 g.

597. TUNA AND OLIVES PIZZA WAFFLE

Preparation time: 5 min.
Cooking time: 10 min.
Servings: 2 pizza waffles
Ingredients:

- 1 egg
- 1/2 c. mozzarella cheese
- 1/4 tsp. garlic powder
- 1 can of tuna, drained
- 1 tbsp. black olives, pitted
- 2 tbsp. tomato sauce
- 2 tbsp. mozzarella cheese

Directions:
Heat up the waffle maker and preheat the oven to 400° F.

Add the egg, garlic, and mozzarella cheese to a small mixing bowl and combine well.

Pour 1/2 of the batter in the waffle maker and cook for about 4 min. until golden brown. Repeat with the rest of the batter to make another waffle.

Top each waffle with tomato sauce, mozzarella cheese, tuna, and a few black olives.

Place in the oven on a baking sheet and broil the pizza for approx. 2 min. so that cheese begins to bubble and brown.

Remove from oven.

Serve and enjoy!

Nutrition:
Calories: 197
Fats 5.86 g.
Carbs: 5.28 g.
Protein: 29.99 g.

598. PARMESAN PIZZA WAFFLE

Preparation time: 5 min.
Cooking time: 13 min.
Servings: 2 waffles
Ingredients:

- 1/2 c. shredded mozzarella cheese
- 1 tbsp. almond flour
- 1/2 tsp. baking powder
- 1 egg, beaten
- 1/4 tsp. garlic powder
- A pinch of salt and pepper

For pizza topping:

- 2 tbsp. low-carb pasta sauce
- 2 tbsp. mozzarella cheese, shredded
- 1 tbsp. parmesan cheese, shredded
- 1/4 tsp. fresh basil

Directions:
Heat up the waffle maker.

Add all the waffle ingredients to a small mixing bowl and combine well.

Pour half of the batter into the waffle maker and cook for about 4 min. until golden brown. Repeat with the rest of the batter to make another waffle.

Once both waffles are cooked, place them on the baking sheet of the toaster oven.

Put 1 tbsp. low-carb pasta sauce on top of each waffle.

Sprinkle 1 tbsp. shredded mozzarella and 1 tbsp. shredded parmesan on top of each one. Season with fresh basil.

Bake at 350° F in the toaster oven for about 5 min., until the cheese is melted.

Serve and enjoy!

Nutrition:
Calories: 298
Fats 6.11 g.
Carbs: 10.28 g.
Protein: 50.86 g.

599. BACON AND ZUCCHINI PIZZA WAFFLE

Preparation time: 5 min.
Cooking time: 10 min.
Servings: 2 waffles
Ingredients:
For the waffles:

- 1/2 c. shredded mozzarella cheese
- 1 tbsp. almond flour
- 1/2 tsp. baking powder
- 1 egg, beaten
- A pinch of salt

For topping:

- 2 tbsp. low-carb pasta sauce
- 2 tbsp. mozzarella cheese, shredded
- 2 tbsp. bacon bits
- 2 tbsp. zucchinis, grated

Directions:
Heat up the waffle maker.

Add all the waffle ingredients to a small mixing bowl and combine well.

Pour half of the batter into the waffle maker and cook for about 4 min. until golden brown. Repeat with the rest of the batter to make another waffle.

Once both waffles are cooked, place them on the baking sheet of the toaster oven.

Put 1 tbsp. low-carb pasta sauce on top of each waffle.

Sprinkle 1 tbsp. shredded mozzarella cheese on top of each one.

Top with bacon bits and zucchinis.

Bake at 350° F in the toaster oven for about 2 min., until the cheese is melted.

Serve and enjoy!

Nutrition:
Calories: 312
Fats 7.22 g.
Carbs: 9.8 g.
Protein: 52.15 g.

600. TUNA AND ONION PIZZA WAFFLE

Preparation time: 5 min.
Cooking time: 13 min.
Servings: 2 waffles
Ingredients:
For the waffles:

- 1 egg, beaten
- 1/2 c. mozzarella cheese, shredded
- A pinch of salt

For pizza topping:

- 2 tbsp. tomato sauce
- 2 tbsp. mozzarella cheese, shredded
- 1 can of tuna, drained
- 1 tbsp. onion, browned and chopped
- 1 tsp. dried oregano

Directions:
Heat up the waffle maker and preheat the oven to 400° F.

Add all the waffle ingredients to a small mixing bowl and stir until well combined.

Pour 1/2 of the batter in the waffle maker and cook for about 4 min. until golden brown. Repeat with the rest of the batter to make another waffle.

Top each waffle with tomato sauce, mozzarella cheese, tuna, and onions. Season with oregano.

Place in the oven on a baking sheet and broil the pizza for approx. 2 min. so that cheese begins to bubble.

Serve and enjoy!
Nutrition:
Calories: 356
Fats 5.69 g.
Carbs: 9.64 g.
Protein: 65.82 g.

601. HAM AND PARMESAN PIZZA WAFFLE

Preparation time: 5 min.
Cooking time: 13 min.
Servings: 2 pizza waffles
Ingredients:
For the waffles:
- 1/2 c. shredded mozzarella cheese
- 1 tbsp. almond flour
- 1/2 tsp. baking powder
- 1 egg, beaten

For topping:
- 2 tbsp. low-carb pasta sauce
- 2 tbsp. mozzarella cheese
- 1 tbsp. parmesan cheese
- 2 slices of ham

Directions:
Heat up the waffle maker.
Add mozzarella cheese, baking powder, egg, and almond flour to a medium mixing bowl and combine well.
Pour half of the batter into the waffle maker and cook for about 4 min. Repeat with the rest of the batter to make another waffle.
Once both waffles are cooked, place them on the baking sheet of the toaster oven.
Put 1 tbsp. low-carb pasta sauce on top of each pizza waffle.
Sprinkle 1 tbsp. shredded mozzarella cheese on top of each one.
Top with a slice of ham and sprinkle with parmesan cheese.
Bake at 350° F in the toaster oven for about 5 min., until the cheese is melted.
Serve and enjoy!

Nutrition:
Calories: 151
Fats 6.84 g.
Carbs: 4.08 g.
Protein: 18.33 g.

602. BROCCOLI PIZZA WAFFLE

Preparation time: 5 min.
Cooking time: 10 min.
Servings: 2 waffles
Ingredients:
For the waffles:
- 1/2 c. shredded mozzarella cheese
- 1 tbsp. almond flour
- 1/2 tsp. baking powder
- 1 egg, beaten
- 1/2 tsp. garlic powder
- A pinch of salt

For topping:
- 2 tbsp. low-carb pasta sauce
- 2 tbsp. mozzarella cheese, shredded
- 2 tbsp. broccoli, boiled and chopped

Directions:
Heat up the waffle maker.
Add all the waffle ingredients to a small mixing bowl and combine well.
Pour half of the batter into the waffle maker and cook for about 4 min. until golden brown. Repeat with the rest of the batter to make another waffle.
Once both waffles are cooked, place them on the baking sheet of the toaster oven.
Put 1 tbsp. low-carb pasta sauce on top of each waffle.
Sprinkle 1 tbsp. shredded mozzarella cheese on top of each one.
Top with broccoli.
Bake at 350° F in the toaster oven for about 2 min., until the cheese is melted.
Serve and enjoy!

Nutrition:
Calories: 289
Fats 5.41 g.
Carbs: 8.25 g.
Protein: 49.81 g.

603. VEGGIE PIZZA WAFFLE

Preparation time: 5 min.
Cooking time: 13 min.
Servings: 2 waffles
Ingredients:

- 1/2 c. shredded mozzarella cheese
- 1 tbsp. almond flour
- 1/2 tsp. baking powder
- 1 egg, beaten
- 1/4 tsp. garlic powder
- A pinch of salt and pepper

For pizza topping:

- 2 tbsp. low-carb pasta sauce
- 2 tbsp. mozzarella cheese, shredded
- 1/2 tbsp. onion, browned and chopped
- 1/2 tbsp. mushrooms, chopped
- 1/2 tbsp. zucchini, grated
- 1/4 tsp. fresh basil

Directions:
Heat up the waffle maker.
Add all the waffle ingredients to a small mixing bowl and combine well.
Pour half of the batter into the waffle maker and cook for about 4 min. until golden brown. Repeat with the rest of the batter to make another waffle.
Once both waffles are cooked, place them on the baking sheet of the toaster oven.
Put 1 tbsp. low-carb pasta sauce on top of each waffle.
Sprinkle 1 tbsp. shredded mozzarella on top of each one. Season with fresh basil.

Top the waffle with onions, zucchinis, and mushrooms.
Bake at 350° F in the toaster oven for about 5 min., until the cheese is melted.
Serve and enjoy!
Nutrition:
Calories: 289
Fats 5.43 g.
Carbs: 10.3 g.
Protein: 50.29 g.

604. HAM AND ZUCCHINI PIZZA WAFFLE

Preparation time: 5 min.
Cooking time: 10 min.
Servings: 2 waffles
Ingredients: For the waffles:

- 1/2 c. shredded mozzarella cheese
- 1 tbsp. almond flour
- 1/2 tsp. baking powder
- 1 egg, beaten
- A pinch of salt

Ingredients: for topping:

- 2 tbsp. low-carb pasta sauce
- 2 tbsp. mozzarella cheese, shredded
- 2 slices of ham
- 2 tbsp. zucchini, grated

Directions:
Heat up the waffle maker.
Add all the waffle ingredients to a small mixing bowl and combine well.
Pour half of the batter into the waffle maker and cook for about 4 min. or until golden brown. Repeat with the rest of the batter to make another waffle.
Once both waffles are cooked, place them on the baking sheet of the toaster oven.

Put 1 tbsp. of low-carb pasta sauce on top of each waffle.

Sprinkle 1 tbsp. of shredded mozzarella cheese on top of each one.

Top with a slice of ham and zucchinis.

Bake at 350° in the toaster oven for about 2 min., until the cheese is melted.

Serve and enjoy!

Nutrition:

Calories: 303,

Fats 6.19 g.,

Carbs: 8.03 g.,

Protein: 53.8 g.

605. MINI KETO PIZZA WAFFLE

Preparation time: 5 min.
Cooking time: 10 min.
Servings: 2 Mini Keto Pizzas
Ingredients:

- 1/4 tsp. basil
- 2 tbsp. mozzarella cheese
- 1 tbsp. almond flour
- 1/4 tsp. garlic powder
- 1 egg
- 1/2 tsp. baking powder
- 2 tbsp. low-carb pasta sauce
- 1/2 c. Shredded Mozzarella cheese

Directions:

Reheat the mini waffle maker until hot.

Add all the ingredients except pasta sauce and shredded mozzarella to a bowl and mix well.

Grease the waffle maker and put half of the batter onto the waffle maker, spread across evenly.

Cook until golden, about 4 min.

Gently remove from the waffle maker and let it cool.

Repeat with the remaining batter.

Once they are cooked, place them on the baking lined sheet in the toaster oven.

Top each pizza crust with 1 tbsp. each of pasta sauce.

Sprinkle with 1 tbsp. each of shredded mozzarella cheese.

Bake at 350 °F for 5 min., until the cheese is a little melted.

Remove from the oven and let it cool.

Serve and Enjoy!

Nutrition:

Calories 195

Net carbs 2 g.

Fat: 14 g.

Protein: 13 g.

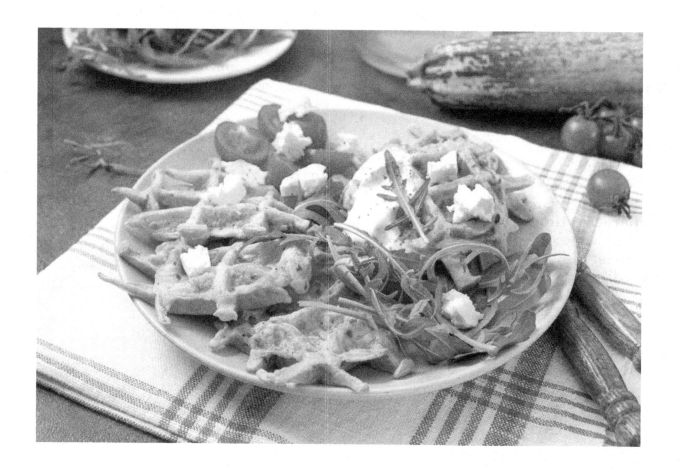

606. ZUCCHINI BACON WAFFLES

Preparation time: 10 min.
Cooking time: 12 min.
Servings: 2
Ingredients:

- 1 c. grated zucchini
- 1 tbsp. bacon bits (finely chopped)
- 1/4 c. shredded mozzarella cheese
- 1/2 c. shredded parmesan
- 1/2 tsp. salt or to taste
- 1/2 tsp. ground black pepper or to taste
- 1/2 tsp. onion powder
- 1/4 tsp. nutmeg
- 2 eggs

Directions:

Add 1/4 tsp. salt to the grated zucchini and let it sit for about 5 min.

Put the grated zucchini in a clean towel and squeeze out excess water.

Plug in the waffle maker and preheat it. Spray it with non-stick spray.

Break the eggs into a mixing bowl and beat.

Add the grated zucchini, bacon bits, nutmeg, onion powder, pepper, salt, mozzarella and the parmesan cheese.

Mix until the ingredients are well combined.

Fill the preheated waffle maker with the batter and spread out the batter to the edge to cover all the holes on the waffle maker.

Close the waffle maker lid and cook until the waffle is golden brown and crispy. The zucchini waffle may take longer than other waffles to get crispy.

After the baking cycle, use a plastic or silicone utensil to remove the waffle from the waffle maker.

Repeat step 8–10 until you have cooked all the batter into the waffles.

Serve and enjoy.

Nutrition:

Calories 216 Cal
Total Fat: 13.6 g.
Saturated Fat: 5.4 g.
Cholesterol 183 mg.
Sodium 903 mg.
Total Carbohydrate 4.7 g.
Dietary Fiber 0.9 g.
Total Sugars 1.6 g.

607. CHOCO PEANUT BUTTER WAFFLE

Preparation time: 5 min.
Cooking time: 10 min.
Servings: 2
Ingredients:
Filling:

- 3 tbsp. all-natural peanut butter
- 2 tsp. swerve sweetener
- 1 tsp. vanilla extract
- 2 tbsp. heavy cream

Waffle:

- 1/4 tsp. baking powder
- 1 tbsp. unsweetened cocoa powder
- 4 tsp. almond flour
- 1/2 tsp. vanilla extract
- 1 tbsp. granulated swerve sweetener
- 1 large egg (beaten)
- 1 tbsp. heavy cream

Directions:
For the waffle:

Plug the waffle maker and preheat it. Spray it with a non-stick spray.

In a large mixing bowl, combine the almond flour, cocoa powder, baking powder and swerve.

Add the egg, vanilla extract and heavy cream. Mix until the ingredients are well combined and you form a smooth batter. Pour some of the batter into the preheated waffle maker. Spread out the batter to the edges of the waffle maker to cover all the holes on the waffle iron.

Close the lid of the waffle iron and bake for about 5 min. or according to the waffle maker's settings.

After the baking cycle, use a plastic or silicone utensil to remove the waffle from the waffle maker.

Repeat step 4–6 until you have cooked all the batter into the waffles.

Transfer the waffles to a wire rack and let the waffles cool completely.

For the filling: combine the vanilla, swerve, heavy cream and peanut butter in a bowl. Mix until the ingredients are well combined.

Spread the peanut butter frosting over the waffles and serve.

Enjoy.

Nutrition:

Calories 560 Cal
Total Fat: 43.2 g.
Saturated Fat: 8.8 g.
Cholesterol 124 mg.
Sodium 168 mg.
Total Carbohydrate 32 g.
Dietary Fiber 8.1 g.
Total Sugars 9 g.

608. GARLIC BREAD WAFFLE

Preparation time: 5 min.
Cooking time: 15 min.
Servings: 2
Ingredients:

- 1 tbsp. + 1 tsp. almond flour
- 1 egg
- 1/4 tsp. baking powder
- 1/2 tsp. garlic powder
- 1/8 tsp. Italian seasoning
- 1 tbsp. finely chopped cooked beef liver
- 1/4 tsp. garlic salt
- 3 tsp. unsalted butter (melted)
- 1/2 c. shredded mozzarella cheese
- 2 tbsp. shredded parmesan cheese

Garnish:

- Chopped green onion

Directions:

Preheat the oven to 375°F and line a baking sheet with parchment paper.

Plug the waffle maker to preheat it and spray it with non-stick spray.

In a mixing bowl, combine the almond flour, baking powder, Italian seasoning, garlic powder, beef liver and mozzarella cheese. Add the egg and mix until the ingredients are well combined.

Fill the waffle maker with appropriate amount of the batter and spread the batter to the edges of the waffle maker to cover all the holes on the waffle iron.

Close the lid of the waffle maker and cook for about 3–4 min. or according to the waffle maker's settings.

Meanwhile, whisk together the garlic salt and melted butter in a bowl.

After the cooking cycle, remove the waffle from the waffle iron with a plastic or silicone utensil.

Repeat step 4, 5 and 7 until you have cooked all the batter into the waffles.

Brush the butter mixture over the face of each waffle.

Top the waffles with parmesan cheese and arrange them into the line baking sheet.

Place the sheet in the oven and bake for about 5 min. or until the cheese melts.

Remove the bread waffles from the oven and leave them to cool for a few minutes. Serve warm and top with chopped green onions.

Nutrition:
Calories 218 Cal
Total Fat: 18 g.
Saturated Fat: 6.6 g.
Cholesterol 112 mg.
Sodium 840 mg.
Total Carbohydrate 4.5 g.
Dietary Fiber 1.6 g.
Total Sugars 0.9 g.

609. KETO AVOCADO WAFFLE TOAST

Preparation time: 5 min.
Cooking time: 8 min.
Servings: 1
Ingredients:
For the topping::
- 1 tbsp. butter
- 1 green bell pepper (finely chopped)
- 1/2 c. shredded feta cheese
- 1/2 avocado
- 1 tsp. lemon juice
- 1/4 tsp. nutmeg
- 1/4 tsp. onion powder
- 1/2 tsp. ground black pepper or to taste

Waffle:
- 1/2 mozzarella cheese
- 1 egg (beaten)
- 1 tbsp. Almond flour
- 1 tsp. cinnamon
- 1/2 tsp. baking soda

Directions:
Plug the waffle maker to preheat it and spray it with a non-stick spray.
In a mixing bowl, combine the mozzarella, almond flour, baking soda and cinnamon. Add the egg and mix until the ingredients are well combined and you form a smooth batter.

Fill the waffle maker with appropriate amount of the batter and spread the batter to the edges of the waffle maker to cover all the holes on the waffle iron.

Close the lid of the waffle maker and cook for about 3–4 min. or according to the waffle maker's settings.

Meanwhile, dice the avocado into a bowl and mash until smooth. Add the bell pepper, nutmeg, onion powder, ground pepper and lemon juice. Mix until well combined.

After the baking cycle, remove the waffle the waffle maker with a silicone or plastic utensil.

Repeat step 3, 4 and 6 until you have cooked all the batter into the waffles.

Brush the butter over the waffles. Spread the avocado mixture over the waffles. Top with the shredded feta cheese.

Serve and enjoy.

Nutrition:
Calories 820 Cal
Total Fat: 68.6 g.
Saturated Fat: 26.7 g.
Cholesterol 268 mg.
Sodium 1716 mg.
Total Carbohydrate 31 g.
Dietary Fiber 13 g.
Total Sugars 11.5 g.

610. HAM WAFFLE

Preparation time: 5 min.
Cooking time: 5 min.
Servings: 1
Ingredients:
• 1 large egg
• 4 tbsp. chopped ham steak
• 1 scallion (chopped)
• 1/2 c. shredded mozzarella cheese
• 1/4 tsp. garlic salt
• 1/8 tsp. Italian seasoning
• 1/2 jalapeno pepper (chopped)
Directions:
Plug the waffle maker to preheat it and spray it with a non-stick spray.
In a mixing bowl, combine the cheese, Italian seasoning, jalapeno, scallion, ham and garlic salt. Add the egg and mix until the ingredients are well combined.
Fill the waffle maker with an appropriate amount of the batter. Spread the batter to the edges of the waffle maker to cover all the holes on it.
Close the waffle maker and cook for about 4 min. or according to the waffle maker's settings.
After the cooking cycle, remove the waffle from the waffle maker with plastic or silicone utensil.
Serve and enjoy.
Nutrition:
Calories 178 Cal
Total Fat: 10.6 g.
Saturated Fat: 4.1 g.
Cholesterol 213 mg.
Sodium 598 mg.
Total Carbohydrate 4.3 g.
Dietary Fiber 1.1 g.
Total Sugars 1.2 g

611. WAFFLES WITH KETO ICE CREAM

Preparation time: 10 min.
Cooking time: 14 min.
Servings: 2
Ingredients:
• 1 egg, beaten
• 1/2 c. finely grated mozzarella cheese
• 1/4 c. almond flour
• 2 tbsp. swerve confectioner's sugar
• 1/8 tsp. xanthan gum
• Low-carb ice cream (flavor of your choice) for serving
Directions:
Preheat the waffle iron.
In a medium bowl, mix all the ingredients except the ice cream.
Open the iron and add half of the mixture. Close and cook until crispy, 7 min.
Transfer the waffle to a plate and make second one with the remaining batter.
On each waffle, add a scoop of low-carb ice cream, fold into half-moons and enjoy.
Nutrition:
Calories: 89 Cal
Total Fat: 6.48 g.
Saturated Fat: 0 g.
Cholesterol: 0 mg.
Sodium: 0 mg.
Total Carbs: 1.67 g.
Fiber: 0 g.
Sugar: 0 g.

612. STRAWBERRY SHORTCAKE WAFFLE BOWLS

Preparation time: 10 min.
Cooking time: 28 min.
Servings: 4
Ingredients:
• 1 egg, beaten
• 1/2 c. finely grated mozzarella cheese

- 1 tbsp. almond flour
- 1/4 tsp. baking powder
- 2 drops cake batter extract
- 1 c. cream cheese, softened
- 1 c. fresh strawberries, sliced
- 1 tbsp. sugar-free maple syrup

Directions:

Preheat a waffle bowl maker and grease lightly with cooking spray.

Meanwhile, in a medium bowl, whisk all the ingredients except the cream cheese and strawberries.

Open the iron, pour in half of the mixture, cover, and cook until crispy, 6–7 min..

Remove the waffle bowl and put onto a plate and set aside.

Make a second waffle bowl with the remaining batter.

To serve, divide the cream cheese into the waffle bowls and top with the strawberries.

Drizzle the filling with the maple syrup and serve.

Nutrition:

Calories: 235 Cal
Total Fat: 20.62 g.
Saturated Fat: 0 g.
Cholesterol: 0 mg.
Sodium: 0 mg.
Total Carbs: 5.9 g.
Fiber: 0 g.
Sugar: 0 g.

613.   WAFFLE CANNOLI

Preparation time: 15 min.
Cooking time: 28 min.
Servings: 4
Ingredients:
For the waffles:
- 1 large egg
- 1 egg yolk
- 3 tbsp. butter, melted
- 1 tbsp. swerve confectioner's

- 1 c. finely grated Parmesan cheese
- 2 tbsp. finely grated mozzarella cheese

For the cannoli filling:
- **1/2 c. ricotta cheese**
- **2 tbsp. swerve confectioner's sugar**
- **1 tsp. vanilla extract**
- **2 tbsp. unsweetened chocolate chips for garnishing**

Directions:

Preheat the waffle iron.

Meanwhile, in a medium bowl, mix all the ingredients for the waffles.

Open the iron, pour in 1/4 of the mixture, cover, and cook until crispy, 7 min.

Remove the waffle onto a plate and make 3 more with the remaining batter.

Meanwhile, for the cannoli filling: beat the ricotta cheese and swerve confectioner's sugar until smooth. Mix in the vanilla.

On each waffle, spread some of the filling and wrap over.

Garnish the creamy ends with some chocolate chips.

Serve immediately.

Nutrition:

Calories: 308 Cal
Total Fat: 25.05 g.
Saturated Fat: 0 g.
Cholesterol: 0 mg.
Sodium: 0 mg.
Total Carbs: 5.17 g.
Fiber: 0 g.
Sugar: 0 g.

614.   NUTTER   BUTTER WAFFLES

Preparation time: 15 min.
Cooking time: 14 min.
Servings: 2
Ingredients:
For the waffles:

- 2 tbsp. sugar-free peanut butter powder
- 2 tbsp. maple (sugar-free) syrup
- 1 egg, beaten
- 1/4 c. finely grated mozzarella cheese
- 1/4 tsp. baking powder
- 1/4 tsp. almond butter
- 1/4 tsp. peanut butter extract
- 1 tbsp. softened cream cheese

For the frosting:
- 1/2 c. almond flour
- 1 c. peanut butter
- 3 tbsp. almond milk
- 1/2 tsp. vanilla extract
- 1/2 c. maple (sugar-free) syrup

Directions:
Preheat the waffle iron.
Meanwhile, in a medium bowl, mix all the ingredients for the waffles until smooth.
Open the iron and pour in half of the mixture.
Close the iron and cook until crispy, 6–7 min.
Remove the waffle onto a plate and set aside.
Make a second waffle with the remaining batter.
While the waffles cool, make the frosting: pour the almond flour in a medium saucepan and stir-fry over medium heat until golden.
Transfer the almond flour to a blender and top with the remaining frosting ingredients.
Process until smooth.
Spread the frosting on the waffles and serve afterward.

Nutrition:
Calories: 239 Cal
Total Fat: 15.48 g.
Saturated Fat: 0 g.
Cholesterol: 0 mg.
Sodium: 0 mg.
Total Carbs: 17.42 g.
Fiber: 0 g.
Sugar: 0 g.

615. WAFFLED BROWNIE SUNDAE

Preparation time: 12 min.
Cooking time: 30 min.
Servings: 4
Ingredients:
For the waffles:
- 2 eggs, beaten
- 1 tbsp. unsweetened cocoa powder
- 1 tbsp. erythritol
- 1 c. finely grated mozzarella cheese

For the topping:
- 3 tbsp. unsweetened chocolate, chopped
- 3 tbsp. unsalted butter
- Low-carb ice cream for topping
- 1 c. whipped cream for topping
- 3 tbsp. sugar-free caramel sauce

Directions:
For the waffles:
Preheat the waffle iron.
Meanwhile, in a medium bowl, mix all the ingredients for the waffles.
Open the iron, pour in 1/4 of the mixture, cover, and cook until crispy, 7 min.
Remove the waffle onto a plate and make 3 more with the remaining batter.
Plate and set aside.
For the topping:
Meanwhile, melt the chocolate and butter in a medium saucepan with occasional stirring, 2 min.
To **Servings:**
Divide the waffles into wedges and top with the ice cream, whipped cream, and swirl

the chocolate sauce and caramel sauce on top.
Serve immediately.

Nutrition:
Calories: 165 Cal
Total Fat: 11.39 g.
Saturated Fat: 0 g.
Cholesterol: 0 mg.
Sodium: 0 mg.
Total Carbs: 3.81 g.
Fiber: 0 g.
Sugar: 0 g.
Protein: 12.79 g.

616. BRIE AND BLACKBERRY WAFFLES

Preparation time: 15 min.
Cooking time: 36 min.
Servings: 4
Ingredients:
For the waffles:
- 2 eggs, beaten
- 1 c. finely grated mozzarella cheese

For the topping:
- 1 1/2 c. blackberries
- 1 lemon, 1 tsp. zest and 2 tbsp. juice
- 1 tbsp. erythritol
- 4 slices Brie cheese

Directions:
For the waffles:
Preheat the waffle iron.
Meanwhile, in a medium bowl, mix the eggs and mozzarella cheese.
Open the iron, pour in 1/4 of the mixture, cover, and cook until crispy, 7 min..
Remove the waffle onto a plate and make 3 more with the remaining batter.
Plate and set aside
For the topping:
Preheat the oven to 350 °F and line a baking sheet with parchment paper.

In a medium pot, add the blackberries, lemon zest, lemon juice, and erythritol. Cook until the blackberries break and the sauce thickens, 5 min. Turn off the heat.
Arrange the waffles on the baking sheet and place two Brie cheese slices on each. Top with blackberry mixture and transfer the baking sheet to the oven.
Bake until the cheese melts, 2–3 min.
Remove from the oven, allow cooling and serve afterward.

Nutrition:
Calories: 576 Cal
Total Fat: 42.22 g.
Saturated Fat: 0 g.
Cholesterol: 0 mg.
Sodium: 0 mg.
Total Carbs: 7.07 g.
Fiber: 0 g.
Sugar: 0 g.
Protein: 42.35 g

617. CEREAL WAFFLE CAKE

Preparation time: 5 min.
Cooking time: 8 min.
Servings: 2
Ingredients:
- **1 egg**
- **2 tbsp. almond flour**
- **1/2 tsp. coconut flour**
- **1 tbsp. melted butter**
- **1 tbsp. cream cheese**
- **1 tbsp. plain cereal, crushed**
- **1/4 tsp. vanilla extract**
- **1/4 tsp. baking powder**
- **1 tbsp. sweetener**
- **1/8 tsp. xanthan gum**

Directions:
Plug in your waffle maker to preheat.
Add all the ingredients in a large bowl.
Mix until well blended.

Let the batter rest for 2 min. before cooking.

Pour half of the mixture into the waffle maker.

Seal and cook for 4 min..

Make the next waffle using the same steps.

Nutrition:

Calories: 154 Cal

Total Fat: 21.2 g.

Saturated Fat: 10 g.

Cholesterol: 113.3 mg.

Sodium: 96.9 mg.

Potassium: 453 mg.

Total Carbohydrate: 5.9 g.

Dietary Fiber: 1.7 g.

Protein: 4.6 g.

Total Sugars: 2.7 g.

618. HAM, CHEESE AND TOMATO WAFFLE SANDWICH

Preparation time: 5 min.

Cooking time: 10 min.

Servings: 2

Ingredients:

- 1 tsp. olive oil
- 2 slices ham
- 4 basic waffles
- 1 tbsp. mayonnaise
- 2 slices Provolone cheese
- 1 tomato, sliced

Directions:

Add the olive oil to a pan over medium heat.

Cook the ham for 1 min. per side.

Spread the waffles with mayonnaise.

Top with the ham, cheese and tomatoes.

Top with another waffle to make a sandwich.

Nutrition:

Calories: 198 Cal

Total Fat: 14.7 g.

Saturated Fat: 6.3 g.

Cholesterol: 37 mg.

Sodium: 664 mg.

Total Carbohydrate: 4.6 g.

Dietary Fiber: 0.7 g.

Total Sugars: 1.5 g.

Protein: 12.2 g.

Potassium: 193 mg.

619. WAFFLE WITH SAUSAGE GRAVY

Preparation time: 5 min.

Cooking time: 15 min.

Servings: 2

Ingredients:

- 1/4 c. sausage, cooked
- 3 tbsp. chicken broth
- 2 tsp. cream cheese
- 2 tbsp. heavy whipping cream
- 1/4 tsp. garlic powder
- Pepper to taste
- 2 basic waffles

Directions:

Add the sausage, broth, cream cheese, cream, garlic powder and pepper to a pan over medium heat.

Bring to a boil and then reduce heat.

Simmer for 10 min. or until the sauce has thickened.

Pour the gravy on top of the basic waffles Serve.

Nutrition:

Calories 212 Cal

Total Fat: 17 g.

Saturated Fat: 10 g.

Cholesterol: 134 mg.

Sodium: 350 mg.

Potassium: 133 mg.

Total Carbohydrate: 3 g.

Dietary Fiber: 1 g.

Protein: 11 g.

Total Sugars: 1 g.

620.   BACON AND CHICKEN RANCH WAFFLE

Preparation time: 5 min.
Cooking time: 8 min.
Servings: 2
Ingredients:

- 1 egg
- 1/4 c. chicken cubes, cooked
- 1 slice bacon, cooked and chopped
- 1/4 c. cheddar cheese, shredded
- 1 tsp. ranch dressing powder

Directions:

Preheat your waffle maker.

In a bowl, mix all the ingredients.

Add half of the mixture to your waffle maker.

Cover and cook for 4 min.

Make the second waffle using the same steps.

Nutrition:

Calories: 200 Cal
Total Fat: 14 g.
Saturated Fat: 6 g.
Cholesterol: 129 mg.
Sodium: 463 mg.
Potassium: 130 mg.
Total Carbohydrate: 2 g.
Dietary Fiber: 1 g.
Protein: 16 g.
Total Sugars: 1 g.

621.   CHEESEBURGER WAFFLE

Preparation time: 15 min.
Cooking time: 15 min.
Servings: 2
Ingredients:

- 1 lb. ground beef
- 1 onion, minced
- 1 tsp. parsley, chopped
- 1 egg, beaten
- Salt and pepper to taste
- 1 tbsp. olive oil
- 4 basic waffles
- 2 lettuce leaves
- 2 cheese slices
- 1 tbsp. dill pickles
- Ketchup for topping
- Mayonnaise for topping

Directions:

In a large bowl, combine the ground beef, onion, parsley, egg, salt and pepper.

Mix well.

Form 2 thick patties.

Add olive oil to the pan.

Place the pan over medium heat.

Cook the patty for 3–5 min. per side or until fully cooked.

Place the patty on top of each waffle.

Top with lettuce, cheese and pickles.

Squirt ketchup and mayo over the patty and veggies.

Top with another waffle.

Nutrition:

Calories: 325 Cal
Total Fat: 16.3 g.
Saturated Fat: 6.5 g.
Cholesterol: 157 mg.
Sodium: 208 mg.
Total Carbohydrate: 3 g.
Dietary Fiber: 0.7 g.
Total Sugars: 1.4 g.
Protein: 39.6 g.

Potassium: 532 mg

622. MAPLE ICED SOFT GINGERBREAD COOKIES WAFFLE

Preparation time: 5 min.
Cooking time: 10 min.
Servings: 2
Ingredients:
Waffles ingredients
• 1 egg
• 1-oz. cream cheese softened to room temperature
•   2 tsp. melted butter
•   1 tbsp. Swerve Brown sweetener
•   1 tbsp. almond flour
•   2 tsp. coconut flour
•   1/4 tsp. baking powder
•   3/4 tsp. ground ginger
•   1/2 tsp. ground cinnamon
•   Generous dash ground nutmeg
Icing ingredients
2 tbsp. powdered sweeteners such as Swerve or Lakanto
1 1/2 tsp. heavy cream
1/8 tsp. maple extract
Water as needed to thin the frosting
Directions:
Heat mini Dash waffle iron until thoroughly hot.
Beat all the waffle ingredients together into a small bowl until smooth.
Add a heaping 2 tbsp. of the batter to the waffle iron and cook until done about 4 min..
Repeat to make 2 waffles. Let cool on wire rack.
Maple Icing **Directions:**
In a small bowl, whisk together sweetener, heavy cream, and maple extract until smooth.

Add enough water to thin to a spreadable consistency.
Spread icing on each waffle and sprinkle with additional ground cinnamon, if desired.
Nutrition:
Calories: 161 Cal
Total Fat: 12.5 g.
Cholesterol: 117.5 mg.
Sodium: 86.6 mg.
Total Carbohydrate: 7.6 g.
Dietary Fiber: 1.9 g.
Sugars: 1.3 g.
Protein: 5.2 g.

623. KETO REUBEN WAFFLES

Preparation time: 15 min.
Cooking time: 28 min.
Servings: 4
Ingredients:
For the waffles:
•   2 eggs, beaten
•   1 c. finely grated swiss cheese
•   2 tsp. caraway seeds
•   1/8 tsp. salt
•   1/2 tsp. baking powder
For the sauce:
•   2 tbsp. sugar-free ketchup
•   3 tbsp. mayonnaise
•   1 tbsp. dill relish
•   1 tsp. hot sauce
For the filling:
•   6 oz. pastrami
•   2 swiss cheese slices
•   1/4 c. pickled radishes
Directions:
For the waffles:
Preheat the waffle iron.
In a medium bowl, mix the eggs, swiss cheese, caraway seeds, salt, and baking powder.
Open the iron and add 1/4 of the mixture. Close and cook until crispy, 7 min..

Transfer the waffle to a plate and make 3 more waffles in the same manner.

For the sauce: in another bowl, mix the ketchup, mayonnaise, dill relish, and hot sauce.

To assemble:

Divide on two waffles; the sauce, the pastrami, swiss cheese slices, and pickled radishes.

Cover with the other waffles, divide the sandwich in halves and serve.

Nutrition:

Calories 316

Fats 21.78 g.

Carbs: 6.52 g.

Net carbs 5.42 g.

Protein: 23.56 g.

624.   CREAMY WAFFLE

Preparation time: 5 min.

Cooking time: 5 min.

Servings: 2

Ingredients:

- 1 egg, whisked
- 2 tbsp. stevia
- 1 tbsp. heavy cream
- 1/2 tsp. almond extract
- 1 tsp. almond flour
- 1/2 tsp. baking soda

Directions:

In a bowl, mix the egg with the cream, stevia, and the other ingredients and whisk well.

Preheat the waffle iron at medium-high, pour half of the batter, close the iron, cook the waffle for 4 min. and transfer to a plate.

Repeat with the rest of the batter and serve warm.

Nutrition:

Calories: 66

Fat: 4.5

Fiber: 1

Carbs: 2

Protein: 7.4

625.   BERRY WAFFLE

Preparation time: 5 min.

Cooking time: 5 min.

Servings: 2

Ingredients:

- 1 egg, whisked
- 2 tbsp. stevia
- 1 tsp. coconut flour
- 4 strawberries, chopped
- 1/2 tsp. baking powder
- 1 tsp. cream cheese, soft

Directions:

In a bowl, mix the strawberries with the egg, stevia, and the other ingredients and whisk well.

Heat up the waffle iron over medium-high heat, pour half of the batter, close the waffle maker, cook for 5 min. and transfer to a plate.

Repeat with the other half of the batter and serve the waffles warm.

Nutrition:

Calories: 58

Fat: 5

Fiber: 1.2

Carbs: 2

Protein: 3.2

626. HERBED PIZZA WAFFLE

Preparation time: 5 min.
Cooking time: 8 min.
Servings: 2
Ingredients:
- 1 egg, whisked
- 1/2 tsp. oregano, dried
- 1/2 tsp. basil, dried
- 1/2 tsp. parsley flakes
- 1/2 tsp. garlic powder
- 2 tbsp. tomato passata
- 1 c. mozzarella shredded, shredded

Directions:
In a bowl, mix the egg with the herbs, the garlic and half of the mozzarella and stir well.
Preheat the waffle iron over medium-high heat, pour half of the waffle mix, cook for 4 min. and transfer to a plate.
Repeat with the rest of the batter, spread the tomato passata and the rest of the cheese over the waffles and serve.

Nutrition:
Calories 252
Fat: 11 g.
Fiber: 3.2 g.
Carbs: 5 g.
Protein: 11.2 g.

627. SPINACH PIZZA WAFFLE

Preparation time: 5 min.
Cooking time: 6 min.
Servings: 2
Ingredients:
- 1 egg, whisked
- 1/2 c. mozzarella, shredded
- 1 tbsp. cheddar, shredded
- 2 tbsp. cream cheese, soft
- 1 tsp. onion powder
- 1/4 c. spinach, torn
- 1/2 tsp. garlic powder
- 2 tbsp. tomato passata

Directions:
In a bowl, mix the eggs with the mozzarella and the other ingredients except the cheddar, spinach and passata and stir.
Preheat the waffle iron over medium-high heat, pour half of the waffle mix, cook for 6 min. and transfer to a plate.
Repeat with the rest of the batter; then top the waffles with the cheddar, spinach and tomato passata and serve.

Nutrition:
Calories: 252
Fat: 8.3 g.
Fiber: 4.2 g.
Carbs: 5 g.
Protein: 11.2 g

628. ROASTED PEPPERS PIZZA WAFFLE

Preparation time: 5 min.
Cooking time: 5 min.
Servings: 2
Ingredients:
- 1 egg, whisked
- 1/2 c. cheddar cheese, shredded
- 1/4 c. roasted peppers, chopped
- 1/2 tsp. oregano, dried
- 1/2 tsp. garlic powder
- 2 tbsp. tomato passata

Directions:
In a bowl, mix egg with the cheese and the rest of the ingredients except the peppers and passata and stir.
Preheat the waffle iron over high heat, pour half of the waffle mix, cook for 5 min. and transfer to a plate.

Repeat with the rest of the batter; spread the remaining ingredients over the waffles and serve.

Nutrition:
Calories: 202 g.
Fat: 12.3 g.
Fiber: 4.2 g.
Carbs: 5 g.
Protein: 11.2 g.

629. MUSHROOM WAFFLE

Preparation time: 5 min.
Cooking time: 6 min.
Servings: 2
Ingredients:
- 2 eggs, whisked
- 1/2 c. mozzarella, shredded
- 1/2 c. mushrooms, sliced
- 1 tsp. coriander, ground
- 1/2 tsp. rosemary, dried
- 1/2 tsp. cayenne pepper
- 2 tbsp. tomato passata

Directions:
In a bowl, mix the eggs with the mozzarella, coriander, rosemary and cayenne and stir well.

Preheat the waffle iron over medium-high heat, pour half of the waffle mix, cook for 6 min. and transfer to a plate.

Repeat with the rest of the batter, spread the passata and the mushrooms over the waffles and serve.

Nutrition:
Calories: 202
Fat: 9.3 g.
Fiber: 3.2 g.
Carbs: 5 g.
Protein: 8.4 g.

630. KETO CHOCOLATE TWINKIE COPYCAT WAFFLE

Preparation time: 5 min.
Cooking time: 12 min.
Servings: 3
Ingredients:
- 2 tbsp. of butter (melted and cooled)
- 2 oz. cream cheese softened
- 2 large egg room temperature
- 1 tsp. of vanilla essence
- 1/4 c. Lakanto confectionery sweetner
- 1 tsp. cinnamon
- Pinch of pink salt
- 1/4 c. almond flour
- 2 tbsp. coconut flour
- 2 tbsp. cocoa powder
- 1 tsp. baking powder

Directions:
Preheat the Waffle maker.
Melt the butter for a minute and let it cool.
Whisk the eggs in the butter until smooth.
Add cream cheese, cinnamon, sweetener and blend well.
Add almond flour, coconut flour, cocoa powder, baking powder and salt.
Blend until well embedded.
Fill each well with ~2 tbsp. of the batter and spread evenly.
Close the lid and let it cook for 4 min.
Lift from the rack and let it cool.

Nutrition:
Calories: 104
Total Fat: 6.2 g.
Cholesterol: 67.1 mg.
Sodium: 485.5 mg.
Total Carbohydrate: 5.3 g.
Dietary Fiber: 1.7 g.
Sugars: 1.6 g.
Protein: 4.4 g.

631. KETO CORNBREAD WAFFLE

Preparation time: 5 min.
Cooking time: 5 min.
Servings: 2
Ingredients:

- 1 egg
- 1/2 c. + ½ tbsp. shredded cheddar cheese (or mozzarella cheese)
- 5 slices Jalapeno freshly picked
- 1 tsp. of Frank's Red-Hot Sauce
- 1/4 tsp. corn extract (an essential secret ingredient!)
- Pinch of salt

Directions:
Preheat the mini waffle makers and beat the eggs into a small bowl.
Combine with the beaten egg the remaining ingredients.
Put 1 extra tbsp. shredded cheese into the waffle maker for 30 sec. before pouring the waffle mixture. This will create a very clean and friendly crust!
Then pour in the waffle maker half of the mixture.
Cook for a total of 3–4 min, until crunchy, Enjoy it served warm!

Nutrition:
Calories: 150
Total Fat: 11.8 g.
Cholesterol: 121 mg.
Sodium: 1399.4 mg.
Total Carbohydrate: 1.1 g.
Dietary Fiber: 0 g.
Sugars: 0.2 g.
Protein: 9.6 g.

632. MAPLE PUMPKIN KETO WAFFLE

Preparation time: 5 min.
Cooking time: 4 min.
Servings: 2
Ingredients:

- 3/4 tsp. baking powder
- 2 eggs
- 4 tsp. heavy whipping cream
- 1/2 c. mozzarella cheese, shredded
- 2 tsp. Liquid Stevia
- Pinch of salt
- 3/4 tsp. pumpkin pie spices
- 1 tsp. coconut flour
- 2 tsp. pumpkin puree (100% pumpkin)
- 1/2 tsp. vanilla

Directions:
Preheat the mini waffle maker.
Whisk the eggs in a bowl; then add the cheese and mix well.
Stir in the remaining ingredients.
Scoop 1/2 of the batter into the waffle maker, spread across evenly.
Cook 3–4 min., until done as desired (or crispy).
Gently remove from the waffle maker and let it cool.
Repeat with the remaining batter.
Top with sugar-free maple syrup or keto ice cream.
Serve and Enjoy!

Nutrition:
Calories: 201
Net carbs: 2 g.
Fat: 15 g.
Protein: 12 g.

633. KETO ALMOND BLUEBERRY WAFFLE

Preparation time: 5 min.
Cooking time: 5 min.
Servings: 5
Ingredients:

- 1 tsp. baking powder
- 2 eggs
- 1 c. of mozzarella cheese
- 2 tbsp. almond flour
- 3 tbsp. blueberries
- 1 tsp. cinnamon
- 2 tsp. of Swerve

Directions:

Preheat the mini waffle maker.

Whisk the egg in a bowl and add the cheese, then mix well.

Stir in the remaining ingredients.

Grease the preheated waffle maker with non-stick cooking spray.

Scoop 1/2 of the batter into the waffle maker, spread across evenly.

Cook until a bit browned and crispy, about 4 min.

Gently remove from the waffle maker and let it cool.

Repeat with the remaining batter.

Top with keto syrup, if desired.

Serve and Enjoy!

Nutrition:

Calories: 116
Net carbs: 1 g.
Fat: 8 g.
Protein: 8 g.

634. SWEET CINNAMON "SUGAR" WAFFLE

Preparation time: 5 min.
Cooking time: 4 min.
Servings: 1
Ingredients:

- 10 drops of liquid stevia
- 1 tbsp. almond flour
- 2 large eggs
- A splash of vanilla
- 1/2 c. mozzarella cheese
- 1/2 tsp. cinnamon (for topping)
- 1 tbsp. melted butter

Directions:

Preheat the waffle maker.

Whisk the egg in a bowl; then add the cheese and mix well.

Stir in the remaining ingredients (except cinnamon).

Scoop 1/2 of the batter onto the waffle maker, spread across evenly.

Cook 3–4 min., until done as desired.

Gently remove from the waffle maker and let it cool

Repeat with the remaining batter.

Top with melted butter and a sprinkle of cinnamon.

Serve and Enjoy!

Nutrition:

Calories: 221
Net carbs: 2 g.
Fat: 17 g.
Protein: 12 g.

635. KETO "CINNAMON ROLL" WAFFLES

Preparation time: 5 min.
Cooking time: 10 min.
Servings: 3
Ingredients:
For the waffle:

- 1/2 c. mozzarella cheese
- 1/4 tsp. baking powder
- 1 tsp. Granulated Swerve
- 1 tbsp. almond flour
- 1 tsp. cinnamon
- 1 egg

For the cinnamon roll swirl:

- 2 tsp. confectioners swerve
- 1 tbsp. butter
- 1 tsp. cinnamon

For the Keto cinnamon roll glaze:

- 2 tsp. swerve confectioners
- 1/4 tsp. vanilla extract
- 1 tbsp. cream cheese
- 1 tbsp. butter

Directions:
Preheat the waffle maker.
Add the waffle ingredients into a bowl and combine well.
In another small bowl, add the cinnamon roll swirl ingredients and stir well. Then microwave it for 15 sec. and mix well.
Spray the waffle maker with non-stick spray and add 1/3 of the batter to your waffle maker.
Swirl in 1/3 of the cinnamon roll swirl mixture on top of it.
Cook for 3–4 min. Repeat for the remaining batter.
In a small bowl, add "Keto cinnamon roll glaze ingredients", combine and microwave for 20 sec.
Drizzle on top of the waffles

Nutrition:
Calories: 180
Net carbs: 1 g.
Fat: 16 g.
Protein: 7 g.

636. CINNAMON SUGAR WAFFLE

Preparation time: 10 min.
Cooking time: 20 min.
Servings: 4 mini waffles
Ingredients:

- 4 tbsp. almond flour
- 4 tbsp. erythritol sweetener
- 1/2 tsp. baking powder
- 1 tsp. cinnamon
- 1 tsp. psyllium husk powder
- 1 tsp. vanilla extract, extract
- 1 tbsp. coconut butter, melted
- 1 1/2 c.. shredded mozzarella cheese
- 2 eggs, at room temperature

For the topping::

- 1 1/2 tsp. cinnamon
- 1/2 c./100 g. erythritol sweetener
- 2 tbsp. coconut butter, melted

Directions:
Take a non-stick waffle iron, plug it in, select the medium or medium-high heat setting and let it preheat until ready to use; it could also be indicated with an indicator light changing its color.
Meanwhile, prepare the batter: in a large bowl add almond flour, then stir in sweetener, baking powder, cinnamon, and husk powder until mixed.
Take another bowl, crack the eggs in it and beat it until fluffy; then mix in vanilla, coconut butter and cheese until combined; then stir this mixture into the flour with the spatula until incorporated.

Use a ladle to pour one-fourth of the prepared batter into the heated waffle iron in a spiral direction, starting from the edges, then shut the lid and cook for 5 min. or more until solid and nicely browned; the cooked waffle will look like a cake.

When done, transfer the waffles to a plate with a silicone spatula and repeat with the remaining batter.

Then sprinkle with cinnamon and sweetener, top with butter and eat straight away.

Nutrition:
Cal: 210
Fat: 16.2 g.
Protein: 10.9 g.
Carb: 4.1 g.
Fiber: 2 g.
Net Carb: 2.1 g

637. BANANA FOSTER WAFFLE

Preparation time: 10 min.
Cooking time: 20 min.
Servings: 4 large waffles
Ingredients:
For the waffles:

- 1/8 tsp. cinnamon
- 1/2 tsp. banana extract, unsweetened
- 4 tsp. swerve sweetener
- 1 c./225 g. cream cheese, softened
- 1/2 tsp. vanilla extract, unsweetened
- 8 eggs, at room temperature

For Syrup:

- 20 drops of banana extract, unsweetened
- 8 tsp. swerve sweetener
- 20 drops of caramel extract, unsweetened
- 12 drops of rum extract, unsweetened
- 8 tbsp. unsalted butter
- 1/8 tsp. cinnamon

Directions:
Take a non-stick waffle iron, plug it in, select the medium or medium-high heat setting and let it preheat until ready to use; it could also be indicated with an indicator light changing its color.

Meanwhile, prepare the batter for waffle: in a large bowl, crack the eggs, add sweetener, cream cheese, all the extracts and cinnamon and mix with an electric mixer until smooth; let the batter sit for 5 min.

Use a ladle to pour one-fourth of the prepared batter into the heated waffle iron in a spiral direction, starting from the edges, then shut the lid and cook for 5 min. or more until solid and nicely browned; the cooked waffle will look like a cake.

When done, transfer the waffles to a plate with a silicone spatula, repeat with the remaining batter and let waffles stand for some time until crispy.

Meanwhile, prepare the syrup and for this, take a small heatproof bowl, put butter and microwave on high for 15 sec. until it melts.

Add the remaining ingredients for the syrup and mix until combined.

Drizzle syrup over the waffles and then serve.

Nutrition:
530 Cal
49.7 g. Fat
14.6 g. Protein
15.8 g. Carb
0 g. Fiber
15.8 g. Net Carb

638. FLAXSEED WAFFLE

Preparation time: 10 min.
Cooking time: 20 min.
Servings: 4 medium waffles
Ingredients:

- 2 c. ground flaxseed
- 2 tsp. ground cinnamon
- 1 tsp. of sea salt
- 1 tbsp. baking powder

- 1/3 c. avocado oil
- 5 eggs, at room temperature
- 1/2 c. water
- Whipped cream as needed for topping

Directions:

Take a non-stick waffle iron, plug it in, select the medium or medium-high heat setting and let it preheat until ready to use; it could also be indicated with an indicator light changing its color.

Meanwhile, prepare the batter: in a large bowl, stir flaxseed, salt and baking powder until combined.

Crack the eggs in a separate bowl, pour in avocado oil and water, whisk these ingredients until blended and then stir this mixture into the dry ingredient mixture with the spatula until well incorporated and fluffy.

Let the batter sit for 5 min. and then stir in cinnamon until mixed.

Use a ladle to pour one-fourth of the prepared batter into the heated waffle iron in a spiral direction, starting from the edges, then shut the lid and cook for 5 min. or more until solid and nicely browned; the cooked waffle will look like a cake.

When done, transfer the waffle to a plate with a silicone spatula and repeat with the remaining batter.

Top waffles with whipped cream and then serve straight away.

Nutrition:

Cal: 140
Fat: 11 g.
Protein: 4.7 g.
Carb: 4.5 g.
Fiber: 3.8 g.
Net Carb: 0.7 g

639.   HAZELNUT WAFFLE

Preparation time: 10 min.
Cooking time: 30 min.
Servings: 6 mini waffles
Ingredients:

- 1 c. hazelnut flour
- 1/2 tsp. baking powder
- 2 tbsp. hazelnut oil
- 1 c. almond milk, unsweetened
- 3 eggs, at room temperature

Directions:

Take a non-stick waffle iron, plug it in, select the medium or medium-high heat setting and let it preheat until ready to use; it could also be indicated with an indicator light changing its color.

Meanwhile, prepare the batter: in a large bowl, add hazelnut flour, stir in the baking powder and then mix in hazelnut oil, milk and egg with an electric mixer until smooth.

Use a ladle to pour one-sixth of the prepared batter into the heated waffle iron in a spiral direction, starting from the edges, then shut the lid and cook for 5 min. or more until solid and nicely browned; the cooked waffle will look like a cake.

When done, transfer the waffle to a plate with a silicone spatula and repeat with the remaining batter.

Serve straight away.

Nutrition:

Cal: 192
Fat: 17.1 g.
Protein: 7.5 g.
Carb: 4.7 g.
Fiber: 2.2 g.
Net Carb: 2.5 g.

640.   CHEDDAR WAFFLE

Preparation time: 5 min.
Cooking time: 12 min.
Servings: 4 mini waffles
Ingredients:

- 2 tbsp. almond flour
- 1 c. shredded cheddar cheese
- 2 eggs, at room temperature

Directions:

Take a non-stick mini waffle iron, plug it in, select the medium or medium-high heat setting and let it preheat until ready to use; it could also be indicated with an indicator light changing its color.

Meanwhile, in a large bowl add all ingredients and whisk with an electric mixer until smooth.

Use a ladle to pour one-fourth of the prepared batter into the heated waffle iron in a spiral direction, starting from the edges, then shut the lid and cook for 3 min. or more until solid and nicely browned; the cooked waffle will look like a cake.

When done, transfer the waffles to a plate with a silicone spatula and repeat with the remaining batter.

Serve straight away.

Nutrition:

Cal: 173
Fat: 14.2 g.
Protein: 10.1 g.
Carb: 2.2 g.
Fiber: 0 g.
Net Carb: 2.2 g

641.   JALAPENO   PEPPER WAFFLE

Preparation time: 10 min.
Cooking time: 20 min.
Servings: 4 medium waffles
Ingredients:

- 4 slices of bacon, cooked, crumbled
- 1 jalapeno pepper, deseeded, sliced
- 1 jalapeno pepper, diced
- 3 tbsp. coconut flour
- 1 tsp. baking powder
- 1/4 tsp. of sea salt
- 1 c. shredded cheddar cheese
- 3 eggs, at room temperature
- 1 c. cream cheese, softened

Directions:

Take a non-stick waffle iron, plug it in, select the medium or medium-high heat setting and let it preheat until ready to use; it could also be indicated with an indicator light changing its color.

Meanwhile, in a large bowl add coconut flour, then stir in baking powder and salt until well combined.

Take another bowl, place cream cheese in it and beat with an electric mixer until fluffy.

Crack the eggs in a separate bowl, beat with an electric mixer until fluffy, then add cheddar cheese and 1/2 c. of beaten cream cheese and continue beating until combined.

Add flour mixture into egg-cream cheese mixture, beat with an electric mixer until incorporated, and then fold in diced peppers.

Use a ladle to pour one-fourth of the prepared batter into the heated waffle iron in a spiral direction, starting from the edges, then shut the lid and cook for 5 min. or more until solid and nicely browned; the cooked waffle will look like a cake.

When done, transfer the waffles to a plate with a silicone spatula and repeat with the remaining batter.

Last, top with bacon, jalapeno slices and the remaining cream cheese and serve.

Nutrition:

Cal 336
Fat: 27.6 g.
Protein: 16 g.
Carb 7.5 g.

Fiber 2.9 g.
Net Carb 4.6 g

642.   WAFFLES BENEDICT

Preparation time: 20 min.
Cooking time: 3 min.
Servings: 4
Ingredients:
For the waffles:

- 12 eggs
- 1 c. cheddar cheese, shredded
- 8 slices bacon

For the hollandaise sauce:

3 egg yolks
1 tbsp. lemon juice
2 pinches kosher salt
1/4 tsp. dijon mustard or hot sauce, optional
1/2 c. butter, salted

Directions:

Preheat the waffle maker.

Pour water in a pan and place over medium-high heat.

Take 4 eggs and beat them in a bowl. The remaining eggs are for poaching.

Once the waffle maker is heated up, sprinkle 1 tbsp. of the cheese and let it toast.

Take 1 1/2 tbsp. of the beaten eggs and place them on the toasted cheese.

Once the egg starts cooking, add another layer of sprinkled cheese on top.

Close the lid. Cook for 2–3 min.

Remove the cooked waffle and repeat the steps until you've created 8 waffles.

Fry bacon and set aside for later.

Poach the remaining eggs.

To make the sauce, combine lemon juice, salt, egg yolks, and dijon mustard or hot sauce in a bowl.

In a separate container, melt the butter in the microwave. Let it cool for a few minutes.

Pour the melted butter over the egg yolk mixture. Using an immersion blender, pulse the mixture until it becomes yellow and cloudy. Continue pulsing until the consistency becomes creamy and thick.

To serve, place cooked waffles on a plate.

Place a slice of bacon over each waffle.

Top the bacon with poached egg and drizzle with hollandaise sauce.

Nutrition:
calories: 601
carbohydrates: 1 g.
fat: 51 g.
protein: 34 g.

643.   EGGNOG WAFFLES

Preparation time: 10 min.
Cooking time: 6 min.
Servings: 1
Ingredients:

- 1 egg, separated
- 1 egg yolk
- 1/2 c. mozzarella cheese, shredded
- 1/2 tsp. spiced rum
- 1 tsp. vanilla extract
- 1/4 tsp. nutmeg, dried
- A dash of cinnamon
- 1 tsp. coconut flour

For the icing:

- 2 tbsp. cream cheese
- 1 tbsp. powdered sweetener
- 2 tsp. rum or rum extract

Directions:

Preheat the mini waffle maker.

Beat egg yolks into a small bowl until smooth.

Add the coconut flour, cinnamon, and nutmeg. Mix well.

In another bowl, mix rum, egg white and vanilla. Whisk until well combined.

Add it to the yolk mixture. You should be able to form a thin batter.

Add the mozzarella cheese and combine.

Separate the batter into two batches. Put 1/2 of the batter into the waffle maker and let it cook for 6 min. until its solid.

Repeat until you've used up the remaining batter. In a separate bowl, mix all the icing ingredients. Top the cooked waffles with the icing, or you can use this as a dip.

Nutrition:
Calories: 266
Carbohydrates: 2 g.
Fat: 23 g.
Protein: 13 g.

644. RASPBERRY WAFFLE

Preparation time: 10 min.
Cooking time: 8 min.
Servings: 1
Ingredients:

- 1 large egg (beaten)
- 1 tsp. cinnamon
- 2 tbsp. cream cheese
- 1/2 tsp. vanilla extract
- 2 tbsp. heavy cream
- 2 tbsp. almond flour
- 1/4 tsp. baking powder
- 1/3 c. raspberries
- 2 tsp. swerve sweetener or to taste
- 1/8 tsp. salt

Directions:
Plug the waffle maker to preheat it and spray it with a non-stick spray.
In a medium mixing bowl, combine the cinnamon, almond flour, baking powder, 1 tsp. swerve and salt.
In another mixing bowl, combine the cream cheese, egg and vanilla extract.
Pour the cream cheese mixture into the cheese mixture and mix until well combined and you have formed a smooth batter.
Fold in half of the raspberries.
Fill the waffle maker with an appropriate amount of the batter. Spread out the batter to cover all the holes on the waffle maker.

Close the waffle maker and cook for about 3–4 min. or according to the waffle maker's settings.
After the cooking cycle, use a plastic or silicone utensil to remove the waffle from the waffle maker.
Repeat 6–7 until you have cooked all the batter into the waffles.
In a mixing bowl, combine the remaining swerve and heavy cream. Whisk until you form soft peak.
Spread the cream cheese mixture over the waffles and top with the remaining raspberries.
Serve and enjoy.

Nutrition:
Calories 369 Cal
Total Fat: 30.4 g.
Saturated Fat: 13.4 g.
Cholesterol 249 mg.
Sodium 433 mg.
Total Carbohydrate 16.4 g.
Dietary Fiber 5.4 g.
Total Sugars 3.1 g.

645. CHOCOLATE MELT WAFFLES

Preparation time: 15 min.
Cooking time: 36 min.
Servings: 4
Ingredients:
For the waffles:
• 2 eggs, beaten
• 1/4 c. finely grated Gruyere cheese
• 2 tbsp. heavy cream
• 1 tbsp. coconut flour
• 2 tbsp. cream cheese, softened
• 3 tbsp. unsweetened cocoa powder
• 2 tsp. vanilla extract
• A pinch of salt
For the chocolate sauce:
1/3 c. + 1 tbsp. heavy cream

1 1/2 oz. unsweetened baking chocolate, chopped
1 1/2 tsp. sugar-free maple syrup
1 1/2 tsp. vanilla extract
Directions:
For the waffles:
Preheat the waffle iron.
In a medium bowl, mix all the ingredients for the waffles.
Open the iron and add 1/4 of the mixture. Close and cook until crispy, about 7 min.
Transfer the waffle to a plate and make 3 more with the remaining batter.
For the chocolate sauce:
Pour the heavy cream into saucepan and simmer over low heat, 3 min.
Turn the heat off and add the chocolate. Allow melting for a few minutes and stir until fully melted, 5 min.
Mix in the maple syrup and vanilla extract.
Assemble the waffles in layers with the chocolate sauce sandwiched between each layer.
Slice and serve immediately.
Nutrition:
Calories: 172 Cal
Total Fat: 13.57 g.
Saturated Fat: 0 g.
Cholesterol: 0 mg.
Sodium: 0 mg.
Total Carbs: 6.6 g.
Fiber: 0 g.
Sugar: 0 g.

646. MIDDAY WAFFLE SNACKS

Preparation time: 8 minutes
Cooking Time: 5 Minutes
Ingredients:
- 4 minutes Chaffles
- 2 oz. coconut flakes
- 2 oz. kiwi slice
- 2 oz. raspberry
- 2 oz. almonds chopped
- CHAFFLE Ingredients:
- 1 egg
- 1/2 cup mozzarella cheese
- 1 tsp stevia
- 1 tsp vanilla
- 2 tbsps. almond flour

Directions:
Make 4 minutes chaffles with the chaffle ingredients.
Arrange coconut flakes, raspberries, almonds and raspberries on each chaffle.
Serve and enjoy keto snacks
Nutrition: Protein: 18% 37 kcal Fat: 67% 137 kcal Carbohydrates: 15% 31 kick

647. SIMPLE WAFFLE WITHOUT MAKER

Servings: 2
Cooking Time: 5minutes
Ingredients:
- 1 tbsp. chia seeds
- 1 egg
- 1/2 cup cheddar cheese
- pinch of salt
- 1 tbsp. avocado oil

Directions:
Heat your nonstick pan over medium heat
In a small bowl, mix together chia seeds, salt, egg, and cheese together
Grease pan with avocado oil.
Once the pan is hot, pour 2 tbsps. Chaffle batter and cook for about 1-2 minutes Utes.
Flip and cook for another 1-2 minutes Utes.
Once chaffle is brown remove from pan.
Serve with berries on top and enjoy.
Nutrition: Protein: 19% 44 kcal Fat: % 181 kcal Carbohydrates: 1% 2 kcal

648. HEART SHAPE WAFFLE

Servings: 2
Cooking Time: 5 Minutes
Ingredients:

- 1 egg
- 1 cup mozzarella cheese
- 1 tsp baking powder
- ¼ cup almond flour
- 1 tbsp. coconut oil

Directions:

Heat your nonstick pan over medium heat.

Mix together all ingredients in a bowl.

Grease pan with avocado oil and place a heart shape cookie cutter over the pan.

Once the pan is hot, pour the batter equally in 2 cutters.

Cook for another 1-2 minutes Utes.

Once chaffle is set, remove the cutter, flip and cook for another 1-2 minutes Utes.

Once chaffles are brown, remove from the pan.

Serve hot and enjoy!

Nutrition: Protein: 24% 43 kcal Fat: 6 123 kcal Carbohydrates: 6% 11 kcal

649. CEREAL AND WALNUT WAFFLE

Preparation time: 9 minutes
Cooking Time: 6 Minutes
Ingredients:

- 1 milliliter of cereal flavoring
- ¼ tsp baking powder
- 1 tsp granulated swerve
- 1/8 tsp xanthan gum
- 1 tbsp butter (melted)
- ½ tsp coconut flour
- 2 tbsp toasted walnut (chopped)
- 1 tbsp cream cheese
- 2 tbsp almond flour
- 1 large egg (beaten)

- ¼ tsp cinnamon
- 1/8 tsp nutmeg

Directions:

Plug the waffle maker to preheat it and spray it with a non-stick spray.

In a mixing bowl, whisk together the egg, cereal flavoring, cream cheese and butter.

In another mixing bowl, combine the coconut flour, almond flour, cinnamon, nutmeg, swerve, xanthan gum and baking powder.

Pour the egg mixture into the flour mixture and mix until you form a smooth batter.

Fold in the chopped walnuts.

Pour in an appropriate amount of the batter into the waffle maker and spread out the batter to the edges to cover all the holes on the waffle maker.

Close the waffle maker and cook for about 3 minutes or according to your waffle maker's settings.

After the cooking cycle, use a plastic or silicone utensil to remove the chaffle from the waffle maker.

Repeat step 6 to 8 until you have cooked all the batter into chaffles.

Serve and top with sour cream or heavy cream.

Nutrition: Fat 18.2g 23% Carbohydrate 4.7g 2% Sugars 0.6g Protein 7.1g

650. BROCCOLI WAFFLES

Preparation time: 15 minutes
Servings: 4
Cooking Time: 5 Minutes
Ingredients:

- 1 egg
- 1 cup cheddar cheese
- ½ cup broccoli chopped
- 1 tsp baking powder
- 1 pinch garlic powder
- 1 pinch salt
- 1 pinch black pepper

- 1 tbsp. coconut oil

Directions:

Heat your nonstick pan over medium heat.

Mix together all ingredients in a bowl.

Grease pan with oil.

1.   Once the pan is hot, pour broccoli and cheese batter on greased pan

2.   Cook for 1-2 minutes Utes.

3.   Flip and cook for another 1-2 minutes Utes.

4.   Once chaffles are brown, remove from the pan.

5.   Serve with raspberries and melted coconut oil on top.

6.   Enjoy!

Nutrition: Protein: 20% 40 kcal Fat: 72% 142 kcal Carbohydrates: 7% 15 kcal

CONCLUSION

After reading this book, you will hopefully have a better understanding of how to start cooking the keto waffle recipes. Keep in mind that we never want to force any type of food on our diet—rather, we should be keeping an eye out for foods that are naturally low-carb and keto-friendly. We don't want to get into a routine of depriving ourselves or always feeling like we are doing something wrong. We just need to keep on track with the right general direction and live a healthy lifestyle while maintaining some indulgences. Our goal is not to be perfect, but rather to improve and maintain a healthy lifestyle.

The book will also give you a good idea of various notions on how to prepare and cook waffle recipes. You will learn quite a few things from this book. Once you actually start to cook the recipes, you will see that even though they may seem complicated they aren't nearly as difficult as they may seem at first glance. Use the resources provided in the book and, before long, you will not only be prepared to cook a wide variety of low-carb recipes but also become adept at using many of the cooking utensils available on the market today.

You really can make waffle recipes in your home without having to go out and buy lots of new utensils. If you follow the instructions in this book, you will be able to prepare waffle recipes and actually make a good profit from them, if that is what you are looking to do. Some people are interested in cooking waffle recipes just because they like to try new things. Experimenting with various low-carb foods is a wonderful way to see what you like and what you don't like. It is all a matter of personal taste, but once you find something that you like, it can be yours for life.

There have been many people that have found success with the keto diet and want to share their knowledge with others. The ketogenic diet has also proved to be helpful for people suffering from epilepsy, type 2 diabetes, metabolic syndrome, and many other ailments. If you are interested in learning more about the ketogenic diet or other low-carb foods, you can check out some of our books on diet and nutrition.

All of the recipes in this book were created using a waffle maker and waffle batter. We have taken the time to share all of our recipes with you in an effort to make your keto lifestyle easier. Each recipe has its own unique flavor that is sure to spice up your keto waffle recipes. The ketogenic diet is a way of eating that helps to turn the body into a fat-burning machine through a process called ketosis. It has been used by people for centuries and is still one of the best ways to lose body fat. The ketogenic diet provides the body with the daily dosage of nutrients required for building lean muscle mass, burning fat, and staying healthy. However, as noted earlier, it is not easy to follow and can be very difficult initially, but allows complete flexibility in food choices when you understand how it works.

Now that you know how to prepare waffle recipes, let's talk about the best way to follow the keto lifestyle. In order to stay healthy, you need to eat a diet that consists of high fat, moderate protein, and very low carbohydrates. De-emphasizing carbohydrates is especially important because this is what induces ketosis in your body.

Foods with a high amount of carbohydrates will put your body in an energy state which is dependent on glucose and insulin. Glucose is the easiest form of energy for our bodies to use which they obtain by eating grains, bread, and other starchy foods. Insulin helps our bodies absorb the glucose so that we can use it for energy. Once our bodies are adapted to burning glucose for energy, it creates a dependency and our bodies will start to crave the carbs. The craving becomes a vicious cycle of cravings, binging, and starving which is counterproductive to weight loss.

When following the keto diet, you will be severely limiting your carbohydrate intake since this will help your body induce ketosis. By doing this, you will kick your body out of its sugar-burning state and into its fat-burning state. Insulin levels will drop which helps get rid of excess body fat that has been stored for years in your cells. This diet is great for helping people lose weight because it allows them to eat until they feel full while still losing weight.

Because of all the weight loss support that the keto diet provides, it is a favorite among many people. If you are looking to consume more fat, lose weight, and get fit at the same time then this is definitely the diet for you. The keto waffle recipes in this book will give you a great idea of how to prepare your food and make it delicious while following the ketogenic diet.

Made in the USA
Las Vegas, NV
29 November 2024